# LOW BACK PAIN

## Mechanism, Diagnosis and Treatment

### FOURTH EDITION

# LOW BACK PAIN
## Mechanism, Diagnosis and Treatment

### FOURTH EDITION

**JAMES M. COX, D.C., D.A.C.B.R.**

Director, Low Back Pain Clinic
Fort Wayne, Indiana
Postgraduate Faculty Member
National College of Chiropractic
Lombard, Illinois
President and Director
International Academy on Chiropractic
Low Back Pain Study, Inc.
Diplomate
American Chiropractic Board of Roentgenology

### CONTRIBUTING AUTHOR

**Reuben F. Stevens, D.C., D.A.B.C.O.**

Diplomate, American Board of Chiropractic Orthopedists
National Association of Disability Evaluating Physicians
Member, International Academy on Chiropractic Low Back Pain Study, Inc.

**WILLIAMS & WILKINS**
Baltimore • London • Los Angeles • Sydney

*Editor:* Jonathan W. Pine, Jr.
*Associate Editor:* Victoria M. Vaughn
*Design:* James R. Mulligan
*Illustration Planning:* Reginald R. Stanley
*Production:* Raymond E. Reter

*Made in the United States of America*

**Library of Congress Cataloging in Publication Data**

Cox, James M.
  Low back pain.

  Includes bibliographies and index.
  1. Backache. 2. Chiropractic. I. Title. [DNLM: 1. Backache. 2. Chiropractic. WE 755 C877L]
RZ265.S64C69 1985      617'.56      84-10364
ISBN 0-683-02151-6

Composed and printed at the
Waverly Press, Inc.

# Foreword

The purpose of the foreword to a textbook is to peruse the text and to summarize the goals of the author, to briefly report the impressions and the value of the text, and, finally, to inform the readers as to what they can anticipate upon completion. Is this a reference text? Does the book have a current and extensive bibliography? Is there a review of biomechanics? What about physical examination procedures? Is the work presented in a logical, well-organized manner?

I submit the following opinion regarding Dr. Cox's book, *Low Back Pain: Mechanism, Diagnosis and Treatment*. This text represents current concepts concerning the epidemic phenomenon of low back pain and will be a welcome addition to the private library of all primary care providers. The Doctor of Chiropractic (D.C.) will have particular interest in this text, as it presents a standardized approach leading to a correlative diagnosis and the subsequent management of this type of patient. It is well documented that more than 50% of the patients that seek chiropractic care present with the chief complaint of low back pain.

Both student and practitioner will find this text to be an excellent reference source. The first chapter presents the position of chiropractic. This chapter "opens the door to all who will but enter." It is hoped that in the near future open communication with the allopathic and osteopathic professions will result in intraprofessional dialogue and referrals based on the patient's current health status and need.

Biomechanics of the lumbar spine is next discussed. Special emphasis is given to normal and abnormal structure as it relates to function. The spinal dysarthria, subluxation, so commonly found with this type of case and its diagnosis are discussed, and an interesting array of cases is presented.

Specific discussion of the radiographic biomechanical findings of the lumbar spine and pelvis is augmented by radiographic reproductions. These are preceded by a chapter on the short leg, a topic that is of major interest to the scientific community currently studying low back pain.

Transitional segments, stenosis, and care of the intervertebral disc are presented, with special emphasis given to treatment protocol. Facet syndrome, scoliosis, facet tropism, and spondylolisthesis are discussed in detail. The reader will be exposed to a variety of opinions throughout this book, well documented by an extensive bibliography. The nutritional needs of the intervertebral disc will be of special interest to students of the biochemistry of the lumbar spine.

The chapter on specific low back conditions covers physical examination and x-ray findings, including kinesiology, as they relate to diagnosis and treatment. Dr. Cox has pioneered the specific treatment known as "flexion distraction manipulation." This approach is clearly reviewed. The indications and contraindications will be helpful in the physician's treatment selection, and review of physical therapy applications will be helpful to both doctor and assistant.

The final chapter presents the research findings on 576 patients receiving chiropractic manipulation. This study was conducted by the International Academy on Chiropractic Low Back Pain Study, Inc., with special funding from the Foundation for Chiropractic Education and Research (F.C.E.R.).

The Academy was founded in July 1981 and has continued to grow and develop. The data-gathering forms are completed by doctors of chiropractic and submitted to Indiana University-Purdue University for processing. Scott Schreiner, Ph.D., serves as consultant on this most worthwhile research project. The initial studies will be published in the *Journal of Manipulative and Physiological Therapeutics* (*JMPT*).

In closing, I quote a statement by Ernest G. Napolitano, D.C., President of the New York College of Chiropractic: "It is not in the nature of science to give final and complete answers about many problems and this is surely true of the science of Chiropractic. It is, however, characteristic of the scientific intellect to communicate all new and beneficial material to the scientific community as a continuing effort to develop a greater and more workable discipline."

**Allen Parry, D.C.**

*Director*
*Postdoctoral & Related Professional Education*
*Logan College of Chiropractic*
*Chesterfield, Missouri*

# Preface to the Fourth Edition

Chiropractic has had a major interest in low back pain for the past 90 years, and it has also represented the strongest voice for its conservative care. There has been a paucity of writings by the profession but a vast acceptance of its benefits in relieving pain. This has further resulted in the failure of proper credit being given for the contributions that it has made and that are being made by this profession.

Patients with low back pain are primarily treated conservatively, with a very small percentage requiring surgery. The techniques employed by chiropractors have changed and are far different from the forceful adjustments of 20 or 30 years ago. The manipulative technics of this text incorporate osteopathic long lever maneuvers with the classic specific facetal manipulation of chiropractic. The popular motion palpation concept of diagnosis and treatment of joint dysfunction is presented.

One fact must be recognized—there is so much not known about low back pain.

The best of diagnosis often results in empirical therapy, simply because the mechanical facts are not always logical and decisive. The knowledge that conservative care is the least invasive and damaging provides some security, therefore, when the exact course of care is undecided. Certainly, there are those patients whose greatest relief results from a combination of conservative and surgical care. The future will mandate close work between the chiropractor and his surgical colleagues.

As you read this text, my ideas may insinuate bias concerning the approach to a condition. The technics are not my original ideas, however; rather, they are a marriage of prior workable technics into a hopefully new clinical regimen. They are the results of 20 years of study during which, slowly, educated uncertainty was transformed into clinical prowess.

**James M. Cox, D.C.**

# Acknowledgments

So often it would have been easier and less stressful to have stopped this publication; however, there are individuals and events that produce a need and a purpose.

In 1966, while in postgraduate diagnostic roentgenology study, Dr. Joseph Howe, a mentor to me and now Director of Roentgenology at Los Angeles College of Chiropractic, introduced me to some advanced authors in low back pain and urged me to write a paper on 25 cases of low back and leg pain that I had compiled. That was the beginning of the clinical data collection that has evolved today into a complex research project in low back pain which is discussed in the last chapter of this book. To Dr. Howe I owe the stimulus for this work. His example of stewardship has meant a great deal to me and to his profession.

The National College of Chiropractic, under the now President Emeritus Joseph Janse, D.C., instilled the knowledge and clinical awareness of chiropractic principles of healing that formed the foundation for this work.

Deep appreciation must go to Drs. Allen Parry and Daniel Komesch, Directors of the International Academy on Chiropractic Low Back Pain Study, Inc., as well as to its membership who supported my ideas and added encouragement when it was needed most.

In the everyday toil of collecting and assembling material for this text, one person deserves special credit, Phyllis White, chiropractic assistant and certified x-ray technician, who coped with the stress I generated and ultimately typed and helped assemble this text. Your efforts are appreciated.

Lastly, the sacrifices of my family need to be mentioned. My wife, Judy, is too tolerant. She accepted my absence and the tension of my presence in this book's preparation. She took my place with the children when this project came first. There is no way to be deserving of that kind of love and sacrifice except to acknowledge it.

# Contents

## CONTENTS

CHAPTER 1

# The Position of Chiropractic

## EXTENT OF THE PROBLEM OF LOW BACK PAIN

Back pain, particularly in the low back, has plagued mankind for thousands of years. Descriptions of lumbago and sciatica are found in the Bible and in the writings of Hippocrates (1). It is estimated that today in the United States 75 million people suffer from back pain and there are 7 million new victims each year. Of these, 5 million are partly disabled and 2 million are unable to work at all. Eighty percent of the people in the United States will suffer from this affliction some time in their lives (2).

The financial cost of low back pain is enormous. Five billion dollars will be spent in the United States this year on the diagnosis and treatment of low back pain, and another $10 billion will be spent on disability compensation, lawsuits, and workmen's compensation. The cost for treatment of low back pain is higher than the cost for treatment of heart disease or the cost for treatment from traffic accidents. Ninety-three million work days will be lost annually in the United States due to low back pain. The incidence of low back pain increases faster than that of any other ailment of mankind (3).

It has been estimated that patients with low back complaints comprise the second largest diagnostic group seeking care from family physicians and make up one third of all orthopedic out-patient visits (4). Breen (5) points out that of patients seeking chiropractic care for the first time, 53% complained of low back pain; 20%, of lower leg pain; and 18%, of thigh and knee pain. Yet, no universally recognized treatment exists for this common problem. Consequently, patients with low back pain not only frequently seek assistance from more than one specialist but also often receive conflicting advice as to the appropriate management of their condition (6).

## FACTORS ASSOCIATED WITH THE DIAGNOSIS AND TREATMENT OF LOW BACK PAIN

### Congenital Anomalies

Many authors discuss the incidence of congenital anomalies in association with low back pain. Montgomery (7), who performed a thorough search of the literature, states that the use of pre-employment x-rays has been based upon the hypothesis that developmental abnormalities predispose to an increased incidence of low back injuries. The preponderance of evidence, however, indicates that this hypothesis is not substantiated. Snook et al. (8) point out that the common selection technics such as medical histories, examinations, and x-rays are not an effective control for low back injuries. Employers who use these selection techniques have just as high an incidence of injuries as have employers who use no selection technics.

Finneson (9) states that there is no higher incidence of transitional vertebrae in the backs of those seeking care for low back pain than there is in the normal population. Wigh and Anthony (10) point

1

out that of 200 patients operated on for lumbar disc herniations, 42 had a lumbosacral transitional vertebra. In none of the 42 patients was there myelographic evidence of herniation of such a disc. This certainly raises the question, addressed in the chapter on transitional segments, of how best to treat Bertolotti's syndrome (11). Semon and Spengler (12) point out that there is no significant difference in time loss between athletes with spondylolysis and those without it. Lenz (13) found that 86.6% of patients with spondylolisthesis showed favorable results under chiropractic manipulation of a flexion-distraction type.

Stenosis, it is believed, enhances the symptoms of disc protrusion and necessitates surgery in patients with a prolapsed disc (14). Martin (15) found, however, that back pain preceded leg pain in only 3 of 16 patients with a prolapsed disc. Furthermore, in patients with a recurring prolapsed disc necessitating repeat surgery, stenosis was found at the level of surgery. This raises two questions: Does back pain preceding leg pain indicate protrusion, and does leg pain without back pain indicate prolapse? Rothman and Simeone (16) state that in patients with a prolapsed disc there may be a sudden onset of sciatica without back pain and, at the time of extrusion of the fragment, there may be a sudden onset of sciatica and a sudden abatement of the back pain. It is not clear what role stenosis, lateral recess, and central stenosis play in the etiology of neurogenic intermittent claudication. Eisenstein (17) points out that the lower limit of the sagittal diameter of the vertebral canal is 15 mm. Ullrich et al. (18) point out that the smallest normal sagittal canal diameter is 11.5 mm with stenosis. Therefore, some differing opinion exists as to the lowest normal sagittal diameter of the vertebral canal.

## Facet Involvement

The question as to what causes the onset of pain and instability, the facet or the disc, remains unanswered. Mooney and Robertson (19) performed lumbar facet injection on 100 consecutive patients with lumbago and sciatica and found that one fifth of these patients received long-term

relief and one third received partial relief. Carrera et al. (20) point out that the distance between adjacent points in articular facets of 40 apparently normal joints was 2 to 4 mm. They, therefore, considered a joint space of less than 2 mm diagnostic of articular cartilage thinning. Carrera (21) injected anesthetic and steroid into the facet joints of 20 patients and found that 6 patients reported continued relief of pain after 6 to 12 months, 7 experienced complete return of pain several days to 6 months later, and 7 derived no benefit from the block. Dory (22) found that when anesthetic or steroid was injected into 70 lumbar joints in 27 patients, the articular capsule nearly always burst and the leaking medium provided an explanation of how the injected anesthetics and steroids worked in the relief of low back pain. The leakage occurred in the lateral aspect of the joints where the branches of the posterior ramus of the spinal nerve pass, and medially where it enters the epidural space and, sometimes, the intervertebral foramen.

Chynn et al. (23) report that in spinal stenosis the superior articular process is more sagittally oriented. Furthermore, their study indicates that plain films are of great usefulness in the diagnosis of lumbar spinal stenosis, contrary to the opinion of some authorities who believe that such plain films are of little value. In many cases, clinical presentation and the careful analysis of plain films are sufficient to reach an almost certain diagnosis.

Lora and Long (24) found that radicular radiation of pain is not generated by stimulation of the nerves in and around the facets, but widespread referral of sensation even into the leg is possible. This referral of sensation, however, characteristically has a diffuse nonradicular character, is difficult for the patient to localize, and did not go below the knee in any patient.

## Hypermobility

Van Akkerveeken et al. (25) found that when the annulus fibrosus and posterior longitudinal ligament were unstable due to tearing or stretching, there was a posterior and rotatory displacement of the vertebral bodies upon one another on extension. We utilize this technic in our diagnosis to determine the stability of facet syndrome, and we correlate it with those people having recurrent and totally relievable low back pain.

## Tropism

In a study of 82 patients with low back and sciatic pain, Cox (26) found that 23% revealed tropism at the level of the disc lesion. Ehni and Weinstein (27) state that 20% of the normal population have stenosis. Cyron and Hutton (28) state that articular tropism results in the manifestation of lumbar instability as joint rotation, with this rotation occurring toward the side of the more oblique facet where it will create additional stress on the annulus fibrosus which is on the side of the nuclear protrusion.

## Straight Leg and Well Leg Raising Signs

Breig and Troup (29) state that medial hip rotation is associated with increased tension and neurological dysfunction of the lumbosacral roots. We apply medial hip rotation with the straight leg raising sign to make this evaluation. Furthermore, Hudgins (30) states that the crossed straight leg raising (well leg raising) sign is indicative of a herniated lumbar disc in 97% of the patients, even with a negative myelogram. We also apply this sign for clarification.

## Rotational Motion of the Lumbar Spine

Farfan (31) points out that in the laboratory, as little as 3° forced rotation of the intervertebral joint produces damage to the disc and facets. The outer fibers of the annulus are stretched and may be torn off of the end plate. The inner annulus becomes separated and loose if forced rotation is continued. Virgin (32) observed that compression was not a factor in causing nuclear protrusion. He found that when a longitudinal incision was made in the posterolateral part of the annulus all of the way to the nucleus, under compression the nucleus did not change its shape or escape. It was only under rota-

tion that the loud snapping sounds were heard as the annular fibers tore. These sounds were similar to the loud snapping sounds known to occur with the sudden onset of backache. Lumsden and Morris (33) found that approximately 6° of rotation occurred at the lumbosacral joint during maximal rotation and that rotation at the lumbosacral joint was not measurably affected by tropism. Maigne (34) states that no rotation is possible in the lumbar spine because of facet orientation and form, and that flexion and extension are essentially all that are permitted in the lumbar spine.

The ultimate role of rotation in chiropractic practice must, therefore, be fully evaluated. Certainly it is a problem, as most disc injuries coming to malpractice are the result of various lumbopelvis moves given in the side posture position (35).

## Lateral Bending Studies versus Myelography

Gainer and Nugent (36) state that lumbar disc herniation is one of the most common causes of back pain and leg pain and is usually easily diagnosed by a history and physical examination. The use of lateral bending studies of the lumbar spine is extremely important to the chiropractic physician in the differentiation between medial and lateral discs as well as in the establishment of postreduction findings of improvement. Weitz (37) states that the lateral bending studies have diagnostic reliability equal to that of myelography.

## Treatment Procedures

Ultimately, the clinical result is what matters. What, then, are the results of various treatments and therapies?

Aitken (38) points out that 25% of those patients with ruptured discs and 46% of those without ruptured discs at surgery never returned to work. Wood (39) states that only about 10% to 30% of patients who are operated on become pain-free and return to their original work. The first two discs to cause problems are those at the L4-L5 and L5-S1 levels.

For decades, traction has been the popular form of treatment for low back pain. Kessler (40) has demonstrated, however, that static traction should be avoided during the acute stage of a disc prolapse. The imbibition of fluid into the nucleus can increase intradiscal pressure and exacerbate pain. He believes that specific segmental manual distraction technics are to be preferred, as they will decrease the slack of the posterior longitudinal ligament and the annular fibers overlying the disc bulge and will create a centripetal movement of the disc material away from the pain-sensitive periphery. Furthermore, the avoidance of sitting is recommended. Fahrni (41) states that a tribe in India who squat rather than sit have a zero incidence of back pain or lumbar disc narrowing. Nachemson's (42) intradiscal pressure measurements also support Fahrni's research and the adverse effects of sitting.

Only 5% of patients with acute lumbosacral radiculopathy require surgery (43).

In an article from China entitled, "Treatment of Lumbar Disc Protrusion by Automatic Chiropractic Traction Instrument" (44), it is stated that 400 patients were treated with a specially built chiropractic instrument. (Interestingly, the description of the table is quite similar to that of the Cox distraction instrument used in flexion distraction manipulation and reduction of nuclear disc protrusion.) Of these 400 patients, 290 were completely cured, 48 were greatly improved, 42 experienced some improvement, and 20 patients did not respond to treatment. According to the article, observers viewed x-ray films taken during distraction manipulation of the patient and witnessed the intervertebral disc space widen 1.5 to 2 mm. They often saw a protruded disc return spontaneously to its proper place when the lumbar vertebra was lifted at surgical operation. In other cases, they saw the defect of the vertebra disappear after treatment with the traction instrument. They concluded that traction widened the intervertebral disc space and, by the negative pressure created, caused extension of the annular ring and posterior ligament, thereby reducing the disc protrusion. Furthermore, they believed that it loosened adhesions of the nerve roots.

Szepesi (45) points out that degeneration and herniation of the disc at the L5-S1 level should be treated promptly to prevent degeneration in the sacroiliac joints. He believes that sacroiliac joint degeneration is probably a result of abnormal posture following disc problems.

## Clinical Considerations

In a 2-year statistical study of 194 patients with acute disc syndrome, Valentini (46) found that 171 were successfully treated by chiropractic manipulation and 23 failed to respond to treatment. He believed that in patients with acute disc syndrome the aim of treatment should be the earliest possible reduction of the disc protrusion or adaptation of the protrusion and nerve root to a more specific co-existence. The treatment used was a side posture rotary adjustment performed in the free and painless direction toward the opposite side of the antalgic posture. In 71% of these patients he also utilized a distraction technic.

Tindall (47) states that 200,000 lumbar disc operations are performed by neurosurgeons each year and that this represents the most common operation performed by the majority of neurosurgeons. Concerning the use of the electromyogram (EMG), he believes that it virtually never influences the decision involving the management of the patient and does not establish the diagnosis of a herniated lumbar disc. He also believes that protrusion or rupture of the nucleus pulposus is usually preceded by degenerative changes characterized structurally by radiating cracks in the annulus that weaken its resistance to nuclear herniation. The characteristic clinical features of back and leg pain are related to irritation and stretching of the sinuvertebral nerve by the bulging annulus and by direct pressure on the nerve root, respectively.

Eagle (48) states that among the world's 2 million doctors there are only 20 who have devoted their careers exclusively to researching back pain. With a permanent pool of 2 billion patients who might benefit from advice or ministrations, the scope for further research is almost unlimited.

Cookson (49) wrote rather pointedly that when the patient with low back pain is examined, three questions must be kept in mind; for us the most important of these is: "Is this a disc lesion or one of the uncommon causes of backache?" The list of authors who state that 90% of low back pain is caused by the intervertebral disc is quite lengthy.

At the 1975 Symposium on the Research Status of Spinal Manipulative Therapy, Nachemson (50) stated that with some frequency in the medical field, new types of treatment for low back pain are introduced, tried for some time, and then proven or disproven by clinical trials in various places around the world. No such attempts have been made by chiropractors or osteopaths for nearly 100 years.

Goldstein (51) states that studies on the scientific basis of manipulative therapy should not be misread to mean only basic science studies. Studies on the scientific basis of manipulative therapy clearly include both basic studies in areas such as biomechanics and clinical studies in areas such as the reliability of clinical diagnosis and the efficacy of therapy; "clinical studies are considered as much a part of research on the scientific basis of any therapy as is the understanding of the fundamental mechanisms underlying therapy."

### Perspectives of Patients to Chiropractic

Patient acceptance of chiropractic care is demonstrated in a report by Parker and Tupling (52). Of 84 patients visiting a chiropractor for the first time, 82% had received previous treatment and failed to respond, nearly 60% gave a desire for pain relief as the sole reason for their visit, and two thirds affirmed that they visited the chiropractor as a last resort. At 10-week follow-up, however, all but 11% reported some improvement, and 74% were sufficiently satisfied with their treatment to affirm that they would return to a chiropractor if their condition recurred.

Parker and Tupling also found that at the initial consultation, patients who were asked to compare medical doctors and chiropractors with regard to interpersonal attitudes, technical skills, and social characteristics stated that they considered the chiropractor to be more expensive, less available, and less regarded by society than are general practitioners. At follow-up, however, patients judged chiropractors to be equal to general practitioners in technical competence but somewhat superior with regard to interpersonal characteristics. Parker and Tupling conclude that the chiropractor fulfills an emerging cultural need for a less technocratic medical system with an emphasis on holistic natural therapies and consideration of interpersonal needs. They suggest that "the chiropractor may be more attuned to the total needs of the patient than his medical counterpart."

### BACK SURGERY: AN EVALUATION

### Chronology of the Study of Back Pain

Modern studies of the lumbar spine date back to the 1820s. In 1858, von Luschka described the anatomy of the disc (53). Dandy (54) in 1929 performed surgery on a lumbar spine from which he removed free fragments of herniated disc that had compressed the cauda equina; he noted that the lesion afforded explanation of low back and leg pain. Mixter and Barr (55) in 1934 reported on the role of herniation of a lumbar disc in the etiology of sciatica. Their classic paper marked the beginning of the trend toward use of surgery in the relief of low back and leg pain. This trend has continued to the present, and as late as 1976, 450,000 back operations were performed in the United States in that year (56).

### Effects on and Cost to Patients

Dommisse and Grahe (57) state that 48% of 7,391 patients operated on by 17 surgeons and reported in 23 publications had recurrence of symptoms (backache, sciatica, or both) within a year after back surgery (57). Burton (58) states that the long-term failure rate of back surgery has been variously reported as being between 10% and 40%. The number of persons with the failed back surgery syndrome (FBSS) characterized by intractable pain and functional incapacitation must be significant. He concludes by stating that lumbar arachnoiditis, a definable pathological entity, appears to be present in failed back surgery syndrome patients to a much higher degree than was previously thought.

"If for no other reason that the mere existence of lumbar arachnoiditis, it is clear that a major reappraisal of the present medical and surgical approach to lumbar disc disease is called for. The introduction of foreign bodies into the subarachnoid space for diagnostic determinations invariably involves some patient risk. Emphasis must be placed on the most innocuous myelographic agents. Emphasis must also be placed on the development of non-invasive means of diagnosing disease of the lumbar spine" (59).

In a study by the California Health Data Corporation, it is reported that in 1974 in California, 72,645 patients were admitted to the hospital for backache. Fifty percent of these patients were diagnosed as having discogenic disease, and 27% underwent surgery. When the cost of the surgical and medical treatment of these 72,645 patients was extrapolated to a national scale, it was estimated that for 1974 the national cost for hospitalization of patients with backache was $1.38 billion. This does not include the expense for outpatient care or loss of income for those patients who were disabled (60).

With surgery, however, the patient's chance for returning to work is even slimmer than it is without surgery. Each additional surgical procedure and each month of additional inactivity further reduce the chance for return to employment. For instance, in Wisconsin each year it is estimated that 75% of compensation claims are paid to back-injured patients who represent only 3% of the total compensation claims. Once an individual has surgery, medical expenses mount rapidly. One 32-year-old woman recently reported medical, surgical, and hospital costs of $160,000 over the previous 8 years

(61). Shealy of the University of Minnesota Pain and Rehabilitation Center also states that this country is struggling currently with a virtual epidemic of chronic back pain in large extent due to the unique amount of back surgery being done in the United States (62). The typical low back pain patient coming to his clinic has had 4 operations on his back, has suffered pain for 4 to 10 years, and has run up a medical bill of around $75,000. Less than 1 in 10 of the 50,000 lumbar disc surgeries performed annually in this country are warranted, he states; furthermore, if one such surgery is ineffective, a second, third or more will not improve the situation. Conventional physicians are helpless with patients like these. In the treatment of chronic low back pain the American Medical profession is at its weakest.

## Need for Back Surgery

Barr, who was Professor of Orthopedic Surgery at Harvard Medical School from 1947 to 1964 and the first doctor to isolate the disc as the cause of low back and leg pain in 1934, stated at the Officers Club, San Diego Naval Hospital, in May 1961:

"Some of the people here think that open surgery for disc lesions will probably be primarily a thing of the past. This seems incredible but I suspect that it may be true. I hope it is true. But if you can shrink the lesion and stabilize the spine. . . [,] the surgeon is going to have to fold up his tent and silently steal away. I think this could be true. Discs are 90% water. Why should we have to bail them out with surgical instruments? It seems to me a little ridiculous. I don't know how we are going to do it but I believe it can be done and I think it will be done" (63).

Marshall (64) states that at the present time a patient is frequently given the bleak alternative of an operation or is advised to

"live with the problem. Most honest operators will not promise more than a 50-50 chance of success from surgery. As a result . . . patients frequently turn for help to unqualified operators in this field, and some patients obtain complete relief and some obtain partial relief [from pain,] and this situation . . . is constantly eroding faith in the medical profession" (64).

Wood (65) in 1979 wrote:

"Numerous papers have been published on the results of surgical therapy, and even that approach is a discouraging proposition. Those who become pain-free and return to their original work make up about 10% to 30% of cases in which operations were done. This is a consistent finding in almost all of the papers published."

In several reports during the last decade, it has been concluded that for 99% of the patients with low back pain and one- or two-level disc degeneration, the best treatment is not disc removal or fusion. By now we also know that chymopapain is not the proper treatment either. The results of this treatment have been satisfactory in only 50% to 60% of the patients, which is not as good as the results that can be obtained through conservative measures without the high number of multiply-operated surgical cripples (42).

The period of sickness is longer for back pain patients than for other patients. For instance, in a Swedish study (66) the average sickness period for the back pain patients in 1972 was 39 days, which is considerably longer than the 19 days which was the average duration for all sickness absence.

Mooney (67) reported that surgical care of patients with a failed previous surgery seldom is rewarding. In patients with failed back surgery syndrome, the physician searches for specific hard findings to suggest that relief could be achieved by either stabilization or excision of bony fragments impinging on nerve roots. By and large, however, the sources of pain following surgery are ill-defined, do not correspond to anatomical pathways, and must be referred to as bizarre pain patterns. In these situations, the assumption must be that the sources of pain are secondary to postsurgical scarring or scarring from myelograms and will not be relieved by additional surgery, which merely would create another opportunity for scarring (67).

In a survey of 886 patients who had lumbar disc surgery, 56% showed good results, with 63% of these returning to their former occupation (68).

Smith (69) states that he

"has done a thousand laminectomies and never liked doing them. In contrast to other surgery, when you do back surgery you're fooling around with nerve roots that control the patient's lower extremities and bladder. The possibility of serious complications is higher than in other procedures performed by an orthopedic surgeon. It's a bloody surgery, and there is danger of hemorrhage and infection. I quit doing back surgery several years ago."

## Summary

Surgical and technological changes have had a strong impact on the diagnosis and treatment of the protruding intervertebral disc of the lumbar spine. Our generation has witnessed the change from radical complete laminectomy followed by bone transplant fusion, to partial or no laminectomy for removal of disc fragments with no fusion, to the recent use of microsurgical techniques to minimize damage to the spine, to chemonucleolysis and percutaneous nuclectomy without incision. Controversy concerning diagnostic methods has resulted in questioning of what were once accepted diagnostic maneuvers.

The scientific explanation of the source of low back and leg pain was first stated in 1934 in the classic paper of Mixter and Barr; these investigators delineated prolapse of the intervertebral disc as the agent in the production of back and leg pain (55). It now is commonly acknowledged that derangement of the intervertebral disc produces the majority of cases of back pain and sciatica.

Roentgen evaluation of disc lesions has been debated for years, until today the thinking of many leading neurosurgeons is aligned with that of leading chiropractic physicians. Myelography is limited in the diagnosis of disc lesions. Nearly a quarter of all disc protrusions at L5 cannot be seen on the myelogram. Moreover, myelography has shown that one third of patients not complaining of low back pain have large spinal defects which have never caused any trouble (70). Myelography admittedly has a large error factor which can be conservatively stated to be between 30% and 40%; this has resulted in near abandonment of the procedure by some in the evaluation of sciatica induced by disc protrusion. Semmes, Professor of Neurosurgery at the University of Tennessee Medical School, has performed more than 6,000 disc operations and has utilized myelography in less than 3% of the last 350. According to Semmes (71), to subject the patient to the risk of a myelogram merely to confirm a diagnosis that can be made without it is unwarranted.

## CHIROPRACTIC: AN ANSWER TO THE PROBLEM

### Biomechanical Causes of Disc Disease

Intervertebral disc disease represents one of the most complex of medical disorders. It has been hypothesized that when ancestral man traded his arboreal existence for that of an erect biped, the stage may have been set for the later development of intervertebral disc disease. Apparently, the human is not designed to withstand the stresses and strains created by the erect posture and centered on the lumbosacral spine. Repeated small traumatic insults add to the increased susceptibility of the spine and discs to degeneration. Yamada (72, 72a) studied intervertebral disc herniation in biped rats and mice. He noted that when there was a change in the mode of locomotion from the quadriped stance to the bipedal stance, that is, walking on the hind legs, the animals developed degenerated lumbar discs within 12 to 24 months. No degeneration occurred in the control group, however. Yamada also showed that there were great mechanical stresses on the sacroiliac portion of the spinal column in bipedal animals, which, he believed, resulted in intervertebral disc herniation.

Turek (73) describes well the pathophysiology of the continuous and progressive degenerative changes of the intervertebral disc. The process may begin in a young person of 15 with the onset of concentric cracking and cavitation of the annular fibers, proceed in the mature adult in the third decade of life to swollen granular changes in the nucleus pulposus, and culminate in the middle and later years of life with the disc becoming a sodden mass. Turek further describes the thinning of the annular fibers to a thin fibrous ring which is torn by the slightest force (73).

In addition to the stresses caused by erect posture during locomotion and by degeneration of the disc, there is the stress produced by lifting weight. Strait et al. (74) demonstrated that tremendous low back strain may be involved in forward trunk flexion. A 180-lb man flexed 60° at the trunk from vertical and holding 50-lb weight in his hands exerts a 850-lb compression force on the fifth lumbar vertebra.

### The Role of Chiropractic

Over half the patients seen by the chiropractic physician complain of low back pain. When this low back pain is associated with sciatic neuralgia, the chiropractic physician must determine whether there is a disc protrusion, the level of its involvement, and the therapeutic approach to be instituted. It behooves our profession, therefore, to develop an approach to the problem of disc protrusion that encompasses diagnosis without the use of contrast medium and therapy without the use of surgical repair, tempered by the possibility that ultimately a surgical approach may be necessary in a few cases.

We in chiropractic have an opportunity to demonstrate that we have "an idea whose time has arrived," namely, that the best treatment for the patient with low back pain caused by disc protrusion is the conservative approach of chiropractic manipulation as described in this textbook. For many years we have heard much about the diagnosis of disc protrusion from routine x-ray study of the low back. As is true in most other diseases of humans, diagnosis cannot and does not depend on x-ray study alone—it requires the use of clinical, laboratory, x-ray, and special procedures to achieve the highest degree of accuracy, and yet this use so often is found wanting. The diagnosis of disc protrusion is no different—it requires careful clinical, orthopedic, neurological, and roentgen findings to determine the site, type, and severity of the lesion.

## Lind Autotraction

Practically all medical authors give fairly detailed examination procedures, and almost all discuss rest, exercise, drugs, some form of heat, bracing and, ultimately, surgery in the treatment of low back pain, but few, if any, discuss the use of manipulation. Lind (75) provides probably the most thorough and detailed analysis of conservative treatments for low back pain. She states that patients who had received physiotherapy or chiropractic treatment recovered slower with the use of her autotraction device than did those who had received no treatment. She, therefore, questioned the advisability of these therapies. Of course, we take exception to this, especially since this text outlines a much different approach to treatment of disc disease than conventional torsion chiropractic adjustment. It is to be emphasized here that the reduction of subluxation following disc reduction is extremely beneficial to many patients.

Lind used autotraction to treat 20 patients who had confirmed disc lesions and were awaiting surgical repair. All 20 patients had had previous treatment including rest, analgesics, physiotherapy, sacral injections, short wave therapy, radiotherapy, and chiropractic. Within 1 week, all but 4 of the 20 were rid of their back and leg pain. Lind used myelograms before, during, and after many of these treatments and demonstrated reduction of the disc protrusion. She states that patients not improving following surgery, or suffering a relapse, respond with more difficulty to autotraction, probably due to ligament damage and the inability to exert enough pressure at traction to bring about a reduction. Lind further states that laterorhizal herniation is easier to repair than mediorhizal herniation and that autotraction may prove futile in the repair of sequestration of a disc. She believes that the use of analgesics and long periods of bed rest are undersirable also, since their use slows recovery by autotraction (75).

Lind quotes such authorities as Cyriax (76) on the effects of plane traction, stating that it temporarily separated the lumbar vertebra on the dorsal side and the stretched ligaments help to squeeze the protrusion back into place. Traction exerts suction on the disc herniation (77, 78), and repeated traction induces a push-pull pumping effect on the blood and lymph in the tissues surrounding the disc and apophyseal joints (79).

The Lind treatment (75) incorporates a multiplane autotraction table, designed by her, which generates the tractive force as the patient pulls with his arms against a fixed pelvic traction apparatus. The direction of traction can be changed by placement of the traction belt around the waist and by the choice of appropriate combinations of table adjustment. This table has two sections which can be rotated in a longitudinal and a transverse axis.

Lind (75) reports that of 1,023 patients treated by autotraction for low back pain and/or sciatica, 929 had a satisfactory response, and of these, 90.8% had an excellent response; 4.1%, a good response; 4.3%, a fair response; and 0.08%, a poor response. As pointed out previously, Lind reported a 70% recovery rate for patients with myelographically confirmed disc herniation who underwent autotraction.

## Stoddard's Observations

Stoddard (80) states that all too often patients are subjected to surgery with disastrous results. Surgical intervention is warranted in only a very small percentage of these patients, but all patients require the most careful definitive diagnosis and management. Furthermore, manipulation should be attempted on all patients, since the chance for success is great. Stoddard uses the straight leg raising sign as a guide to prognosis. If the patient is able to raise the leg 30° or less, with the leg held straight out, the sign is positive and the prospect of success is distinctly limited. If the patient is able to raise the leg 45°, the prospect of success is 50%. (Later we will compare this with our statistics.)

Stoddard (80) believes that the criteria for advising surgery are (1) irreversible severe pain which is intolerable with no relief from conservative measures, (2) recurrent crippling attacks affecting the livelihood of the patient or the patient's family, and (3) symptoms of cauda equina pressure. The use of sustained traction is justifiable in some patients, but physiologically, sustained traction has an adverse effect on the supportive ligaments, especially if excessive weights are used. Intermittent sustained traction is physiologically better, if it will provide the same benefits as sustained traction.

When nuclear material has escaped into the spinal canal and become wedged between the nerve root and intervertebral foramen, Stoddard believes (80), manipulation can sometimes alter the site of pressure or shift the prolapsed material to another site where there is less irritation of the nerve roots. If the manipulative techniques are sufficiently gentle to avoid further damage, they are well worth attempting because the attempt succeeds in roughly half of the patients. Even if the attempt is successful, the patient must still use caution, and it is hoped that the prolapsed material will in time shrink and cause less trouble. If the attempt is unsuccessful and the technique was designed to avoid further damage, the patient is no worse off and, if necessary, can still take advantage of surgical procedures.

## Results of a Study by Nashold and Hrubec

Nashold and Hrubec (81), in a 20-year follow-up study on lumbar disc disease on 1,123 patients with low back pain and sciatica, found that of those patients on whom a record was kept, 45% had left leg pain and 36% had right leg pain. They also found that 60.2% of these patients leaned toward the side opposite the pain, whereas 39.8% leaned toward the same side as the pain. The average age of the surgical patient was 29, and the average age of the nonsurgical patient was 30. Interestingly, these statistics contrast with those of Lind who states that 10 of 20 patients she kept records on were between ages 40 and 49, 7 were between ages 50 and 59, and the remaining 3 were in other age groups (75). Nashold and Hrubec (81) state that of 1,123 patients, 55.3% still had pain following surgery and 65.1% had pain following conservative care. The conservative care consisted of bed rest, drugs, and therapies. Specifically, of 400

patients operated on, 5% had complete relief, 12% had relief from leg pain, 18% had relief from back pain, and 52.2% still had both leg pain and back pain following surgery (81).

## Cyriax's Conclusions

Cyriax (82) in his textbook entitled, *Soft Tissue Lesions*, states that small and very recent nuclear herniations sometimes respond well to manipulation, provided that the technique is changed from the jerk to sustained pressure. Interestingly, he also discusses the co-existence of back pain and sciatica. He believes that a central protrusion impinging first upon dura mater creates back pain before sciatica sets in, whereas lateral disc protrusion creates sciatica without back pain. In practice, he found that about two thirds of all patients prove amenable to manipulative reduction. Patients with a nuclear protrusion for whom no treatment existed except prolonged rest in bed or laminectomy now fall within the scope of conservative treatment for the first time. As a result, his laminectomy rate, which used to be 1 in 40, has fallen to 1 in 200. Cyriax (82) states that the effects of sustained traction and its attendant distraction are (1) increase in the interval between the vertebral bodies, thus enlarging the space into which the protrusion must recede; (2) tautening of the joint capsule, which allows the ligaments joining the vertebral bodies to exert centripetal force all around the joint, thus tending to squeeze the pulp back into place; and (3) suction.

## Results of Cox Closed Reduction

Chiropractic closed reduction was used on 100 patients with lumbar disc protrusion and prolapse at the Chiropractic Associates Diagnostic and Treatment Center in Fort Wayne, Indiana. Table 1.1 shows

**Table 1.1.**
**Results of Disc Protrusion Study**

|  | Required Surgery | Responded to Chiropractic |
|---|---|---|
| Medial disc protrusions | 9 | 34 |
| Lateral disc protrusions | 2 | 55 |

**Table 1.2.**
**Facet Facings of the Involved Disc Level**

| Closed Reduction (Nonsurgical) | | Open Reduction (Surgical) | |
|---|---|---|---|
| Coronal facets | 72 | Medial | 9 |
| Sagittal facets (19.1%) | 17 | Sagittal (64%) | 6 |
| Total nonsurgical disc cases | 89 | Coronal | 3 |
| | | Lateral (both sagittal) | 2 |
| | | Total surgical disc cases | 11 |

**Table 1.3.**
**Response to Nonsurgical Treatment of Disc Protrusion**

| Nashold and Hrubec | Lind Autotraction | Cyriax Traction | Cox Closed Reduction |
|---|---|---|---|
| 67% with conservative care | 70% of 20 cases scheduled for surgery and 929 of 1023 ambulatory cases with low back pain and/or sciatica had satisfactory result | ⅔ response | 79.5% medial disc 96.5% lateral disc |

the results of this treatment, and Table 1.2 breaks down these results into the type of facet involvement. These results reveal that (1) patients with a lateral disc protrusion with coronal facet involvement respond most favorably to chiropractic reduction, and (2) patients with a medial disc protrusion with sagittal facet involvement most often require surgery.

Table 1.3 gives an estimate of the results of the various nonsurgical approaches used today.

Concerning Lind's statement that chiropractic treatment made autotraction more difficult, we must state that the chiropractic utilized in those cases was probably the side-posture torsional technique. We don't use this technique in the treatment of the patient with an acute disc; however, it is best to wait until symptoms of sciatica have disappeared before specific adjustive corrections to reduce subluxations are made. Admittedly the subluxations are often found to be reduced following Cox closed reduction. We do agree with Lind that the use of drugs such as muscle relaxants along with prolonged bed rest make the condition more difficult to treat due to the destruction of ligament tone and musculature, with the resultant slow healing involved. Lind (75) quoting from Lidstrom and Zachrisson (83) states that "physiotherapy may be not only ineffective but actually detrimental."

Herlin (84) states that the lateral disc protrusion is most commonly seen in patients with short-term sciatica, and Lind states that lateral disc protrusion is easier to treat than medial disc protrusion. Our statistics certainly confirm these statements. One point of disagreement between Lind and myself concerns treatment of the postsurgical patient. Although we have not treated as many patients as has Lind, we have had very little difficulty in treating the postsurgical patient. Why this is so I do not know. Perhaps there is a variation in surgical techniques between our two countries.

## References

1. Hippocrates: *Hippocrates*, with an English translation by Dr ET Withington. London, vol 3, 1944. In Lind G: *Auto-Traction, Treatment of Low Back Pain and Sciatica*. Linkoping, 1974, p 19. (Private publication available from library of author, JM Cox.)
2. Toufexis A: That aching back. *Time* July 14, 1980, p 30 (col 3).
3. *Medical Bulletin*, April 21, 1981. Globe International Group, Box 21, Rouses Point, NY 12979.
4. Hall H: Logical approach to diagnosis of back pain. *Can Fam Physician* 21:79–83, 1975.
5. Breen AC: Chiropractors and the treatment of back pain. *Rheumatol Rehabil* 16(1):48, 1977.
6. Zylbergold RS, Piper MC: Lumbar disc disease: comparative analysis of physical therapy treatments. *Arch Phys Med Rehabil* 62:176, 1981.
7. Montgomery CH: Preemployment back x-rays. *J Occup Med* 18:495–498, 1976.
8. Snook SH, Campanelli RA, Hart JW: A study of

three preventive approaches to low back injury. *J Occup Med* 20(7):480, 1978.

9. Finneson B: *Low Back Pain*, ed 2. Philadelphia, JB Lippincott, 1980.

10. Wigh RE, Anthony HF: Transitional lumbosacral discs: probability of herniation. *Spine* 6(2):168, 1981.

11. Keim HA, Kirkaldy-Willis WH: Clinical symposia. *Ciba Found Symp* 32(6):89, 1980.

12. Semon RL, Spengler D: Significance of lumbar spondylolysis in college football players. *Spine* 6(2):172, 1981.

13. Lenz WF: Spondylolisthesis and spondyloptosis of the lower lumbar spine: a macrostudy. *ACA J Chiropractic* 15:S107, 1981.

14. Ramani PS: Variations in the size of the bony lumbar canal in patients with prolapse of the lumbar intervertebral discs. *Clin Radiol* 27:301–307, 1976.

15. Martin G: Recurrent disc prolapse as a cause of recurrent pain after laminectomy for lumbar disc lesion. *NZ Med J* 91:206, 1980.

16. Rothman RH, Simeone FA: *The Spine.* Philadelphia, WB Saunders, 1975, vol 1, p 452.

17. Eisenstein S: Measurement of the lumbar spinal canal in two racial groups. *Clin Orthop* 115:43–46, 1976.

18. Ullrich CG, Binet EF, Sanecki MG, Keiffer SA: Quantitative assessment of the lumbar spinal canal by computed tomography. *Radiology* 134:137–143, 1980.

19. Mooney V, Robertson J: The facet syndrome. *Clin Orthop* 115:149–156, 1976.

20. Carrera GF, Haughton VM, Syvertsen A, Williams AL: Computed tomography of the lumbar facets. *Radiology* 134:145–148, 1980.

21. Carrera CG: Lumbar facet joint injection in low back pain and sciatica. *Radiology* 737:665–667, 1980.

22. Dory MA: Arthrography of the lumbar facet joints. *Radiology* 140:23–27, 1981.

23. Chynn KY, Altman I, Shaw WI, Finley N: The roentgenographic manifestations and clinical features of lumbar spinal stenosis with special emphasis of the superior articular process. *Neuroradiology* 16:378–380, 1978.

24. Lora J, Long D: So-called facet denervation in the management of intractable back pain. *Spine* 1(2):121–126, 1976.

25. Van Akkerveeken PF, O'Brien JP, Park W: Experimentally induced hypermobility of the lumbar spine. *Spine* 4(3):236–241, 1978.

26. Cox JM: Low back pain: recent statistics and data in its mechanism, diagnosis and treatment from chiropractic manipulation. *ACA J Chiropractic* 13:S125–S138, 1979.

27. Ehni G, Weinstein P: *Lumbar Spondylosis.* Chicago, Year Book Medical Publishers, 1977, p 19.

28. Cyron BM, Hutton WC: Articular tropism and stability of the lumbar spine. *Spine* 5(2):168–172, 1980.

29. Breig A, Troup JDG: Biomechanical considerations in the straight leg raising sign. *Spine* 4(3):242–250, 1979.

30. Hudgins WR: The crossed straight leg raising test: a diagnostic sign of herniated disc. *J Occup Med* 21(6):407–408, 1979.

31. Farfan H: A reorientation in the surgical approach to degenerative lumbar intervertebral joint disease. *Orthop Clin North Am* 8(1):9–21, 1977.

32. Virgin WJ: Experimental investigation into the physical properties of the intervertebral disc. *J Bone Joint Surg* 33B:607, 1951.

33. Lumsden RM, Morris JM: An in vivo study of axial rotation immobilization at the lumbosacral joint. *J Bone Joint Surg* 50A:1591, 1968.

34. Maigne R: Low back pain of thoracolumbar origin. *Arch Phys Med Rehabil* 61:389–394, 1980.

35. Harrison J: *Malpractice Alert* 2(2): December 1981.

36. Gainer JV, Nugent GR: The herniated lumbar disk. *Am Fam Pract* 127–131, September 1964.

37. Weitz EM: The lateral bending sign. *Spine* 6(4):388–397, 1981.

38. Aitken AP: Rupture of the intervertebral disc in industry: further observations and end results. *Am J Surg* 84:261–267, 1982.

39. Wood K: New approaches to treatment of back pain. *West J Med* 130(4):394–398, 1979.

40. Kessler RM: Acute symptomatic disc prolapse. *Phys Ther* 59:978–987, 1979.

41. Fahrni WH: Conservative treatment of lumbar disc degeneration: our primary responsibility. *Orthop Clin North Am* 6(1):93–103, 1975.

42. Nachemson A: The lumbar spine, an orthopaedic challenge. *Spine* 1(1):59–69, 1976.

43. Johnson EW, Fletcher FR: Lumbosacral radiculopathy: review of 100 consecutive cases, *Arch Phys Med Rehabil* 62:321–323, 1981.

44. Anonymous: Treatment of lumbar disc protrusion by automatic chiropractic traction instrument. Translated at the National College, 1982. (Available from library of author, JM Cox.)

45. Szepesi Z: Prevent sacroiliac degeneration. *Aches Pains* 2(9):15, 1981.

46. Valentini E: Acute lumbar disc syndromes under chiropractic care: a two year statistical study. Swiss Chiropractic Association, 51 Avenue Du Casino, 1820 Montreux, Switzerland, September 1979.

47. Tindall GT: Clinical aspects of lumbar intervertebral disc disease. *J Med Assoc Ga* 70:247–253, 1981.

48. Eagle R: A pain in the back. *New Scientist* 170–173, October 18, 1979.

49. Cookson JC: Orthopedic manual therapy. An overview. Part II—The spine. *Phys Ther* 59(3):259–267, 1979.

50. Nachemson A: A critical look at the treatment of low back pain. In: *The Research Status of Spinal Manipulative Therapy.* Bethesda, MD, National Institute of Neurological and Communicative Disorders and Stroke, NINCDS Monograph No 15, DHEW No 76-998, 1975, pp 287–292.

51. Goldstein M: Research in spinal manipulation—reflections on processes, priorities and responsibilities. *J Manip Physiolog Ther* 3(1):41, 1980.

52. Parker G, Tupling H: The chiropractic patient: psychosocial aspects. *Med J Aust* 2:373–376, 1976.

53. Von Luschka H: *Die Holgelenke des Neuschlichen Korpes.* Berlin, George Reimer, 1858.

54. Dandy WE: Loose cartilage from intervertebral disc simulating tumor of the spinal cord. *Arch Surg* 19:660, 1929.

55. Mixter WJ, Barr JS: Rupture of the intervertebral disc with involvement of the spinal canal. *N Engl J Med* 211:210–215, 1934.

56. Nordby E: *Am Med News* October 3, 1977.

57. Dommisse GF, Grabe RP: The failures of surgery for lumbar disc disorders. In Helfet AJ, Gruebel-Lee DM (eds): *Disorders of the Lumbar Spine.* Philadelphia, JB Lippincott, 1978, p 202.

58. Burton CV: Lumbar arachnoiditis. *Spine* 3(1):24–29, 1978.

59. Burton CV, Wiltse LL: Guest editors comments. *Spine* 3(1):1–23, 1978.

60. Pheasant HG: Backache. Its nature, incidence and cost. *West J Med* 126:330–332, 1977.

61. Shealy CN: Facets in back and sciatic pain. *Minn Med* 199:200, 1974.

62. Shealy CN, Freese AS: *Occult Medicine Can Save Your Life: A Modern Doctor Looks at Unconventional Healing.* New York, Dial Press, 1975.

63. Barr JS: Lumbar disk lesions in retrospect and prospect. *Clin Orthop* 4(8):129, 1977.

64. Marshall LL: The management of intervertebral disc lesions. *Med J Aust* 662, June 1978.

65. Wood K: New approach to treatment of back pain. *West J Med* 130:394, 1979.

66. Anderson G: Low back pain in industry: epidemiological aspects. *Scand J Rehabil Med* 11:163–168, 1979.

67. Mooney V: Surgery and postsurgical management of the patient with low back pain. *Phys Ther* 59(8):1000–1006, 1979.

68. Salenius P, Laurent LE. Results of operative treatment of lumbar disc herniation. A survey of 886 patients. *Acta Orthop Scand* 48:630–634, 1977.

69. Smith L: Bad times for the bad back. *Drug* 168–174, November 1978.

70. Cyriax J: Dural symptoms. *Lancet* 1:919–921, 1978.

71. Semmes ER: *Ruptures of the Lumbar Intervertebral Disc.* Springfield, IL, Charles C Thomas, 1964, pp 13, 17, and 18.

72. Yamada K: The dynamics of experimental posture. Experimental study of intervertebral disc herniation in bipedal animals. *Tokushima J Exp Med* 8:350–361, 1962.

72a. Yamada K: The dynamics of experimental posture. Experimental study of intervertebral disc herniation in bipedal animals. *Clin Orthop* 25:20–31, 1962.

73. Turek S: *Orthopaedics—Principles and Their Applications.* Philadelphia, JB Lippincott, 1956, chap 27, p 748.

74. Strait LA, Inman VT, Ralston HJ: Sample illustrations of physical principles selected from physiology and medicine. *Am J Physics* 15:375–382, 1947.

75. Lind G: *Auto-Traction, Treatment of Low Back Pain and Sciatica, An Electromyographic, Radiographic and Clinical Study.* Linkoping, 1974, pp 108, 109, 111, 114, 118, 120, 121, and 125. (Private publication available from library of author, JM Cox.)

76. Cyriax J: The pros and cons of manipulation. *Lancet* 1:571–573, 1964.

77. Schachtschneider H: Der hintere Bandscheibenprolaps seinen Auswirkungen. *Fortschr* 107–129, 1936.

78. Wyss T, Ulrich SP: Festigkeitsuntersuchungen und gezielte Extensionsbehandlung der Lendenwirbensaule unter Berucksichtigung des Bandscheiben—Vorfalles Vierenljahrs-schrift der Naturforschenden Gesellschaft in Zurich. Zurich, Beiheft Nr 3/4, September 30, 1954.

79. Cyriax J: *The Elements of Kellgren's Manual Treatment.* London, John Bale, Sons & Danielsson, 1903.

80. Stoddard A: *Manual of Osteopathic Technic.* New York, Harper & Row, 1969, chap 1, pp 25–27; chap 2, p 56; chap 3, pp 137, 140, and 141.

81. Nashold BS, Hrubec Z: *Lumbar Disc Disease, A Twenty-Year Clinical Follow-up Study.* St Louis, CV Mosby, 1971, chap 3, p 11; chap 5, p 34, chap 7, pp 65 and 66.

82. Cyriax J: *Soft Tissue Lesions,* ed 3. London, Paul B Hoeber, 1903, pp 450, 453, 454, and 457.

83. Lidstrom A, Zachrisson M: Physical therapy on low back pain and sciatica. *Scand J Rehabil Med* 2:37–42, 1970.

84. Herlin L: *Sciatic and Pelvic Pain due to Lumbosacral Nerve Root Compression.* Springfield, IL, Charles C Thomas, 1966, chap 4, p 10.

# CHAPTER 2

# Biomechanics of the Lumbar Spine: Physiological and Aberrant

International authorities differ in their opinions concerning the role that the intervertebral disc plays in the production of sciatica. Some state that only 5% of the cases of sciatica are due to lesion of the intervertebral disc, while others state that over 90% are due to this lesion. Rees (1) states that the slipped disc syndrome is the cause of more disability than is any other single affliction on earth. Rothman and Simeone (2) state that the most common cause of acute sciatica with low back pain involves herniation of lumbar disc material. Henry Feffer, Professor of orthopedic surgery at George Washington University, says that disc problems, by far, are the most common cause of back ailments (3). And Cyriax (4) states that "lumbar disc lesions are responsible for well over 90% of all organic symptoms attributable to the lower back."

Incomplete studies concerning the intervertebral disc date back to the first description by Vesalius in 1555. Two to three centuries later such men as Virchow and von Luschka published more detailed descriptions of the structure of the disc. Sicard, in 1916, correlated irritation of the intraspinal roots of the sciatic nerve with the production of sciatica. Description of the clinical syndrome of sciatica can be found in the writings of Dominico Cotunio as early as 1764. It was not until the 1920s and 1930s, however, that clinical and pathological manifestations of the disc lesion were documented into a syndrome by Schmorl, Dandy, Mixter, and Barr. The purpose of this brief historical reminder is to explain the relative infancy of the study of the lumbar disc lesion in the production of sciatica. The period from Mixter and Barr's work until today is barely 50 years, and these five decades have been filled with controversy and inaccuracy, proof that more research in the study of the disc lesion must be undertaken.

Authorities have also given opposing opinions on the use of myelography. Day (5) says that there is need for improvement in the diagnosis and treatment of the lumbar disc disease. Furthermore, the diagnosis can be made on the basis of history and physical examination alone. He believes that myelography has grave shortcomings, since it provides indirect evidence by the indentations of the Pantopaque column. Myelography is reliable only when herniations contact this column. Day advocates use of the discogram over use of the myelogram. Rothman and Simeone (6), however, dislike use of the discogram.

Semmes (7) states that the clinical findings and history are more reliable than myelograms because nearly one third of myelograms are uncertain or misleading. He explains that the myelogram is too frequently used for diagnosis and indication for surgical treatment. It is wholly unnecessary in the diagnosis of the average patient requiring surgery for a ruptured lumbar disc and is hardly justifiable in cases not requiring surgery. He used myelograms in less than 3% of his last 350 surgeries.

In their article concerning lumbar spondylolisthesis with ruptured disc, Scoville and Corkill (8) say that 7 of 17 patients with spondylolisthesis and ruptured disc had negative myelograms.

Abdullah et al. (9) in their article on extreme lateral lumbar disc herniation state that this type of disc herniation is outside the anatomical boundary of the spinal canal and cannot be demonstrated by myelography. The classical clinical manifestations of an extreme lateral lumbar disc lesion are necessary for their diagnosis; and discography often proves helpful. According to the authors, whenever neurological findings suggest upper lumbar nerve root compression, the chances are 4:1 that an extreme lateral disc herniation is responsible. Categorically stated: a systematic diagnostic approach to the disc lesion, up to but not including the use of myelographic exploration, can yield an excellent diagnostic impression about the level and type of disc lesion in relationship to the nerve root it compresses.

Nachemson (10) in discussion of the role of the disc in low back and leg pain concludes:

1. Disc hernia is usually preceded by one or more attacks of low back pain.

2. Following intradiscal injection of either hypertonic saline or contrast media, it is often possible, in patients with complaints of pain as well as in normal subjects, to artificially cause the same type of pain as that which occurs from disc degeneration.

3. Investigations have been performed in which thin nylon threads were surgically fastened to various structures in and around the nerve root. Three to four weeks after surgery these structures were irritated by pulling on the threads, but pain resembling that which the patient had experienced previously could be registered only from the outer part of the annulus and the nerve root.

4. Pathoanatomically radiating ruptures are known to occur in the posterior part of the annulus, reaching out toward the areas in which naked nerve endings are located. Such single ruptures in the lumbar discs are first manifested in people about 25 years old, the same age at which the low back pain syndrome becomes clinically important. Various theories on how these ruptures elicit pain exist.

5. Of all the structures that theoretically could be involved in the pain process, only the disc shows changes that could account for the anatomic changes at such an early age. Such changes in other structures in the region generally show up much later in life and then only secondary to severe disc degeneration.

6. Although a late sign, disc degeneration is noted on radiographs of patients between 50 and 60 years old and has been seen significantly more often in those who have had back pain than in those who have not.

The facet joints have been demonstrated to show histologic signs of arthritis very late in life and always secondary to degenerative changes in the discs.

## DEFINITIONS AND ILLUSTRATIONS OF DISC PROTRUSION AND PROLAPSE

Disc protrusion (Fig. 2.1) is an extension of nuclear material through the annulus into the spinal canal with no loss of continuity of extruded material. Protrusion and herniation are synonymous.

Disc prolapse (Fig. 2.2) occurs when the extruded material loses continuity with the existing nuclear material and forms a free fragment in the spinal canal. Disc prolapse is the most common indication for disc surgery.

Protrusion of disc material (Fig. 2.3) exists when the bulging nuclear material is contiguous with the remaining nucleus pulposus, and the annulus fibrosus is stretched, thinned, and under pressure. Epstein (11) notes that the pressure within the nucleus pulposus is 30 psi and mentions that Nachemson and Morris found that this pressure is 30% less in the standing position than in the sitting position and is 50% less in the reclining position than in the sitting position. Keep in mind, also, that cerebrospinal fluid pressure is 100 to 200 mm of water in the recumbent posture and 400 mm in the sitting posture (12). It is important, therefore, that the patient with a protruding disc avoid sitting.

In people between the ages of 30 and 40 years, the nucleus has a water content of 80% (13). Puschel (14) says this fluid content decreases with age. DePukey (15) found that the average person is 1%

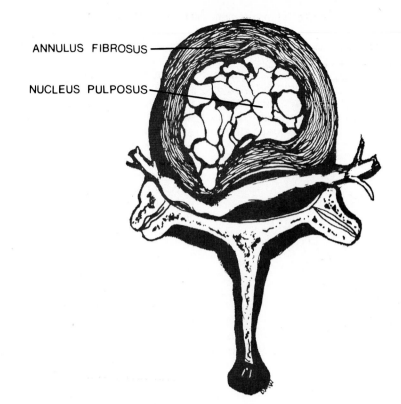

**Figure 2.1.** Nuclear protrusion. The annulus fibrosus is still intact although weakened with nuclear bulge.

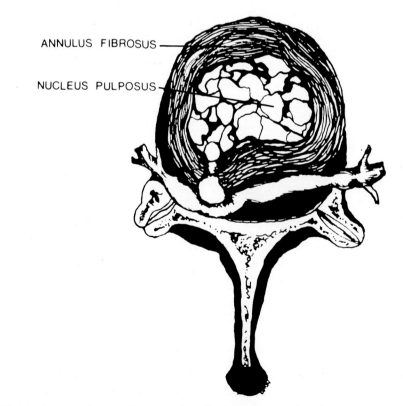

**Figure 2.2.** Nuclear prolapse. The annulus fibrosus is completely torn, allowing nuclear escape into the posterior vertebral canal as a free fragment.

shorter in height at the end of the day than on first arising in the morning. He also found that a person in the first decade of life is 2% shorter at bedtime and a person in the eighth decade of life is 0.5% shorter. This difference he attributes to decreasing water content in the disc which occurs with advancing age.

Hendry (16) believes that the hydrodynamics of the disc result from the gel structure of the nucleus pulposus, enabling it to absorb 9 times its volume of water. No chemical bond influences this water content, as it can be mechanically expressed under pressure; thus, there is the decrease of 1% average height from weight bearing in a day.

The nucleus pulposus occupies about half the disc surface area and bears the vertical load, while the annulus bears the tangential load (17). Because of nuclear degeneration, shift in stress and weight-bearing forces occurs. Bradford and Spurling state that the ratio of the anterior to posterior weight-bearing forces of the body is 15:1; therefore, lifting 100 lb with the arms extended places a total pressure of 1,500 lb on the nucleus pulposus. Even more revealing is the finding of Morris et al. (18) that a 170-lb man lifting 200 lbs exerts a force of 2,071 lb on the L5-S1 disc space.

*Discography* is performed by the injection of contrast material into the nucleus, which normally will accept approximately 1 cc of solution. If the injection duplicates the patients symptoms, disc protrusion, irritating the annulus and/or nerve root, is signified. Figure 2.4 reveals

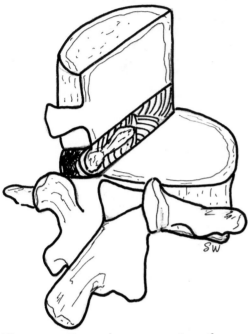

**Figure 2.3.** In nuclear protrusion, the annular fibers are containing the bulging nuclear material.

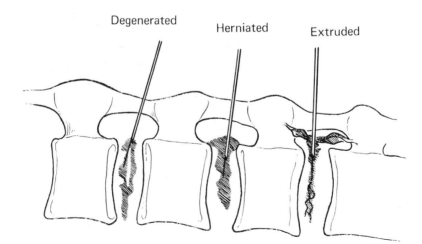

Degenerated     Herniated     Extruded

ABNORMAL

**Figure 2.4.** Some abnormal discogram configurations. (Reproduced with permission from B. E. Finneson: *Low Back Pain*, edition 2. Philadelphia, J. B. Lippincott, 1980, p. 104.)

normal and abnormal nuclear appearances on discography.

Gresham and Miller (19) carried out postmortem discography on 63 fresh autopsy specimens; the patients who came to autopsy ranged in age from 14 to 80 years and had relatively asymptomatic backs. The results of this study are presented in Table 2.1

Abnormalities in the disc reduce its capacity to aid in supporting torsional loads of the spine by about 40% (20).

Degeneration of the intervertebral disc and subsequent changes in adjacent vertebrae and ligaments are termed spondylosis. Fissuring of the annulus fibrosus occurs posteriorly, usually where the common ligament is least strong (21). Finneson (22) describes two disc changes following injury (Fig. 2.5): disc herniation (or protrusion) and spondylosis. He notes that in less than 20% of patients with annular tears or fissures, a large fragment of nucleus bulges forth to compress a nerve root, producing classic disc symptoms. Usually, however, the annulus never completely tears and contains the nucleus within its boundary with only slight protrusion.

Finneson goes on to say that fibrosis of the annulus fibrosus occurs as the annulus loses its sponginess and elasticity. The

**Table 2.1.**
**Results of Postmortem Discography from a Study by Gresham and Miller (Total Autopsies, 60) (19)**

| Group | Age Range (years) | Findings |
|-------|--------------------|----------|
| I | 14–34 | 90% normal discs<br>10% degenerated discs |
| II | 35–45 | 25% normal discs |
| III | 46–59 | 25% normal discs at L3-L4<br>0% normal discs at L5-S1 |
| IV | 60 and over | 5% normal discs<br>0% normal at L5-S1<br>2% normal at L4-L5[a]<br>3% normal at L3-L4[b] |

[a] One autopsy in 60.
[b] Two autopsies in 60.

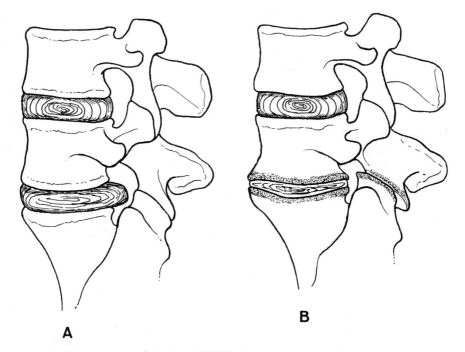

**A**                                         **B**

**Figure. 2.5.** *A:* Herniation of the nucleus pulposus. *B:* Spondylosis. (Reproduced with permission from B. E. Finneson: *Low Back Pain*, edition 2. Philadelphia, J. B. Lippincott, 1980, p. 437.)

disc space thins, with sclerosis of the cartilaginous end plates and new bone formation around the periphery of the contiguous vertebral surfaces occurring. The altered mechanics place stress on the posterior diarthrodial joints, causing them to lose their normal nuclear fulcrum for movement. With the loss of disc space, the plane of articulation of the facet surfaces is no longer congruous. This stress results in degenerative arthritis of the articular surfaces. Complete fibrous ankylosis of the disc and articular surfaces is possible.

Disc prolapse (Fig. 2.6), as stated earlier, exists when the extruded nuclear material loses continuity with the existing nuclear material and forms a free fragment within the spinal canal.

Figure 2.7 illustrates that a disc may protrude either lateral to a nerve root, medial to a nerve root, under a nerve root, or in a central position. When the disc protrudes lateral to the nerve root, the patient assumes an antalgic lean away from the side of disc lesion (Fig. 2.8). When the disc protrudes medial to the nerve root, the patient assumes an antalgic lean into the side of disc lesion or pain (Fig. 2.9). With a central disc lesion, the patient assumes a flexed posture of the lumbar spine with or without lean to either side. With protrusion under the nerve root, the patient may assume no lean.

The dermatome chart (Fig. 2.10) reveals innervation of the sensory nerves of the lower extremity. Ninety percent or more of lumbar disc lesions occur at either the L4-L5 or L5-S1 disc level. The L4-L5 disc usually compresses the fifth lumbar nerve root, resulting in pain sensations down the lower extremity in the fifth lumbar nerve root innervation. The L5-S1 disc usually compresses the first sacral nerve root, resulting in pain distribution down the first sacral dermatome of the lower extremity. Lecuire et al. (23) found that of 641 patients with disc lesion, 307 showed definite S1 dermatome patterns, 267 showed definite L5 dermatome patterns, and 67 showed mixed patterns. Sixty percent of these patients had an antalgic lean. A single disc lesion was noted in 562 patients, with 47% occurring at L5-S1,

39% occurring at L4-L5, and 2% occurring at L3-L4. Myelograms were performed on 238 of the 641 patients prior to surgery. Knowledge of specific innervation of the nerve root is important in deciding which disc is involved. By ascertaining the antalgic posture, the clinician may determine whether the problem is a medial, a central, or a lateral disc protrusion.

Therefore, there are two facts of primary importance in the evaluation of a patient: the side of sciatic pain distribution and the side of antalgic inclination; i.e., whether the patient leans toward or away from the side of pain in relation to the convexity of the sciatic scoliosis (Fig. 2.11).

These two facts establish the location of the disc protrusion in relation to the compressed nerve root. A disc lying medial to the nerve root results in patient lean toward the diseased or painful side. A disc lying lateral to the nerve root results in patient lean toward the healthy side. A central protrusion may result in no antalgic lean.

The author finds that the level of disc involvement usually is the site of vertebral rotational and lateral flexion changes; this level may be observed on visual examination of the patient's spine. Often it is noted only on x-ray examination; x-ray studies are made with the patient in both a recumbent and a standing position, since no difference is noted in these disc cases. The site of lateral flexion and rotation change may be quite noticeable or only very slightly discernible on radiographs; therefore, close correlation with the history and clinical examination is needed to pinpoint the site of disc protrusion. In other cases, the x-ray finding is quite striking regarding the amount of flexion and rotational change that results in a sciatic scoliosis. Some cases of disc prolapse requiring surgery, however, often reveal minimal change in functional spinal unit relationships. Case presentations and x-ray findings demonstrating these cases are given in Chapter 8 on the disc cases. An interesting observation is that sciatic scoliosis often appears as a Lovett failure or as reverse scoliosis; i.e., there is a failure of body rotation or a rotation to the convexity of the scoliosis

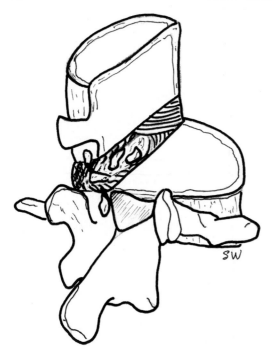

**Figure 2.6.** In nuclear prolapse, the annulus completely tears, allowing escape of free fragments of nuclear material into the vertebral canal or extremely laterally into the intervertebral foramen.

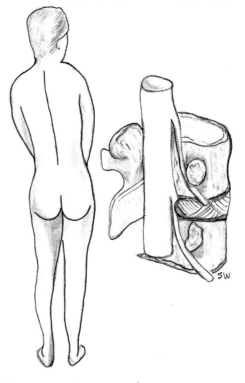

**Figure 2.8.** Sciatic scoliosis in a patient with a right lateral disc protrusion.

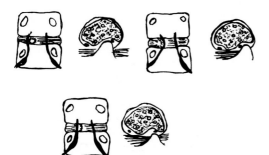

**Figure 2.7.** Nerve root displacement by disc protrusion. *Upper left:* Medial disc displaces nerve laterally. *Upper right:* Lateral disc displaces nerve root medially. *Lower center:* Disc lies directly under nerve root, stretching it.

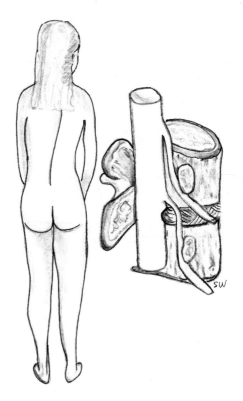

**Figure 2.9.** Sciatic scoliosis in a patient with right medial disc protrusion.

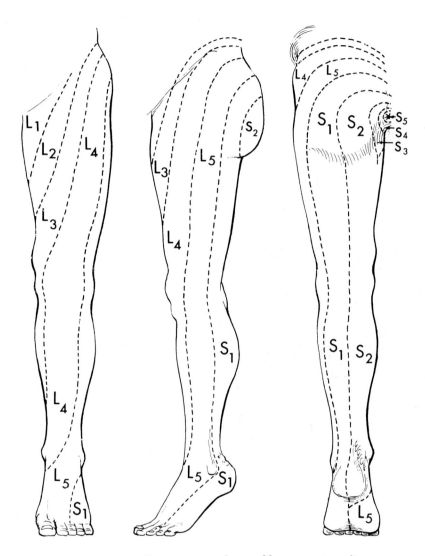

**Figure 2.10.** Dermatome chart of lower extremity.

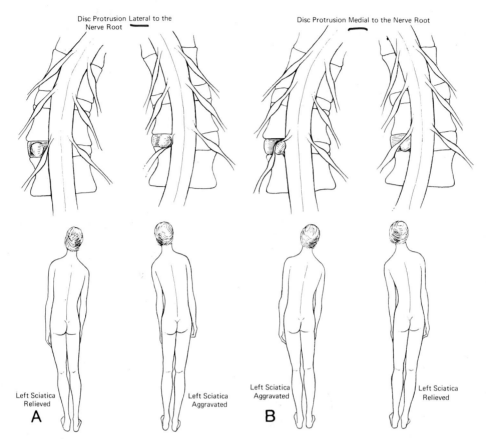

**Figure 2.11.** Relief or aggravation of pain with lateral flexion may indicate whether the disc protrusion is lateral or medial to the nerve root. (Reproduced with permission from B. E. Finneson: *Low Back Pain*, edition 2. Philadelphia, J. B. Lippincott, 1980, p. 302.)

by the vertebral bodies instead of toward the side of concavity. Another point to remember is that a false negative is sometimes reported on myelography when a laterally protruded disc lies too far lateral to the subarachnoid space to impress upon it. Compilation of these findings delineates the nerve root and disc involved.

A discussion of the normal anatomical relationship of the nerve root origin from the dural sac and its ultimate exit via its intervertebral foramen is in order before proceeding. The adult spinal cord ends at the level of L1-L2 at the conus medullaris, continuing caudally as the filum terminale to attach at the back of the coccyx. The filum terminale is encased in dura mater to the level of S2. At each vertebral level, a pair of nerve roots leave the dural sac, with each enclosed by dural nerve

root sleeves. In the lumbar spine these nerve roots pass directly downward, forming the cauda equina surrounding the filum terminale, until their eventual exit from each respective intervertebral foramen. The origin of the nerve root from the dural sac (cauda equina) is about one segment above the exit from its intervertebral foramen (IVF). The nerve root runs down laterally to the IVF from which it exits. Specifically, the fourth lumbar root exits the dural sac at the level of the third lumbar disc to exit the IVF one vertebra below; the fifth lumbar nerve root exits the dural sac at the level of the fourth lumbar disc to exit the IVF one vertebral segment below; the first sacral root exits the dural sac at the fifth lumbar disc level, passing down to the first sacral IVF; and the second sacral nerve root lies medial to S1, originating at the lower border of the fifth lumbar disc.

From Figure 2.12, it can be seen that the L4 nerve root can be compressed at its origin and course by the protrusion of the third lumbar disc, that the L5 nerve root can be compressed by the fourth lumbar disc, and that the S1 and S2 nerve roots can be compressed by the fifth disc protrusion.

## INTERVERTEBRAL DISC BIOMECHANICS

Pressure changes within the nucleus pulposus as they relate to postural and physiological stresses are shown in Figures 2.13, 2.14, and 2.15.

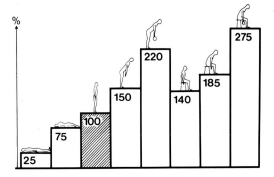

**Figure 2.13.** Relative change in pressure (or load) in the third lumbar disc in various positions in living subjects. (Reproduced with permission from A. L. Nachemson: The lumbar spine, an orthopaedic challenge. Spine 1(1):61, 1976 (10).)

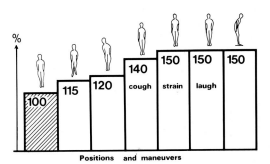

**Figure 2.14.** Relative change in pressure (or load) in the third lumbar disc in various maneuvers in living subjects. (Reproduced with permission from A. L. Nachemson: The lumbar spine, an orthopaedic challenge. Spine 1(1):61, 1976 (10).

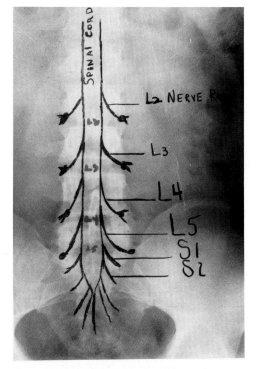

**Figure 2.12.** Schematic overlay of exiting cauda equina nerve roots in relation to the vertebral column and disc level.

**Figure 2.15.** Relative change in pressure (or load) in the third lumbar disc in various muscle-strenghtening exercises in living subjects. (Reproduced with permission from A. L. Nachemson: The lumbar spine, an orthopaedic challenge. Spine 1(1):61, 1976 (10).)

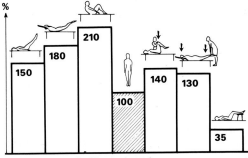

From Figures 2.13 and 2.14, it can be noted that Déjérine's triad and sitting raise the intradiscal pressure 6 times higher than does recumbency.

The intervertebral disc comprises one fourth to one third of the total length of the spinal column and is composed of three distinct parts—the cartilaginous end plate, the nucleus pulposus, and the annulus fibrosus.

## Nucleus Pulposus

The nucleus pulposus is located centrally within the posterior compartment of the disc at the juncture of the central and posterior thirds. It contains various mucopolysaccharides in the form of glucosaminoglycan which has the ability to imbibe fluids to 9 times its own volume. The nucleus fills 40% to 50% of the total disc area, and because of imbibition of fluids, it takes on a stiffness within its cells called turgor. At a person's birth, the water content of a disc is 70% to 90%; the content decreases with increase in the age of the person. The intradiscal pressures drop with loss of fluid; thus, disc herniation occurs most often when the person is between 20 and 50 years old and the intradiscal pressures are their greatest.

## Annulus Fibrosus

The annulus fibrosus contains the nucleus pulposus by concentric laminated bands of fibrous tissue which gradually form at the boundary of the nucleus without a sharp area of differentiation (Fig. 2.16). Sharpey's fibers attach the annular fibers to the end plates in the inner area and to the osseous tissue in the periphery.

## Weight-bearing Changes in the Disc

The disc bears vertical axis weight and distributes it tangentially to the annular fibers. The disc also bears tensile stresses at the annular fibers during rotation motion. The nucleus bears the vertical load and the annular fibers bear the tangential load in a normal disc. Degeneration causes redistribution of the loading mechanism, with the annular fibers bearing most of the vertical load.

On compression loading, the cartilaginous end plate is most susceptible to fracture, allowing rupture of nuclear material into the cancellous bone (Schmorl's nodes). The vertebral body (Fig. 2.17) is next most susceptible to fracture. There is an audible crack as the body gives way, occurring at compression loads of 1,000 to 1,700 lb in young specimens and at as little as 300 lb in older specimens. With the annulus intact, the disc will not compress without vertebral compression (24).

Virgin (as discussed in Ref. 25) also observed that even if posterolateral incisions were made in the annulus fibrosus all the way to the nucleus and then loaded in compression, there would still be very little change in the elastic properties of the annulus and definitely no disc herniation.

## Rotational Changes in the Disc

In the lumbar spine, the axis of rotation is between the articular facets in the arch of the vertebra, with the annular fibers resisting the axial shearing stresses (Fig. 2.18). On flexion and extension, the axis of rotation passes close to or within the nucleus pulposus, so that for the most part the nucleus pulposus can be considered the center of motion in a sagittal plane.

Gregersen and Lucas (26) studied axial rotation of the spine while the trunk was rotated from side to side. Approximately 74° of rotation occurred between T1 and T12, and the average cumulative rotation from the sacrum to T1 was 102°. Very little rotation occurred in the lumbar spine, as compared with that in the thoracic spine; again, this is a reflection of the orientation of the facet joints. Measurements of rotation obtained during walking indicated the following (24):

1. The pelvis and the lumbar spine rotate as a functional unit.

2. In the lower thoracic spine, rotation diminishes gradually up to T7.

3. T7 represents the area of transition from vertebral rotation in the direction of the pelvis to rotation in the opposite direction, that of the shoulder girdle.

4. The amount of rotation in the upper thoracic spine increases gradually from T7 to T1.

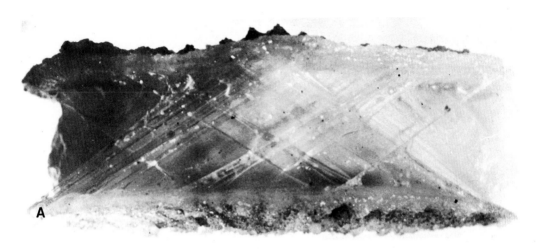

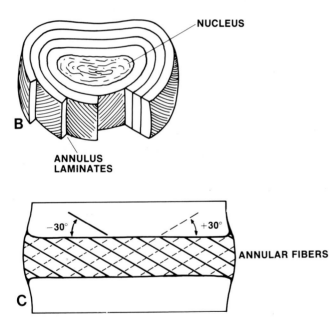

NUCLEUS

B

ANNULUS
LAMINATES

−30°   +30°

ANNULAR FIBERS

C

**Figure 2.16.** Intervertebral disc. A. A photograph of a disc clearly shows the annular fibers and their orientation. B. The disc consists of a nucleus pulposus surrounded by the annulus which is made of concentric laminated bands of annular fibers. In any two adjacent bands the fibers are oriented in opposite directions. C. The fibers are oriented at about ±30° with respect to the placement of the disc. (Photograph courtesy of Dr. Leon Kazarian.) (Reproduced with permission from A. A. White and M. M. Panjabi: *Clinical Biomechanics of the Spine.* Philadelphia, J. B. Lippincott, 1978, p. 3.)

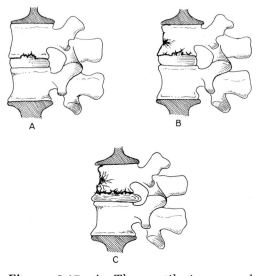

**Figure 2.17.** *A.* The cartilaginous end plates are most susceptible to spinal compression. *B.* The vertebral body is the second most susceptible unit of the spine. *C.* The normal nucleus pulposus and annulus fibrosus are least susceptible to pressure. (Reproduced with permission from B. E. Finneson: *Low Back Pain*, edition 2. Philadelphia, J. B. Lippincott, 1980, p. 39.)

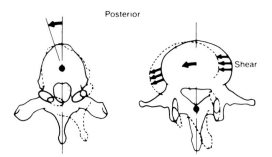

**Figure 2.18.** Mechanism of axial rotation in a thoracic (*left*) and a lumbar (*right*) vertebra. (Reproduced with permission from B. E. Finneson: *Low Back Pain*, edition 2, Philadelphia, J. B. Lippincott, 1980, p. 34 (24).)

Lumsden and Morris (27) measured axial rotation at the lumbosacral level in vivo and found that approximately 6° of rotation occurred at this level during maximum rotation. Approximately 1.5° of rotation occurred during normal walking. They also found that rotation at L5-

S1 was not measurably affected by asymmetrically oriented facets (tropism); it has always been associated with flexion of L5 on the sacrum.

White and Panjabi (28) state that the disc annulus supports two types of stress—the normal or perpendicular and the shearing or parallel. Shear stresses are larger in magnitude, and there is no provision for resisting shear stress in the way that annular fibers resist normal perpendicular stresses by the alternating annular layers. Thus, the risk of disc failure is greater with tensile loading than with compression loading.

When a disc is subjected to torsion, there are shear stresses in the horizontal as well as the axial plane. The magnitude of these stresses varies in direct proportion to the distance from the axis of rotation (Fig. 2.19). The stresses at 45° and 60° to the horizontal are shown in Figure 2.19. Shear stresses that are perpendicular to the fibers direction may produce disc failure.

The application to proper lifting (Fig. 2.20) can be considered with the above tensile stress failures.

## Findings of Various Authorities on Nerve Supply to the Disc

1. Bernini and Simeone (28a) state that the sinuvertebral nerve supplies the posterior longitudinal ligament, annulus fibrosus, and neurovascular contents of the epidural space.

2. Nachemson (10) found that the outer annulus and nerve root were the most pain-sensitive and reproduced the patient's presurgical symptoms when stimulated 3 to 4 weeks postsurgically.

3. Farfan (28b) points out that there is increasing evidence that there are unmyelinated nerve endings, usually associated with pain reception in the posterior annulus and even penetrating the nucleus. The posterior longitudinal ligament is well innervated.

4. Helfet and Gruebel-Lee (28c) have shown that when a radial tear penetrates the outer annulus, there is an attempt at healing by ingrowth of granulation tissue. Naked endings of the sinuvertebral nerve have been identified in this granulation

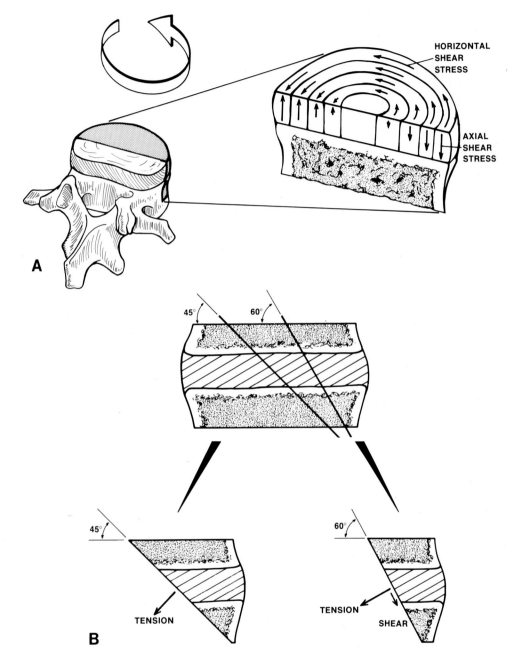

**Figure 2.19.** Disc stresses with torsion. A. Application of a torsional load to the disc produces shear stresses in the disc. These are in the horizontal plane as well as in the axial plane, and both are always of equal magnitude. They vary, however, at different points in the disc in proportion to the distance from the instantaneous axis of rotation. B. At 45° to the disc plane, the stresses are normal (i.e., there are no shear stresses). At 60° to the disc plane, perpendicular to the annular fibers, however, both types of stresses are present, normal as well as shear. The normal stresses are efficiently taken up by the annular fibers. (Reproduced with permission from A. A. White and M. M. Panjabi. *Clinical Biomechanics of the Spine.* Philadelphia, J. B. Lippincott, 1978, p. 16.)

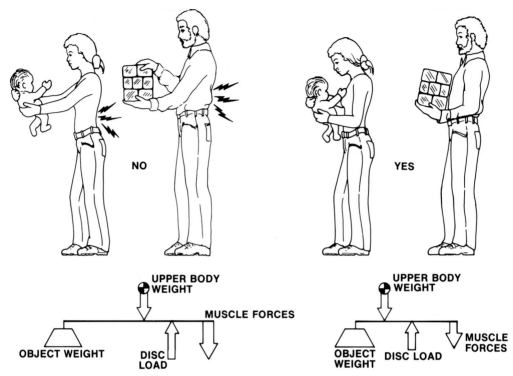

**Figure 2.20.** Diagram of the ergonomics of proper lifting. The load on the discs is a combined result of the object weight, the upper body weight, the back muscle forces, and their respective lever arms to the disc center. On the *left*, the object is farther away from the disc center, compared to the object on the *right*. The lever balances at the *bottom* show that smaller muscle forces and disc loads are obtained when the object is carried nearer to the disc. (Reproduced with permission from A. A. White and M. M. Panjabi: *Clinical Biomechanics of the Spine*. Philadelphia, J. B. Lippincott, 1978, p. 331.)

tissue. These may be pain receptors, which would explain discogenic pain in the absence of herniation.

5. Bogduk (29) says that the sinuvertebral nerve supplies the annulus fibrosus and the posterior longitudinal ligament. It runs up and down two segments, supplying the annulus and posterior longitudinal ligament above and below.

6. Tsukada (28d) and Shinohara (28e) claim that nerve fibers exist not only in the posterior longitudinal ligament but also in the nucleus and notochord. Malinsky (28f) and Hirsch et al. (28g) observed that nerve fibers penetrated into the outer layers of the disc. Tsukada (28d) and Shinohara (28e) found nerve endings in granulation tissue within the inner layers of the annulus and in the nucleus of some degenerated discs. In another article,

Yoshizawa et al. (28k) found profuse free nerve terminals in the outer half of the annulus but no such terminals in the nucleus.

7. Sunderland (28h), at the National Institute of Neurological and Communicative Disorders and Stroke (NINCDS) Conference, 1975, stated that the recurrent meningeal nerve supplies the dura, intervertebral disc, and associated structures.

8. Edgar and Ghadially (28i) say that the sinuvertebral nerve divides into ascending, descending, and transverse branches adjacent to the posterior longitudinal ligament. Lazorthes (28j) states that this nerve supplies the neural laminae, intervertebral disc at the adjacent levels, posterior longitudinal ligament and the internal vertebral plexus, the epidural tissue, and the dura mater. Con-

cerning the tissues supplied by this nerve, however, there is still disagreement; some authorities do not believe that there is such a wide distribution. Tsukada (28d) and Shinohara (28e) found that the outer annulus is innervated in a normal disc but that fine nerve fibers accompany granulation tissue present in a degenerated disc. In one instance, fine fibers were observed in the nucleus. Most of these were naked nerve endings and probably mediated pain sensation. Edgar and Ghadially (28i) found that sinuvertebral nerves supply the anterior dura. In spinal stenosis, therefore, irritation of the sinuvertebral nerve may be the mechanism of claudication pain.

## WELL-SUBSTANTIATED NEUROLOGICAL FACTS

In discussing the lumbar intervertebral disc syndrome, Bogduk (29) states that there are four elements of the nervous system which may be involved in the production of this syndrome: the lumbosacral nerve roots, the spinal nerves, the dorsal rami, and the sinuvertebral nerves. The nerve root is usually irritated because of its being stretched over a protruding or prolapsed disc. The irritation of the spinal nerve may result from arthrosis of the zygapophyseal joints, ligamentum flavum hypertrophy, osteophytes, intervertebral disc protrusion, subluxation, spondylolisthesis, infection, tumor, fracture, Paget's disease, or ankylosing spondylitis. The dorsal rami (which supply the zygapophyseal joints, erector spinae muscles and their related fascia and skin, the periosteum of the vertebral arches, multifidus muscles, the interspinous ligament, and interspinous muscles) are irritated by articular facet arthrosis, subluxation, sacroiliac joint arthrosis, spinous process impingement, strain of the sacral joints, hyperlordosis, scoliosis, myositis, muscle spasm, and reactions secondary to sclerosis or arthrosis of the articular facets. The sinuvertebral nerve, also known as the recurrent meningeal nerve, supplies the posterior longitudinal ligament as well as the annulus fibrosus of the disc. A descending branch runs caudally for a maximum of two segments, supplying the annulus fibrosus and the posterior longitudinal ligament. An ascending branch may also behave similarly. Any lesion of the annulus or posterior longitudinal ligament is capable of setting up pain impulses in the sinuvertebral nerve.

Two basic causes of low back pain are internal derangements of the intervertebral disc and irritation of the zygapophyseal articulation. The ontogeny of low back pain concerns two structures: the disc and facet. Debate continues as to which is the initial lesion and which is a secondary or compensatory change. After study, this author believes that the initial change takes place in the intervertebral disc, which later affects the articular facet. Vernon-Roberts and Pirie (30) state that a direct relationship exists between the degree of disc degeneration, the marginal osteophyte formation on vertebral bodies, and the apophyseal joint change, which suggests that disc degeneration is the primary event leading to the clinical condition of degenerative spondylosis.

## Effects of Rotation on the Intervertebral Disc

Farfan (31) proved that torsional stresses of a magnitude encountered in daily living play a major role in initiating lumbar disc degeneration. He found that in compression loading of the lumbar spine, the nucleus pulposus was the last structure to fracture, with the vertebral body fracturing by compression before the disc would so yield. When experiments were devised to test the effects of rotation on the lumbar spine, the normal range of axial rotation at the lumbosacral joint was less than 9°.

The annulus fibrosus may be subdivided into a peripheral portion of thick, firmly attached well-formed laminations and an inner, softer, less well structured portion surrounding the nucleus pulposus. When the disc is subjected to torsion, the resulting damage is found in the outermost layers of the disc but does not involve the longitudinal ligaments and possibly not the most superficial annular laminae. The inner portions of the annulus remain undisturbed. There is increasing evidence that there are unmyelinated nerve endings (usually associated with pain reception) distributed throughout the posterior annulus and even penetrating the nucleus (32).

Measurement of the degree of rotation occurring at the lumbosacral joint has been as high as 9° but is usually 5° or less (32). During walking, minimum rotation occurs between vertebrae; walking at 3.65 mph results in a total rotation of 11° between T1 and the sacrum, with 0.2° to 0.6° of this occurring at the lumbosacral joint. The lumbosacral joint can be rotated 3° to 13° during twisting to one side.

## TORQUE ROTATION CURVES

Rotation was applied to fresh human lumbar spine specimens at the rate of 3.6°/min. This corresponds to the rate of rotation applied during walking at 3.5 mph (32). The following changes took place at various degrees of rotation:

1. 0° to 3°. During this phase, there was little increase of torque with increasing rotation.

2. 3° to 12°. In this second portion of the curve, a major torque was proportional to the applied rotation. During this phase, much tissue was expressed from the specimen. The fluid seemed to come from the vertebral body bone surfaces adjacent to the disc.

3. 12° to 20°. In this portion of the curve, there was little increase of torque with increase of applied rotation. During this phase the curve showed numerous small dips just prior to failure. These small indentations in the recordings were often accompanied by sharp cracking noises emanating from the specimen. Nothing was observed at the specimen's surface to explain these sounds.

The torque rotational curves were similar for intact whole joints, for the isolated disc, and for facet joint preparations. "The normal range of rotation in the human lumbosacral joint probably is limited to less than 5°. Our experiments suggest that the range may even be 3° or less" (emphasis added). The average torque at failure for intact whole intervertebral joints with normal discs was found to be 750 to 900 inch/lb, nearly twice as high as that for joints with degenerated discs. The average angle of rotation at failure for whole joints with normal discs was 22.6°, while for degenerated discs it was 14.3°. The resistance of the normal disc to this torque is approximately 300 inch/lb, while that of a degenerated disc is about 200 inch/lb. The posterior apophyseal joints also provide resistance to rotation, totaling about 250 inch/lb.

Morris (as discussed in Ref. 26) states that the average cumulative rotation from the sacrum to the first thoracic vertebra is 102°, with 74° of this rotation occurring between the first and the twelfth thoracic vertebra. The rotation at the lumbosacral level in vivo is approximately 6°. Figure 2.21 shows the rotational damage to the intervertebral joints at various degrees of rotation.

Farfan (33) believes that it is possible to state with some certainty that the first pathological changes which occur in the disc occur in the annulus. These take the form of small circumferential separations between the lamellae of the annulus, which have been recorded in children as young as age 10 (34, 35). He states that it is impossible to say whether the process of intervertebral joint degeneration begins in the disc, end plate, or neural arch complex. The changes may occur simultaneously in all three locations. The incidence of disc degeneration is the highest at L5-S1, next highest at L4-L5, and the third highest at L3-L4.

|  | NORMAL DISC | DEGENERATED DISC |
|---|---|---|
| Average angle of rotation at failure | 22.6° | 14.3° |
| Resistance to torque | 300 in-lb. | 200 in-lb. |

**Figure 2.21.** Annular fiber failure in rotation.

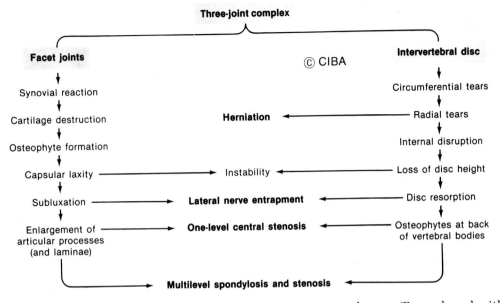

**Figure 2.22.** Pathogenesis of the nerve root entrapment syndrome. (Reproduced with permission from *Clinical Symposia.*© 1980, CIBA Pharmaceutical Company, Division of CIBA-GEIGY Corporation. All rights reserved.)

### Changes in the Intervertebral Disc

Turek (36) states that the annulus fibrosus begins to show concentric cracking and cavitation in children as young as age 15. This dehydration and cracking of the annulus may progress silently for many years, with the nucleus bulging through these cracks, causing the annulus to be thinned and weakened at its periphery. Relatively little force may cause the annulus to tear, allowing the nucleus to burst forth. Ritchie and Fahrni (34) mention that an ingrowth of vascular tissue takes place through the end plates, from the cancellous bone of the vertebral body into the nucleus pulposus. The fluid content of the nucleus decreases with increasing age until approximately 70% of the nucleus is fluid in a person at age 77, as compared with 88% in a newborn. This degeneration of the disc is accompanied by remodeling of the vertebral bodies. Herniation of the nucleus into the vertebral end plate at the site of vascular proliferation is termed Schmorl's node. The rupturing of the nuclear material anteriorly and laterally results in periosteal proliferation or osteophyte formation.

This thinning of the intervertebral disc is accompanied by changes in the facet articulations as well. The facet joints lose their spacing as their articular cartilage shows degenerative changes because of the stress encountered by disc degeneration. The facets lose their gliding motion of one upon another, and the synovium undergoes hypertrophic proliferation, typically known as osteoarthrosis. This former condition involving the loss of intervertebral disc height and the accompanying osteophytic and subchondral sclerotic changes has been termed discogenic spondylosis. The latter condition involving facet arthrosis is consequently termed discogenic spondyloarthrosis. The changes of the two articular facets and the disc (triple joint complex) are outlined in Figure 2.22.

### CHANGES IN THE CLINICAL PICTURE OF DISC DEGENERATION

Yong-Hing and Kirkaldy-Willis (38) describe three clinical stages in the natural history of spinal degeneration.

1. *Stage of Dysfunction.* In the beginning there is little demonstrable pathology. Patient findings are subtle or absent, and conservative care is highly successful. Lumbago and rotatory strain are commonly diagnosed.

2. *Stage of Instability.* Abnormal movement of the motion segment or instability exists. Patient complaints are more severe, and objective findings are present. Conservative care is used and sometimes surgery.

3. *Stage of Stabilization.* Severe degenerative changes of the disc and facets reduce motion, and improvement may be experienced. Stenosis is now very probable.

Nachemson's (10) findings agree with the above second and third stages; he says that histological signs of arthritis have been demonstrated in the facet joints very late in life and always secondary to degenerative change in the disc.

It should be remembered that both the disc and the articular facet are capable of producing low back pain. It is interesting to study the work of Lora and Long (39) who were able to trace scleratogenous pain when various facet levels of the lumbar spine were irritated. L5-S1 facet stimulation resulted in referred pain to the coccyx, hip, posterior thigh, groin, inguinal ligament, and perineum; L4-L5 facet stimulation resulted in pain to the coccyx, posterior hip, and thigh and was less intense than that following irritation of the L5-S1 facets. L3-L4 facet stimulation resulted in pain radiating upward into the thoracic area, flank, and anterior thigh. Irritation of the articular facets at T12, L1, L2, and L3 produced no leg or coccyx sensation.

Arns et al. (40) states that the first stage of disc lesion begins with protrusion of the nucleus pulposus into the outer rings of the annulus fibrosus, resulting in low back pain. This lesion is characterized by local pain which is increased by coughing and sneezing, paravertebral muscle spasm, and antalgia of the lumbar spine. Neurological symptoms are not present. The next stage involves penetration of the nucleus pulposus into the outer rings of the annular fibers, producing pressure on the spinal nerve roots which creates radiating pain down the leg. Neurological signs are now present.

Farfan (33) has defined three stages of disc disease:

1. Annular bulge (protrusion).
2. Facet arthrosis as the disc thins and extrudes.
3. Stenosis if stages 1 and 2 are severe, with tautening of nerve root.

Discal thinning allows the pedicles of the superior vertebra to lower, thus compressing the nerve roots as they course toward the intervertebral foramen for emergence (41, 42). Figure 2.23 shows the normal pedicle nerve root relationship, and Figure 2.24 shows the relationship between the narrowed disc and the pedicle compression of the nerve root. Thus, another reason can be seen for the constant back and sciatic pain before and after a surgical procedure. The reader should note, also, the effect of short, thickened pedicles in conjunction with disc thinning further narrowing the vertebral canal.

## Rotation Not Found in the Low Lumbar Spine

Maigne (43) states that facet orientation at the lumbar spine permits only flexion and extenison. The thoracic spine, by virtue of its facet facings, should have a high degree of mobility, especially rotation. *"No rotation is possible in the lumbar spine by virtue of the facet orientation and form"* (emphasis added). Therefore, the highest degree of rotation and lateral flexion must take place at the level of the thoracolumbar spine.

Helfet and Gruebel-Lee (44) in discussing the instability of the lumbar spine with regard to range of motion point out that rotation injuries affect primarily the intervertebral disc itself.

## Disc or Facet as the Etiology of Back Pain

Vernon-Roberts and Pirie (30) state that there is a direct relationship between the degree of disc degeneration, marginal osteophyte formation on vertebral bodies, and apophyseal joint changes, which sug-

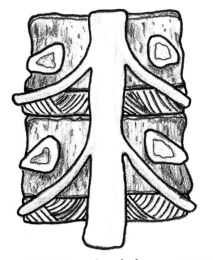

**Figure 2.23.** Normal pedicle to nerve root distance.

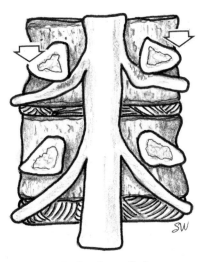

**Figure 2.24.** Tethering of the nerve root as the pedicle settles down upon it and as the disc space narrows or hyperextension subluxation of the superior vertebral arch occurs.

gests that disc degeneration is the primary event leading to the clinical condition of degenerative spondylosis. They also state that they have evidence that enables them to speculate on the role of prolapse in disc degeneration and in the genesis of osteoarthrosis of the apophyseal joints. Nachemson (10) found that arthrosis of the articular facets was always secondary to disc degeneration.

Thus, that internal derangement of the intervertebral disc, namely, the nucleus pulposus, begins the aberrant mobility of the lumbar spine is strongly implicated. The degenerative changes occurring thereafter in the disc spread posteriorly into the arch of the vertebra. We know that both the disc and the facet are pain-producing entities and that specific attention must be given to both of these structures in the treatment of low back pain. Furthermore, it also seems most likely that a combination of surgery and manipulation may be the answer for many people; that is, surgery for the disc prolapse and manipulation for the altered motoricity of the articular facet.

The effects of rotation have been well summarized by Eagle (46) who states that the main cause of severe long-lasting back pain is the damaged intervertebral disc, and once a disc is damaged there is nothing a surgeon can do to repair it. Nor are discs able to repair themselves. Therefore, if we are to prevent back pain, it would be useful to know how much stress the disc fibers can withstand before they give way.

Eagle (46) quotes the work of Hukins and Hickey of Manchester University who state that the most hazardous maneuvers to the low back are bending and twisting. They won the 1979 Volvo Bioengineering Award for their paper proving that annular failure and tearing are caused by torsion and forward bending, causing nuclear protrusion and low back pain. They found that the maximum rotation that will not damage the annular fibers at L5-S1 is 3°.

Miller (47) states that during the lifting of a weight of 200 lb the disc carries an average of 91% of the load and the facet joint carries no more than 12%. Low facet joints put more weight on the disc than do high facet joints. *The facets carry very little weight on compression, but accept large loads on bending.* The amount of load on the facets is 50% on flexion and extension and 30% on torsion.

An in vitro experimental study was carried out to measure the induced loading on human lumbar facets due to varying amounts of compressive axial load (48). Testing was done on the L2-L3 and L4-L5 spinal motion segments obtained from cadavers at autopsy. The compressive loading was applied with the spinal specimens first in a neutral position and then in an extended position. In particular, this study demonstrated that the absolute facet loads remain relatively constant with increasing segmental compressive loads such that the facet load expressed as a percent of the load applied to the segment decreases with increasing axial loads. It also demonstrated that with increasing loads in extension the contact area moves cranially at L2-L3 and caudally at L4-L5. Furthermore, it indicated that after a facetectomy the load on the remaining facet is reduced substantially although peak pressure increases. Finally, this study demonstrated that there is a substantial difference in facet loadings between the L2-L3 and the L4-L5 segments.

A comparison of segments at L2-L3 and L4-L5 at different axial loads in the neutral position shows that the facets at L2-L3 generally take more load than those at L4-L5. The same trend is also observed during extension. Furthermore, the normal load on the facets is always higher in extension than in the neutral position. This holds true for both the L2-L3 and the L4-L5 levels.

Observations based on these data indicate:

1. The average peak pressure for all axial compressive loads is higher in extension than in the neutral position at both the L2-L3 and the L4-L5 levels.

2. The peak pressure is generally higher at the L2-L3 level than at the L4-L5 level in both the neutral and the extended positions.

The facet pressure rather than the facet load, therefore, may be playing a significant role in the degenerative changes of facets.

Contrary to expectations, a unilateral facetectomy causes a significant reduction in the load borne by the remaining facet in both the neutral and the extended positions. This may be explained by the fact that since the facet load on the left side is eliminated by performing a unilateral facetectomy, equilibrium is substantially altered. The superior vertebral body is now free to drift away from the inferior body, thus reducing positive contact at the remaining facets. This phenomenon again reinforces the above observation that pressure rather than load is the precipitating factor in facet degeneration.

A second unexpected phenomenon observed in this study is that in many cases the contact decreases with increasing loads.

## Do Facets Irritate the Nerve Roots to Cause Sciatica?

Mooney and Robertson (49) injected local anesthetic into the facet joints of 100 consecutive patients with "disc syndrome." One fifth had long-term relief and one third had partial relief of lumbago and sciatica. Carrera (50) succeeded in providing some relief to 7 of 20 patients by injection. Dory (51) found that the articular capsule nearly always burst during arthrography and the path of leaking medium provided a possible explanation of how steroids relieve pain on injection. It might be that the injected anesthetic or steroid directly affects the nerve root and can give partial or temporary relief.

## How Do Discs Absorb Compressive Loads?

Discs absorb shock by squeezing fluid out of the nucleus and/or by allowing the fibers of the outer shell to stretch. Studies of disc fibers suggest that they have only limited elasticity and can only stretch to 1.04 times their initial length before suffering irreparable damage. When the disc is compressed, for instance when we lift a heavy object or jump from a great height and land on our feet, this limited elasticity does not present a major problem. Indeed, when we are standing upright, the disc fibers can take 10 times as much compression as can the vertebrae themselves, so a very heavy load will crush bones before it ruptures a disc.

Disc fibers are less able to cope with torsion than with compression because with torsion the stress concentrates at points of maximum curvature. And as the disc shell is made of layers of fibers which lie obliquely to each other in a crisscross pattern, torsion tends to shear one layer from another, further weakening the total structure. As a result, we stand a much greater risk of damaging our discs when we try to lift an object and twist our body around at the same time.

## SITTING AND ITS EFFECTS ON THE INTERVERTEBRAL DISC

The intradiscal pressure within the nucleus pulposus is lowest when the patient is recumbent and is highest when the patient is sitting in a flexed position. Nachemson (10) has measured the relative pressure within the 3rd lumbar disc of people in various positions and has found that these pressures range between 25 and 275 psi as the person moves from the recumbent to the sitting flexed posture.

Fahrni (52) states that he studied a jungle population in India who squat rather than sit and sleep on the ground rather than in beds. These people had no concept of posture principles whatsoever but had a zero incidence of back pain. Furthermore, x-rays of the lumbar spine in 450 of these people of ages 15 to 44 years showed no incidence of disc narrowing. Thus, sitting is to be avoided in treatment of low back pain, especially with intradiscal involvement.

Fromelt et al. (53) found that bending, twisting, and lifting were the most common cause of low back pain and disc injury. The effect of rotational instability on the lateral recess is shown in Fig. 2.25.

## ROENTGEN STUDIES OF THORACOLUMBAR LATERAL FLEXION, UPRIGHT AND RECUMBENT ROTATION

Nine cases are presented to show differing rotation and lateral flexion capabilities in the lumbar spine of patients with transitional segments, disc lesion, tropism, stenosis, or normal spines. The main conclusion is that rotation, whether performed with the patient in the upright or the recumbent position, is slight at L4-L5

and L5-S1 but possible in the upper lumbar spine.

## Upright versus Recumbent Rotation of the Lumbar Spine

**Case 1** is of a 23-year-old white woman who had a history of low back pain but no leg pain. At the time this x-ray study was done, she was being treated only for left shoulder pain; her low back was totally asymptomatic.

Consequently, we performed rotation studies on the spine in order to determine any differences in rotation from the standing to the recumbent non-weight-bearing rotational posture.

The anteroposterior view (Fig. 2.26) reveals that this patient has tropism at L5-S1, with the right facet being sagittal and the left being coronal. The hip and sacroiliac joints are adequate. The lateral view (Fig. 2.27) reveals a moderate increased lumbar lordosis. The disc spaces are normal.

Figures 2.28 and 2.29 were taken with the patient in the standing weight-bearing posture. Figure 2.28 reveals left rotation and Figure 2.29 reveals right rotation. There is lateral flexion of L4 and L5 with actual Lovett reverse rotation of the spinous process at L4 on left lateral flexion and with minimal Lovett positive rotation on right rotation. Normally, the spinous process would deviate to the concave side; instead, it deviates to the left, to the convex side, and this is called a Lovett reverse curve. This may indicate a minimal rotatory capability at L4; there is no rotation at the L5 level.

Figures 2.30 and 2.31 are, respectively, right and left lateral rotation studies of the lumbar spine with the patient in the recumbent position. These films were taken with the patient rotating to each side while in the recumbent position and being supported with foam padding in the thoracic spine as maximum rotation is attained. The purpose of this study is to see whether there is any difference between the muscular contractions causing rotatory change when the patient is in a recumbent position and those causing change when the patient is in a weight-bearing position. As you can see, there is actually no discernible rotation with the patient in the recumbent posture.

This author interprets this to mean that rotation, if possible, is greatest when the patient is in the upright posture. This might also make sense if one considers that most back injuries occur during flexion in the upright posture, with either lifting or rotating in combination motion.

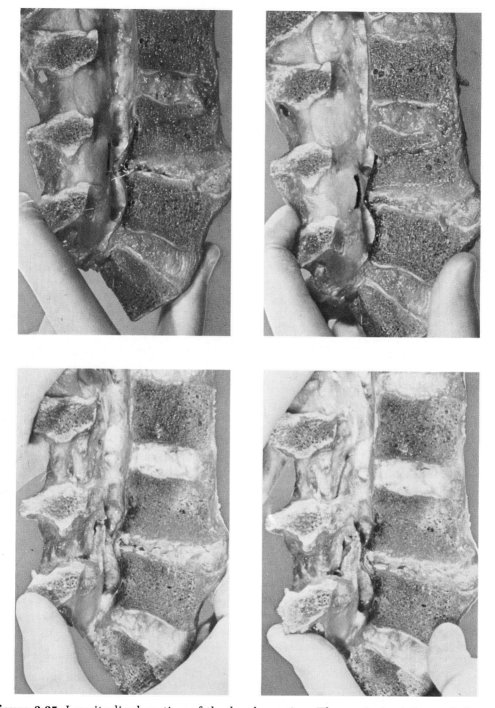

**Figure 2.25.** Longitudinal section of the lumbar spine. The posterior joint and disc at L3-L4 are normal. Those at L4-L5 show marked degenerative changes with rotational instability. *Top left.* Before rotation. The *black line* on the *left* is placed over the front of the superior articular process. Note the size of the lateral recess. *Top right.* Same specimen. The spinous process of L5 has been rotated out of the picture (toward the viewer). This rotation displaces the superior articular process forward with narrowing of the lateral recess. *Bottom left.* Same as *top left*, with the lateral extension of the

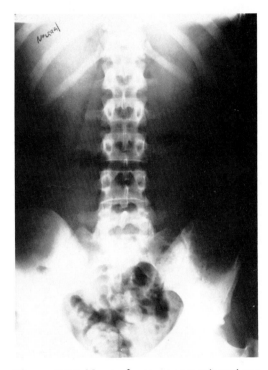

**Figure 2.26.** Neutral anteroposterior view. Tropism is present at L5-S1.

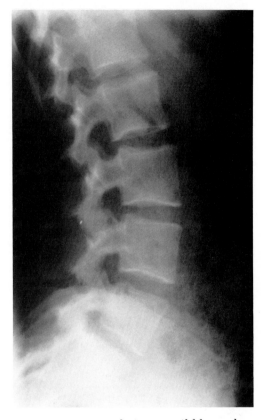

**Figure 2.27.** Lateral view—mild hyperlordosis. The disc spaces are normal.

ligamentum flavum removed. Note the marked degeneration of the posterior joint and disc and the size of the lateral recess. *Bottom right.* Same as *top right*, with the lateral extension of the ligamentum flavum removed. The spinous process of L5 has again been rotated as in *top right*. The posterior joint surfaces are separated. The lateral recess is narrowed by forward displacement of the superior articular process. (Reproduced with permission from K. Yong-Hing, J. Reilly, and W. H. Kirkaldy-Willis: The ligamentum flavum. *Spine* 1(4): 232, 1976.)

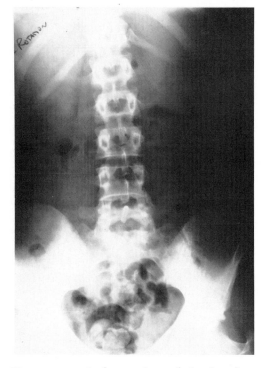

**Figure 2.28.** Left rotation of the lumbar spine in upright posture.

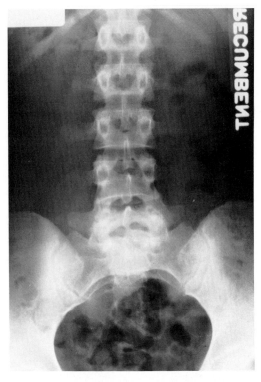

**Figure 2.30.** Right rotation of the lumbar spine in the recumbent supine position.

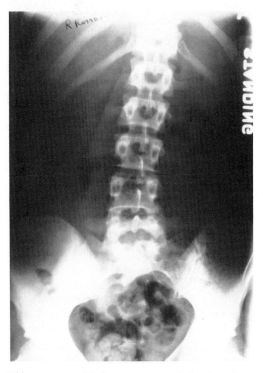

**Figure 2.29.** Right rotation of the lumbar spine in the upright posture.

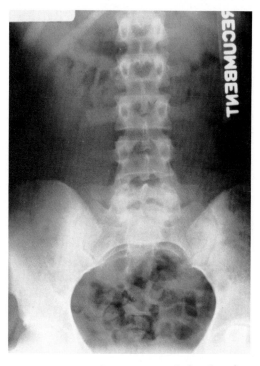

**Figure 2.31.** Left rotation of the lumbar spine in the recumbent supine position.

## Comparison of Lateral Flexion and Rotation of the Lumbar Spine

**Case 2** is of a 34-year-old white woman with low back and left lower extremity pain. She has had numerous episodes of low back pain in the past few years but has had leg pain for only the past 2 weeks.

The rotation movement of the lumbar spine is studied by comparison with lateral flexion movement. Figures 2.32, 2.33, and 2.34 are neutral and lateral bending films showing normal motion. Figures 2.35 and 2.36 reveal a sacral angle of 33° and a lumbar lordosis of 50°. Figure 2.37 shows no stenosis present. Figure 2.38 is a posteroanterior tilt view of the same patient as in Figure 2.32.

Figures 2.39 and 2.40 are, respectively, left and right rotation studies made by having the patient rotate at the waist while holding the pelvis fixed on the bucky. Note that L5 does not rotate measurably and L4 bends laterally but that rotation is no greater than the lateral bendings reveal. There is definite increased rotatory movement of the upper lumbar vertebral bodies, coupled with lateral flexion.

## Lateral Bending and Rotation with Anatomical Short Leg

**Case 3** is of a 39-year-old white man who had low back and left anterior thigh pain. This

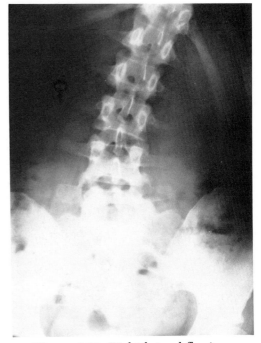

**Figure 2.33.** Right lateral flexion.

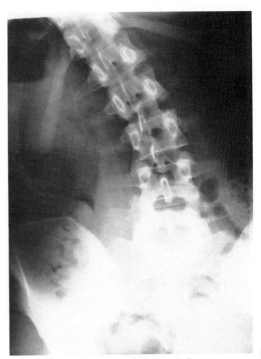

**Figure 2.34.** Left lateral flexion.

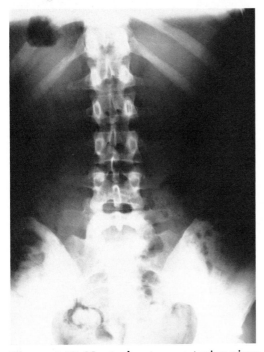

**Figure 2.32.** Neutral anteroposterior view of the lumbar spine and pelvis.

patient had been seen by two orthopedic surgeons who recommended a low back support to him. A chiropractor treated him for a few visits, but he received no relief.

This man is a well developed athlete who

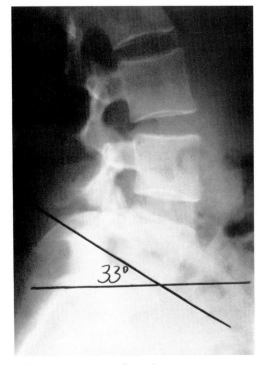

**Figure 2.35.** Sacral angle measurement.

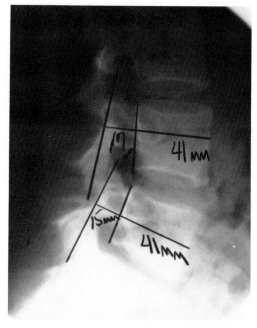

**Figure 2.37.** Eisenstein's measurement for stenosis.

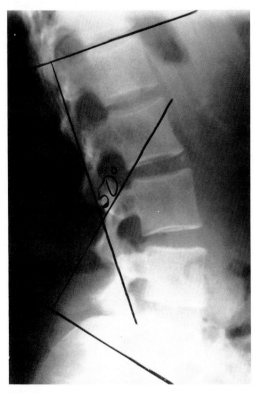

**Figure 2.36.** Lumbar lordosis measurement.

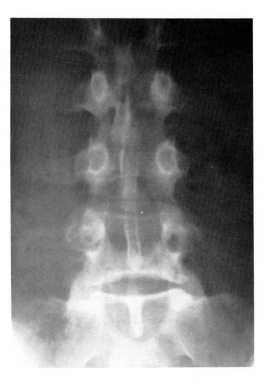

**Figure 2.38.** Posteroanterior tilt view of L5-S1. Note the centered position of the spinous processes.

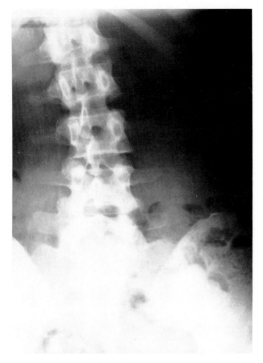

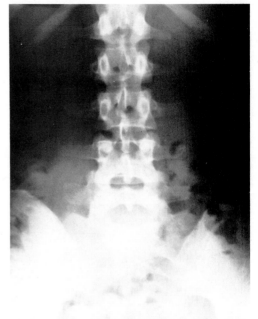

**Figure 2.40.** Right lumbar spine rotation in the upright posture.

**Figure 2.39.** Left lumbar spine rotation in the upright posture.

exercises regularly and takes good care of himself. Both sitting and lying down aggravate his symptoms.

The ranges of motion of the low back are all within normal limits, and the straight leg raising test is negative. Kemp's sign is positive bilaterally. The deep reflexes of the lower extremities are active and equal, and there is hypoesthesia of the left L4 dermatome. Circulation is normal, and muscle strengths are within normal limits.

Figure 2.41 is an anteroposterior view of this spine which reveals a 9-mm inferiority of the left femoral head and hemipelvis with resultant levorotatory scoliosis of the lumbar spine. The sacrum is inferior on the left. The facets at the lower two levels are coronal. Figure 2.42 is a right lateral bending study of the lumbar spine, which is Lovett-positive. Figure 2.43 is a left lateral bending study which reveals that the hemipelvis deviates inferiorly, with less lateral bending of the lumbar vertebrae occurring than occurred in the right lateral bending study.

Figure 2.44 reveals a retrolisthesis subluxation of L5 on the sacrum with approximately a 50% loss of the L5-S1 disc space. There is also minimal lipping and spurring of the anterolateral body plates at L5-S1.

Figure 2.45 reveals a 46-mm body and 12-mm canal, which when corrected for an 80% magnification error would be a 9-mm canal. Therefore, this patient has stenosis at the L5-S1 level, greatly aggravated by the retrolisthesis subluxation of L5 on sacrum.

Figure 2.47 is a left rotation study of the thoracolumbar spine. No rotation of the segments at L4-L5 can be seen on this view in comparison to the neutral view in Figure 2.41.

Figure 2.48 is a right rotation study. Distortion by pelvis movement eliminates valid interpretation of vertebral body rotation.

Thus the diagnosis is:

1. Left 9-mm inferior anatomical short leg.
2. Levorotatory scoliosis of the lumbar spine.
3. Retrolisthesis subluxation of L5 on sacrum with early degenerative disc disease at this level.
4. Femoral nerve radiculopathy.

Treatment consisted of a 9-mm heel and sole lift placed under the left shoe (Fig. 2.46). Flexion distraction manipulation was applied to all levels of the lumbar spine with the patient placed in left rotation and lateral bending during the distractive force. This follows the treatment outlined in Chapter 10, "Scoliosis." Exercises to strengthen the left paravertebral muscles and quadratus lumborum muscles were given. Strengthening exercises were given utilizing the knee-chest position, gluteus

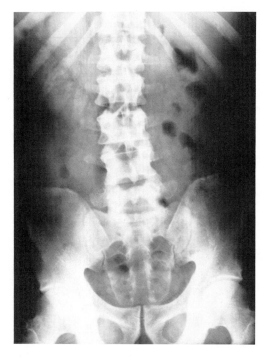

**Figure 2.41.** Anteroposterior view showing 9-mm-short left femoral head and hemipelvis.

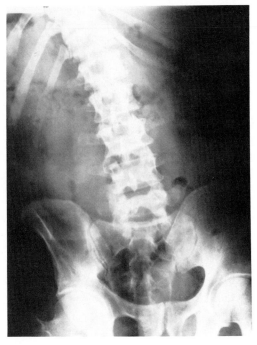

**Figure 2.43.** Left lateral flexion—Lovett positive.

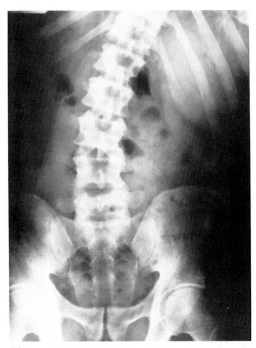

**Figure 2.42.** Right lateral flexion—Lovett positive.

**Figure 2.44.** Lateral view reveals L5 retrolisthesis and L5-S1 disc degeneration.

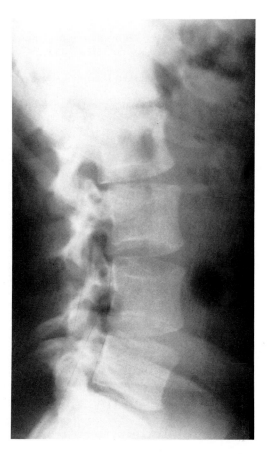

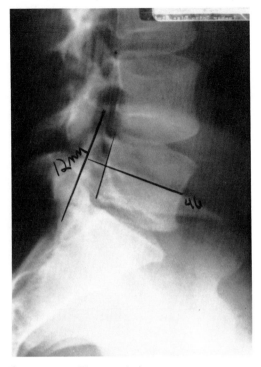

**Figure 2.45.** Eisenstein's measurement reveals L5 stenosis.

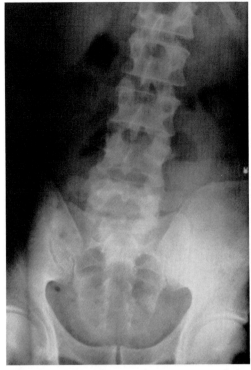

**Figure 2.47.** Left upright rotation of the thoracolumbar spine.

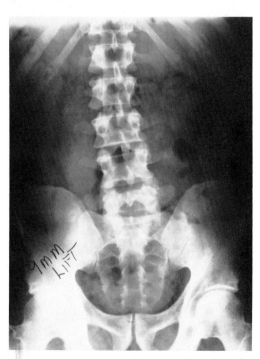

**Figure 2.46.** A 9-mm lift was placed under the left heel and sole to level the pelvis.

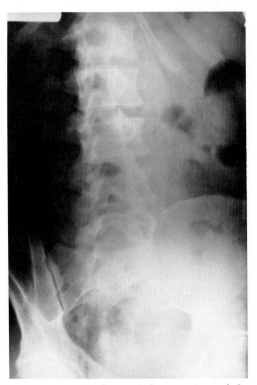

**Figure 2.48.** Right upright rotation of the thoracolumbar spine.

maximus, adductor, abductor, abdominal and extensors of the low back. Stretching of the hamstring muscles was shown. The patient was sent to the Low Back School.

The low back pain was eliminated and the patient continues to follow the directions learned at the Low Back School, while wearing the lift and observing the rules of good spinal hygiene.

## Rotation of the Lumbar Spine

Case 4 is of a 34-year-old woman who had a long history of low back pain but no lower extremity pain. Figure 2.49 is a neutral antero-posterior standing film, Figure 2.50 is a left rotation film, and Figure 2.51 is a right rotation film. Note minimal L5 body spinous process rotation and increasing rotation from L4 ceph-alad.

## Effect of Transitional Segment on Rotation

Case 5 is of a 39-year-old man who has severe low back and right buttock pain after playing racketball.

Figures 2.52 and 2.53 are, respectively, the anteroposterior and lateral views of the low back, revealing a transitional vertebra (sacral-ization). The facet facings are sagittal at L4-L5,

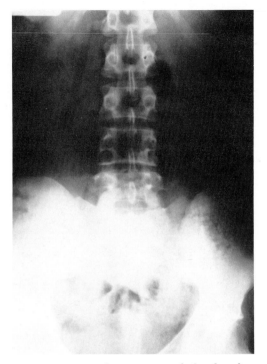

Figure 2.50. Left rotation of the lumbar spine.

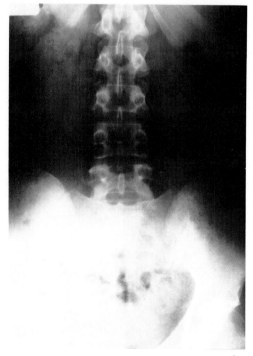

Figure 2.49. Anteroposterior neutral.

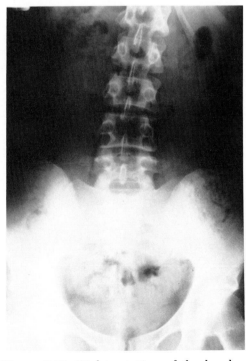

Figure 2.51. Right rotation of the lumbar spine.

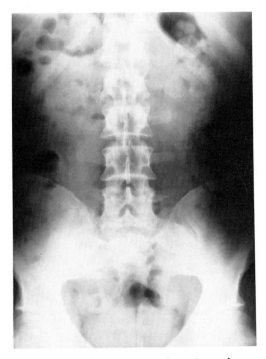

**Figure 2.52.** Anteroposterior view shows fusion of L5 to the sacrum. This sacralization is bilaterally true.

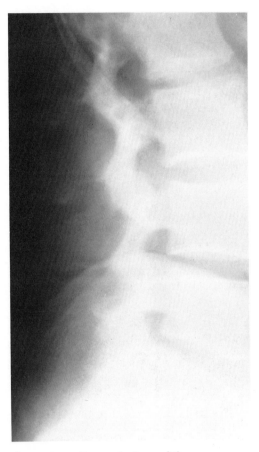

**Figure 2.53.** Lateral view of the same condition shown in Figure 2.52.

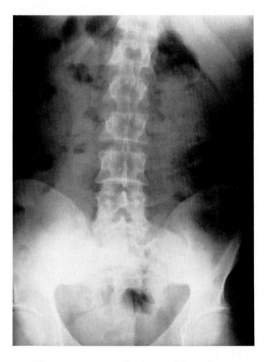 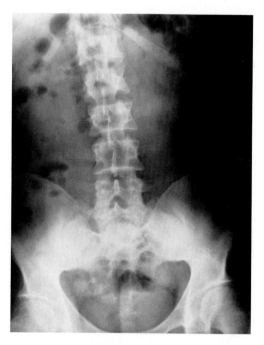

**Figure 2.54.** Right lateral bending.          **Figure 2.55.** Left lateral bending.

and the levels are cephalad. There is thinning of the L5-S1 disc space.

Figures 2.54 and 2.55 are, respectively, right and left lateral bending views showing restriction on the right compared to the left.

Figure 2.56 is a left upright rotation view. Again, there is some pelvic motion to the left, presenting rotational distortion, but rotation is more possible in the midlumbar and upper lumbar spinal units.

Figure 2.57 is a right upright rotation view. There is definitely no rotation at L5 and only a little at L4; most rotation is at the L3 and cephalic segments. True transitional segments allow no lateral flexion and rotation.

## Bilateral True Sacralization in Lateral Flexion and Rotation

**Case 6** is of a 24-year-old white man who has had right low back and buttock pain, with no radiation into the lower extremity, off and on for at least 10 years. In 1979, he was examined and was reported to have only muscle spasms. Two weeks ago, the pain became quite noticeable, and he sought an appointment with us.

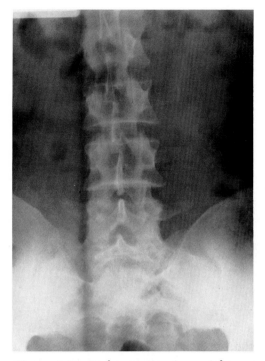

**Figure 2.57.** Right rotation in upright posture.

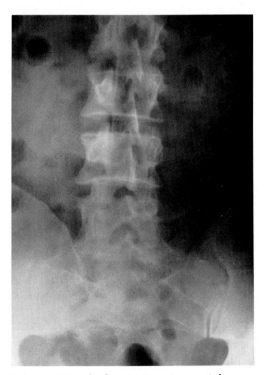

**Figure 2.56.** Left rotation in upright posture.

The range of motion is within normal limits. Kemp's sign is bilaterally positive and more pronounced to the right. The deep reflexes, as is sensory examination of the lower extremities, are normal. Motor strengths are normal. Pain on palpation is marked over the right L5-S1 area and radiates into the ilium. Further questioning revealed that the patient has most of his pain on flexion and bending at his job as a construction worker which entails lifting up to 90 lb a day.

The left lateral bending view (Fig. 2.59) reveals hypermobility of L3 on L4 to the left. Although L4 fails to flex laterally to the right (Fig. 2.60), it does flex laterally to the left. Fusion of the 5th lumbar vertebra transverse processes with the sacrum also is shown, making this a true sacralization (Fig. 2.58). Therefore, Bertolotti's syndrome, a combination of a transitional 5th lumbar segment and a disc involvement at the 4th lumbar level, is present. The lateral view (Fig. 2.61) reveals a hypoplastic disc at the L5-S1 level as well as thinning of the L4-L5 disc with posteriority of L4 on L5 and traction spur formation of the anterior plate of the 5th lumbar vertebral body.

Right and left rotation views (Figs. 2.62 and 2.63, respectively) reveal that rotation is not

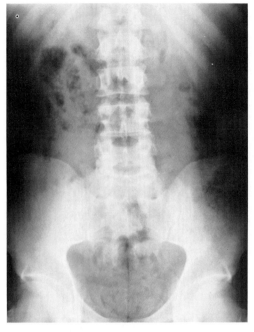

**Figure 2.58.** Anteroposterior neutral view. Note the fusion of L5 to sacrum. This sacralization is bilaterally true.

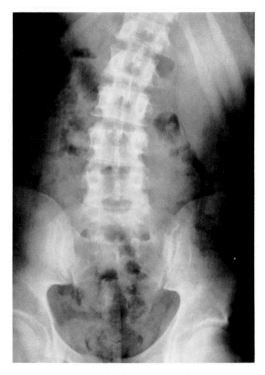

**Figure 2.60.** Right lateral flexion.

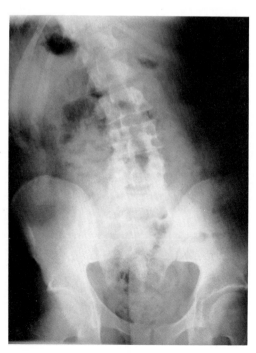

**Figure 2.59.** Left lateral flexion.

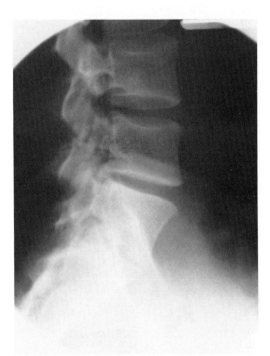

**Figure 2.61.** Lateral projection—discogenic L4-L5 disc disease and rudimentary L5-S1 disc.

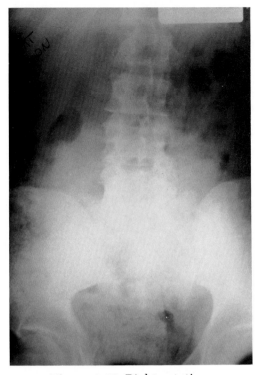

**Figure 2.62.** Right rotation.

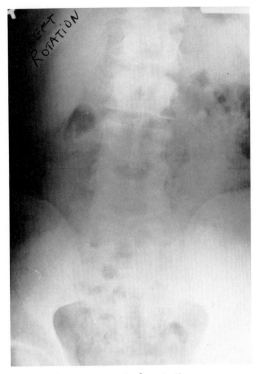

**Figure 2.63.** Left rotation.

present at the L4 level but is increasingly noted cephalad to L4.

Thus the diagnosis is:

1. Transitional sacralization of the 5th lumbar segment, which is bilaterally true.

2. Early discogenic spondylosis of the L4-L5 disc space with posteriority of L4 on L5 (retrolisthesis).

3. Bertolotti's syndrome, namely, the transitional 5th lumbar segment combined with a degenerative change at the L4-L5 disc.

4. Failure of rotation of the lower lumbar spine with the increasing rotational capabilities of the upper lumbar spine.

The patient was instructed that there was no cure for the structural problems of his low back, namely, the transitional segment and the already beginning degeneration of the L4-L5 disc. He was sent to Low Back School to learn to avoid aggravation of his condition, thus enabling him to function with the greatest possible ease in daily living.

Manipulation, specifically flexion distraction, was applied to the lumbar spine, especially the L4-L5 level, and acupressure points B24 through B31 were goaded (see Chapter 8, "Care of the Intervertebral Disc," for explanation of acupressure points). The articulations of L4 cephalad were manipulated through

their physiological ranges of motion. Goading of the right gluteus and iliolumbar ligament was performed as trigger point therapy.

Sending this patient to Low Back School helped him to learn how to avoid activities of daily living that cause back pain. The combination of Low Back School and manipulation provided relief from pain as long as he followed the rules learned at Low Back School.

## Effect of Tropism on Rotation

**Case 7** is of a 29-year-old white man who has right low back pain on jogging.

Figure 2.64 is the neutral anteroposterior view and reveals a straight lumbar spine with five lumbar segments. Tropism is present at L5-S1; i.e., the right facets are sagittal in comparison to the more coronal faced left facets.

Figure 2.65 is a spot lateral view of this patient.

Figure 2.66 is a right lateral flexion view revealing normal motion.

Figure 2.67 is a left lateral flexion view revealing normal motion.

Figure 2.68 is a right rotation view, with rotation occurring primarily in the midlumbar and upper lumbar segments with the bodies rotating right and the spinous processes left.

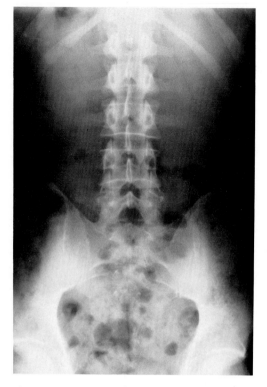

**Figure 2.64.** Neutral anteroposterior view. L5-S1 tropism is present.

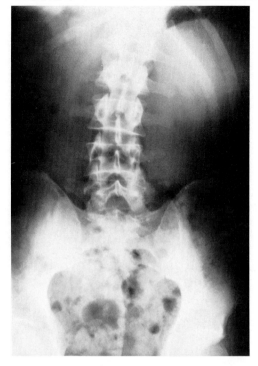

**Figure 2.66.** Right lateral flexion—normal.

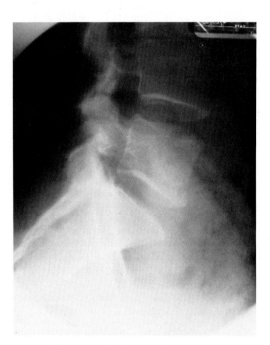

**Figure 2.65.** Lateral spot.

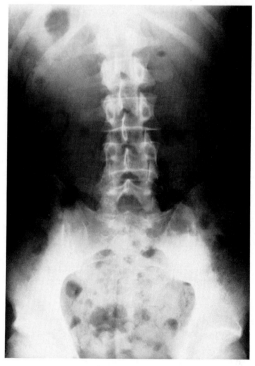

**Figure 2.67.** Left lateral flexion—normal.

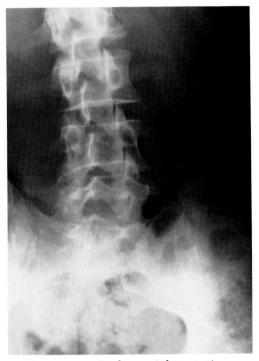

**Figure 2.68.** Right upright rotation.

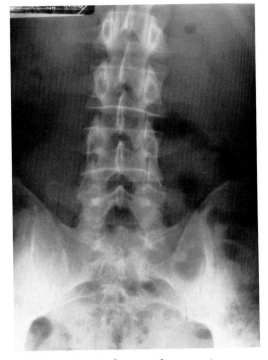

**Figure 2.69.** Left upright rotation—restricted aberrant rotation.

Fig. 2.69 is a left rotation view, with rotation restricted at all levels compared to that shown on the right rotation view.

This patient has marked muscle spasm of the right lumbar spine. Please note the ununited apophysis of the right inferior tip of the 4th lumbar articular facet (Fig. 2.70). Could this act as a pain-producing ossicle?

## Lateral Flexion and Rotation of a Presurgical Patient with L5-S1 Disc Prolapse

**Case 8** is of a patient with low back and left first sacral dermatome sciatica.

Figure 2.71 is a neutral anteroposterior view.

Figure 2.72 is a normal right lateral bending view.

Figure 2.73 is a normal left lateral bending view.

Figures 2.74 and 2.75 are the lateral projection and spot view, respectively, revealing some L5-S1 disc thinning with a traction spur of the inferior anterior L5 plate.

Figure 2.76 is a left rotation of the lumbar spine with the patient in the upright position, revealing increased body rotation from L4 cephalad.

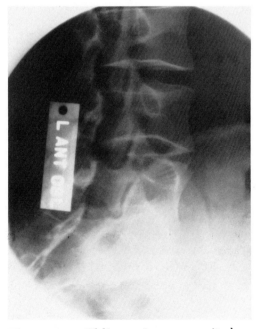

**Figure 2.70.** Oblique view—ununited ossicle at L4 right facet tip.

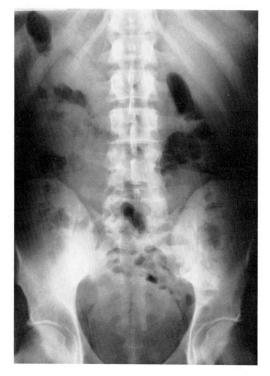

**Figure 2.71.** Neutral anteroposterior projection.

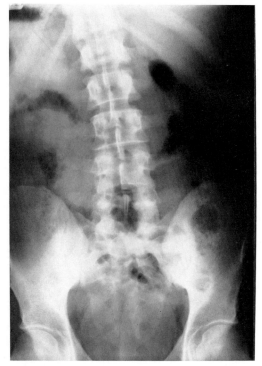

**Figure 2.73.** Left lateral flexion—normal.

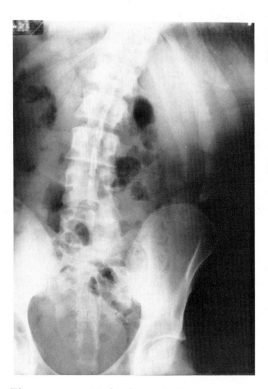

**Figure 2.72.** Right lateral flexion—normal.

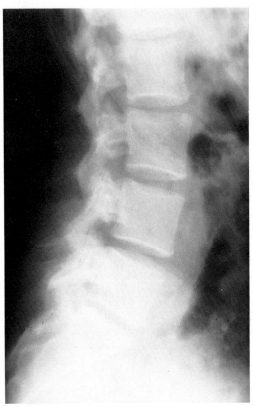

**Figure 2.74.** Lateral view.

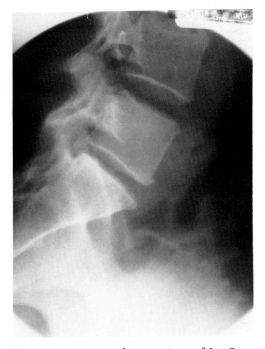

**Figure 2.75.** Lateral spot view of L5-S1—small traction spur at L5-S1.

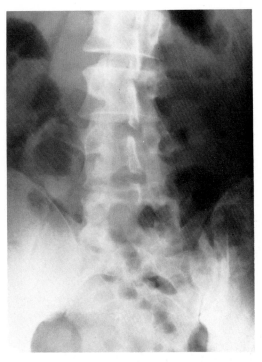

**Figure 2.76.** Left lumbar rotation.

Figure 2.77 is a right rotation view revealing L4 body rotation to the right, which is increasing cephalad in the lumbar spine.

No strong indications of restricted motion are found. This patient had severe sciatic pain due to L5-S1 disc prolapse and underwent surgery within a week of these films.

## Comparison of Normal Lateral Flexion and Abnormal Rotation

**Case 9** is of a 52-year-old white woman who had low back and bilateral leg pain, with pain worse in the left leg. She had been injured in an automobile accident and had been seen by an orthopedic surgeon, a medical doctor, and a chiropractor. She had taken cortisone which provided relief of the leg pain for 3 weeks during its use. Pain returned after discontinuation of the cortisone. She experienced pain in the low back with nonspecific dermatome leg pain at night. Walking aggravated the pain in the leg. She was positive for Déjérine's triad. No myelogram nor EMG had been done.

Vital signs are normal. Range of motion is 90° flexion, 30° extension, 17° right lateral flexion, 15° left lateral flexion, 25° right rotation, and 10° left rotation. The straight leg raising sign is bilaterally positive at 60° and Braggard's sign is positive. Kemp's sign is bilaterally positive. Doppler examination is nor-

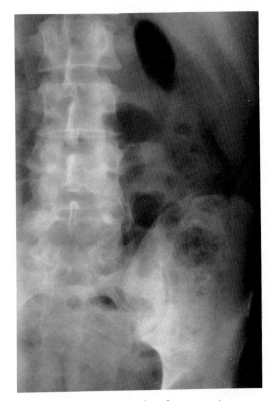

**Figure 2.77.** Right lumbar rotation.

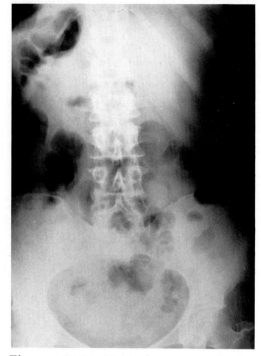

**Figure 2.78.** Neutral anteroposterior view—tropism at L4-L5.

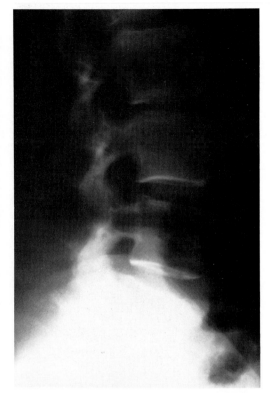

**Figure 2.79.** Lateral view.

mal. Nonorganic physical signs are negative for malingering.

Lateral bending views (Figs. 2.80 and 2.81) reveal normal motion, as is evident in spinous process movement into the concave side of the lean.

The L5-S1 disc shows signs of discogenic spondylosis (Figure 2.79).

Tropism of the L4-L5 facets, the right sagittal and the left coronal, can be seen on Figure 2.78.

Arthrosis of the left L4-L5 facet was present on oblique views (not shown).

The rotation study (Fig. 2.82) with the patient in the upright posture reveals right body rotation with right rotation, especially at the L1, L2, L3, and L4 levels. The left rotation study (Fig. 2.83) reveals much less rotation capability.

Thus the diagnosis is:

1. Tropism at L4-L5.
2. Discogenic spondylosis at L5-S1.
3. Facet arthrosis of the left L4-L5 articulation.
4. Symptoms of intermittent claudication of probable neurogenic variety in the lower extremities, since Doppler examination is normal.

Case 9 is presented mainly to show the differing capabilities of the normal lateral bending study and the rotation study. Case 9

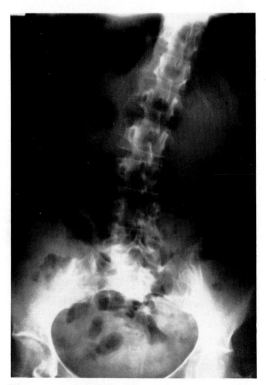

**Figure 2.80.** Right lateral bending—normal.

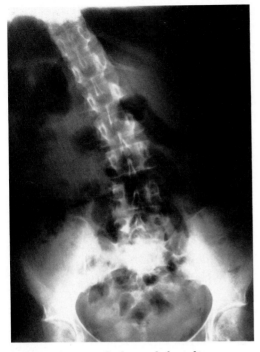

**Figure 2.81.** Left lateral bending—normal.

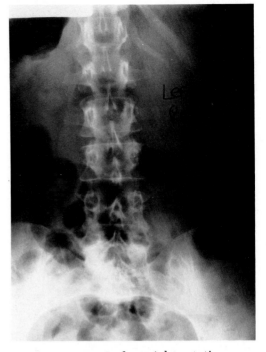

**Figure 2.83.** Left upright rotation.

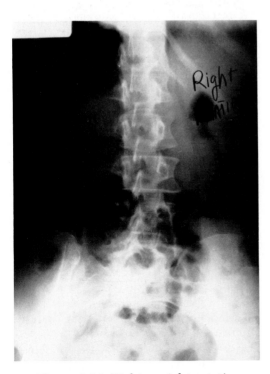

**Figure 2.82.** Right upright rotation.

reveals more rotation of the midlumbar segments than do the other cases presented in this rotation series.

## MECHANICAL FACTORS IN LUMBAR MOTION

In cadaver studies, sustained lordosis produced abnormal loading of apophyseal joints. Forward bending wedged the discs, rendering them vulnerable to fatigue injuries (54). Excessive flexion at some spinal levels caused posterior ligament damage, and a strong contraction of the back muscles then caused prolapse of the intervertebral disc.

The center of rotation for flexion was just anterior to the center of the disc. The average forward bending necessary to damage an intervertebral joint in flexion was 4,938 N (1,097.3 lb). Most resistance came from the disc and capsular ligaments. The supraspinous and interspinous ligaments were slack for the few degrees of flexion but were the first structures to sustain damage at the limit of the physiological range, which averaged 8.4° of flexion. Data on the tensile properties of the apophyseal joint capsule ligaments were used to predict that these ligaments would be damaged after 11.6° of flexion on the average.

On rotation, the center of rotation for axial rotation was poorly defined but was usually located in the posterior annulus or neural arch. Nearly all of the resistance to torsion came from the disc and the facet surfaces in compression, with the percentage from each depending on the location of the center of rotation. On compression, the apophyseal joints of nondegenerated discs sustained damage after only 1° to 3° of rotation, and those in degenerated discs sustained damage after 7° of rotation. Resistance for isolated discs to torque was found to be smooth and reproducible for at least 10°. The authors of these cadaver studies believe that the *disc was not damaged by rotation, since they found that the disc was capable of 10° of rotation.* They also believe that the facet would fracture before the disc would tear. They point out that *flattening or slight flexion of the lumbar curve unloads the facets and compresses the disc which would not be damaged, as is the facet.* They believe that *lordosis is the cause of pain and degeneration of the facets.* Full flexion can distort the lamellae of the disc, giving rise to radial fissures in the annulus which can produce pain and protrusion of the nucleus. Therefore, according to them the order of damage in heavy lifting injuries is:

1. Damage to the supraspinous and interspinous ligaments.
2. Damage to the capsular ligaments of the apophyseal joints.
3. Prolapse of the disc occurring with muscular contraction and hyperflexion of the lumbar spine.

The combination of a degenerated annulus and a turgid nucleus is the most vulnerable to injury. *A slightly protruding nucleus can cause bleeding of the posterior longitudinal ligament that can cause pain.*

The term functional spinal unit (FSU) replaces the term motion segment. Posner et al. (55) defined the FSU as being the ligament, apophyseal joints, and disc joining two adjacent vertebrae. Posner et al. attempted to determine the stability and instability of the lumbar FSU. Seven lumbar spines and sacrums were removed from cadavers within 6 hours of death; the spines were subjected to flexion and extension experiment. In flexion, intertransverse and posterior longitudinal ligaments and the disc failed, with the end plates pulling off the vertebral bodies. In extension, the intertransverse ligament again failed, whereas the apophyseal capsule and the ligamentum flavum pulled off their attachments to bone.

## Effects of Flexion and Extension on the Lumbar Structures

The effects of flexion (Fig. 2.84) on the lumbar spine are:

1. Decrease in the intraspinal protrusion of the lumbar intervertebral disc.
2. Slight increase in the length of the anterior wall of the spinal canal.
3. Significant increase in the length of the posterior wall of the spinal canal.
4. Stretching and a decreased bulge of the yellow ligaments within the spinal canal.
5. Stretching and a decreased cross-sectional area of nerve roots.
6. An overall general increase in spinal canal volume and decreased nerve root bulk.

The effects of extension (Fig. 2.85) are:

1. Bulging of the intervertebral discs into the spinal canal.
2. Slight decrease in the anterior canal length.
3. Moderate decrease in the posterior canal length.
4. Enfolding and protrusion of the yellow ligaments into the spinal canal.
5. Relaxation and an increase in the cross-sectional diameter of the nerve roots.
6. An overall decrease in the volume of the lumbar spinal canal and an increased nerve root bulk.

For these reasons patients seek flexion for relief of back pain, and this is the premise on which the use of flexion distraction manipulation for correction of disc protrusion is based.

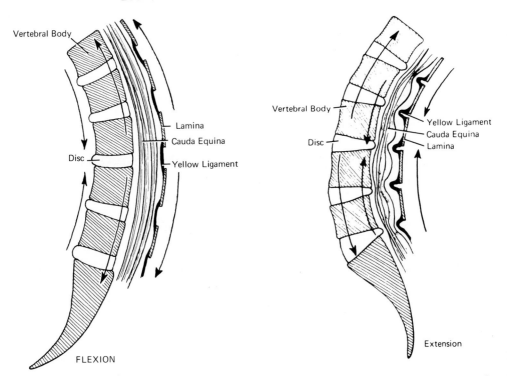

**Figure 2.84.** Increased spinal canal volume and decreased nerve root (cauda equina) bulk with flexion. (Reproduced with permission from B. E. Finneson: *Low Back Pain*, edition 2. Philadelphia, J. B. Lippincott, 1980, p. 432.)

**Figure 2.85.** Decreased spinal canal volume and increased nerve root bulk with extension. (Reproduced with permission from B. E. Finneson: *Low Back Pain*, edition 2. Philadelphia, J. B. Lippincott, 1980, p. 432.)

## Effects of Flexion and Extension on the Lumbar Canal

1. Breig (as discussed in Ref. 55a) has shown that extension of the lumbar spine causes protrusion of the intervertebral disc with dorsal displacement of the cauda equina roots. On myelography, Ehni and Weinstein (55a) showed that extension produces total block and flexion permits the contrast medium to pass through the blocked area. Reaching overhead or bending backward causes the common complaint of painful paresthesia or numbness in both legs.

2. Dyck (55b) showed that extension promotes lumbar stenosis and forward flexion reduces it.

3. Raney (55c) performed a series of myelograms which showed that with flexion of the lumbar spine, the posterior bulge of the posterior annulus and poste-rior longitudinal ligament disappeared as the anterior margin of the vertebral bodies approached each other and the posterior margins separated. The myelographic column became flat, and the dural sac closely approximated the back of the posterior longitudinal ligament and annulus. Even though the force propelling the disc posteriorly is increased by flexion, the tightening of the posterior annulus and posterior longitudinal ligament in flexion improves the barrier to a greater extent, with the net effect being reduction of the posterior protrusion. In prolapse, this relief has not been found. Therefore, the flexed position obliterates the disc bulge and relieves the irritated nerve root in the bulging disc.

4. Pilling (55d), who performed myelography on patients in the upright position, showed that a protrusion is reduced in the flexion position because the poste-

rior longitudinal ligament and annulus are stretched and the disc spaces are widened posteriorly. A prolapse would not show such reduction.

5. With epidurography, Matthews and Yates (55e) showed that with distraction of 120 lb, there is reduction of a disc protrusion.

6. Extension causes the ligamentum flavum, the disc, and the posterior longitudinal ligament to narrow the sagittal diameter of the vertebral canal, whereas flexion reverses this (55b).

7. McNeil and Addison (55g) demonstrated the extensor muscles to be the weakest in the low back. We, therefore, exercise them after the patient has had relief of his low back and leg pain.

8. White and Panjabi (55h) showed that with bending of the spine, the disc bulges on the concave side of the curve and collapses on the convex side of the curve. In flexion, the disc protrudes anteriorly and depresses posteriorly.

9. Finneson (55i) showed disc protrusion on extension and reduction on flexion.

## Criteria for Determining the Level of Disc Involvement

MacGibbon and Farfan (56) give criteria for determining the level of disc degeneration by markings on a plain film study of the lumbar spine (Fig. 2.86). Basically, he states that when the intercrestal line passes through the upper half of the 4th lumbar vertebral body and when the transverse processes of L5 are well developed, the L4-L5 disc degenerates first. If

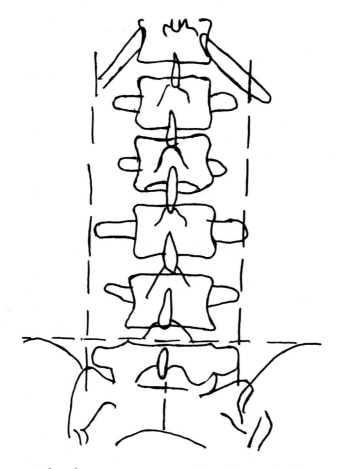

**Figure 2.86.** Intercrestal and transverse process lines drawn for determining probable level of disc degeneration.

the intercrestal line passes through the body of L5 and L5 has short transverse processes, the L5-S1 disc degenerates first. The higher the intercrestal line, the greater is the risk of L4-L5 degeneration; and the lower the intercrestal line, the greater is the risk of L5-S1 degeneration. He further states that if it is assumed that discs are injured and degenerate solely because of torsional strains, the high intercrestal line and long transverse processes become antitorsional devices, protecting the L5-S1 discs and indicating the likelihood of degeneration at L4-L5. Similarly, the low intercrestal line and small transverse processes providing no protection against torsion indicate the likelihood of degeneration at either the L4-L5 or the L5-S1 disc. We would, therefore, expect a high odds ratio for L4-L5 disc degeneration in the protected spines and a more equal odds ratio when there is no protection.

The criteria for probable L4-L5 degeneration is:

1. A high intercrestal line passing through the upper half of L4.
2. Long transverse processes on L5.
3. Rudimentary rib.
4. Transitional vertebra.

The criteria for L5-S1 degeneration is:

1. An intercrestal line passing through the body of L5.
2. Short transverse processes on L5.
3. No rudimentary rib.
4. No transitional vertebra.

Surgical fusion has an effect similar to that of the intercrestal lines described by MacGibbon and Farfan. Fusion places the mobility at the segment above the fusion and can cause disc degeneration at that level. The following case demonstrates this.

The patient was hospitalized for low back and left sciatic pain. Figure 2.87 is the x-ray taken on admission. A spinal fusion was carried out from the 3rd lumbar vertebra through the 2nd sacral vertebra involving a graft along the transverse and spinous processes (Fig. 2.88). For 4 months following surgery, this patient was treated by injection of local anesthesia for back pain. The following month, the patient again underwent low back surgery for the removal of neuromas in the spinal fusion area. She was referred by this surgeon to another doctor for consultation about her pain. The next year, the patient underwent yet another exploration of her fusion from L3 to sacrum. A repair of pseudoarthrosis at L3-L4 and L4-L5 with refusion utilizing right iliac bone and threaded pins and wire fixation was performed. Two months later, another exploration of the spinal fusion was carried out with removal of the metallic pins and wire fixation.

The patient lived in low back pain and leg pain discomfort for 2 years. She then sought chiropractic care. Examination revealed that the patient had left leg 5th lumbar dermatome sciatica and left 4th lumbar medial disc protrusion. Because the fusion had failed to hold up according to the past surgical exploration, traction reduction was applied and very good results were obtained. The sciatic pain was relieved in the 5th lumbar dermatome.

The unique attempt to fuse both the transverse and the spinous processes is a rather shotgun type approach to stabilizing the lumbar spine. Figure 2.89 reveals that at the L2-L3 intervertebral disc space there is a right lateral flexion subluxation of L2 on L3 with marked discogenic spondyloarthrosis present. Normally, 75% of the motion of the lumbar spine occurs at L5-S1 and as that disc degenerates, the motion moves progressively upward, so typically L4-L5 will be the next disc to degenerate. In this patient with attempted fusion from L3 through the sacrum, the point of maximum mobility was changed to L2-L3. The resultant degenerative change, therefore, occurred at the L2-L3 intervertebral disc joint, which was never intended to tolerate such hypermobility. This patient has to be splinted with back support to prevent future pain when lifting, bending, or twisting.

## Immunological Implications of Lumbar Disc Disease

Naylor et al. (57) state that a hypothesis to explain the chemical process of disc prolapse would include the initial change as a disturbance of the normal protein-polysaccharide synthesis-depolymerization equilibrium in favor of increased or unbalanced depolymerization, with the changes in the proteoglycans metabolism being associated with an increased fluid

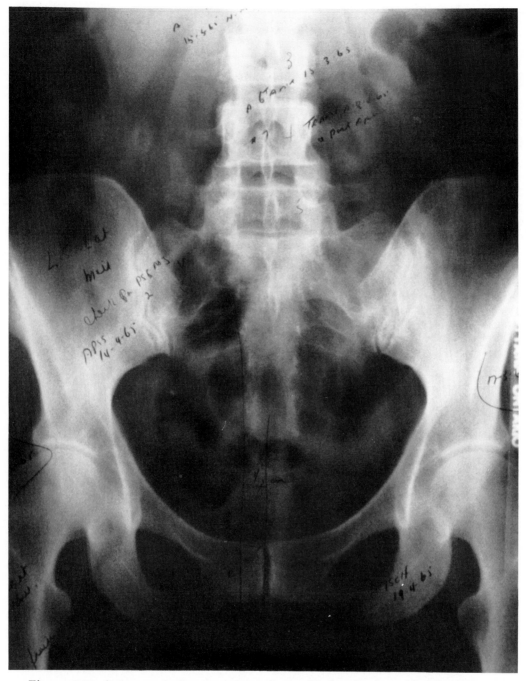

**Figure 2.87.** Anteroposterior x-ray in patient with low back and left leg sciatica.

content and, thus, increased intradisc tension. This could then produce an episode of disc nuclear herniation. Five acid glycerophosphatases have been isolated from disc material. These lysosomal enzymes can be shown to degrade the intervertebral disc. Of these five acid glycerophosphatases isolated in normal nuclei, two have the same activity during prolapse, one has a lower activity, and the others have some deficiencies. The studies of Naylor et al. suggest that lysosomal en-

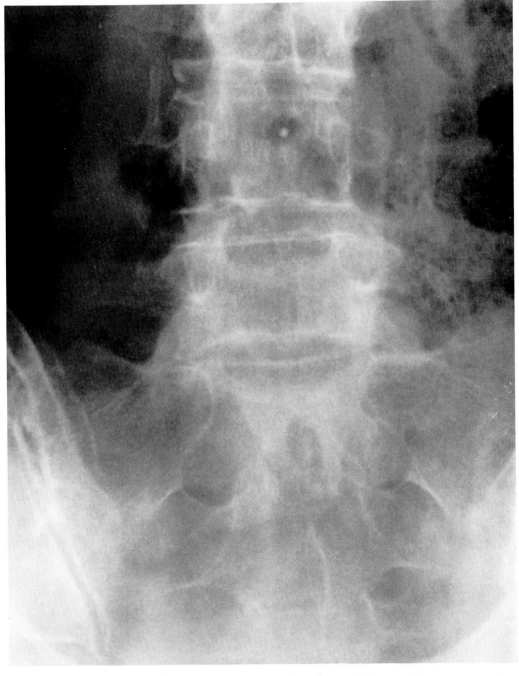

**Figure 2.88.** Intertransverse fusion from L3 to sacrum.

zymes present in the nucleus pulposus of the prolapsed intervertebral disc are capable of degrading the protein-polysaccharide complexes.

Elve et al. (58) studied 12 patients with prolapsed intervertebral discs. All patients had discectomy performed. Eight of these patients had protrusion and 4 had sequestration or prolapse with free fragmentation of the disc. Three of the 4 patients with prolapse showed an immune response to their own disc material. None of those with protrusion gave a positive immune reaction.

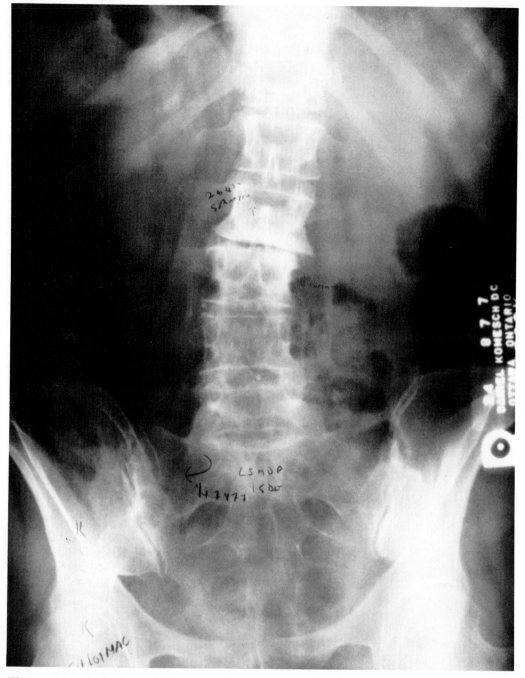

**Figure 2.89.** Right lateral flexion subluxation of L2 on L3 and advanced discogenic spondyloarthrosis of L2-L3. L2-L3 cannot perform all the movements that normally occur at the lower lumbar levels and degenerates severely following lumbar fusion.

Naylor et al. (57) found a significant enhancement of IgM and IgG in patients with lumbar disc prolapse. They suggest that either a nonspecific antigen process or stimulation of an antibody humoral system is the factor in the development of disc prolapse. Gertzbein (59) states that there is evidence for an autoimmune mechanism in the degeneration of the lumbar disc.

It was Falconer (as discussed in Ref. 57) who originally stated that on myelography defects could still be observed in patients whose low back and leg pain had been completely relieved. Thus, there is evidence to support the claim that the pain from disc prolapse is caused by chemical irritation as well as mechanical irritation of nerve roots. Once the degradation products of prolapse are dissipated, the relief of symptoms may be imminent.

Direct chemical analysis, x-ray crystallography, and electron microscopy have shown that disc degeneration shows a fall in the total sulfate, both keratin and chondroitin, although no pH change occurs. In disc herniation, there is a fall in total proteoglycan level, chiefly chondroitin sulfate, and probably in keratosulfate fractions.

The chemical explanation of disc prolapse expressed here is that initially there is a disturbance of the normal protein-polysaccharide synthesis which is associated with an increased fluid content and intradiscal pressure that produces the damage to the annulus, with repeated episodes producing advanced degeneration of the disc. *What creates these changes? The lysosomal enzymes of arthritis and rheumatoid arthritis are similar and may produce the disc changes of herniation.* Ruptured discs have been shown to release *acid phosphatase* which degrades the protein-polysaccharide complexes of the intervertebral disc (57).

Bobechko and Hirsch (as discussed in Ref. 57) showed that the intervertebral disc could act as an antigen, with the common antigenic determinant located in the region of the glycosaminoglycan to the protein core.

*IgM, IgG, and IgA have been isolated in serum of patients with prolapse and not in the serum of normal healthy people (59).* It is primarily IgG and IgM that are elevated in patients with lumbar disc prolapse.

A reaction between IgM and the protein polysaccharide complex has been shown to produce *amyloid* similar to that found in the amyloid-containing tissues of patients with rheumatoid arthritis (57).

Many believe that chronic degeneration of the disc is an autoimmune disease with antibodies directed at components of the nucleus pulposus which normally are shielded from the circulation and the reticuloendothelial system. A highly significant increase of serum IgM was reported in patients with proven Schmorl's nodes, narrowed disc spaces, or neurological signs of disc damage, compared with age-matched controls (60) (Fig. 2.90).

## Summary of Lumbar Mechanics

The bony parts and soft tissues of a cross section of the lumbar spine can be divided into anterior and posterior elements. The dividing line is just behind the vertebral body, with the body, the disc, and the anterior and posterior longitudinal ligaments lying anteriorly. The neural arch with its processes, the intervertebral (apophyseal or facet) joints and the different ligaments attached to the bony elements, lie posteriorly. The back muscles are distributed mainly lateral and posterior to the neural arch, but there are also anterolateral muscles (61).

The division is not merely anatomic but has a functional (mechanical) purpose. The anterior elements provide the major support of the column and absorb various impacts; the posterior structures control patterns of motion. Together they protect the dural content, which is surrounded by the neural arch.

Being synovial in nature, these joints undergo degenerative changes as age progresses. These changes are usually secondary to degeneration of the disc and, therefore, occur later in life. It is obvious that the decrease of intervertebral disc height accompanying degeneration has an effect on the apophyseal joints in stress distribution. It becomes germane, therefore, to postulate on the importance of mechanical factors in degenerative changes. The importance of mechanical factors to these changes is also indicated by the fact that severe osteoarthritis of the apophyseal joints is common in the presence of scoliosis, kyphosis, block vertebrae, spondylolisthesis, and vertebral body collapse.

Normal function of the apophyseal joints is important in stabilizing the motion segment and controlling its movement. The discs and ligaments are thus protected. Loads applied to the lumbar

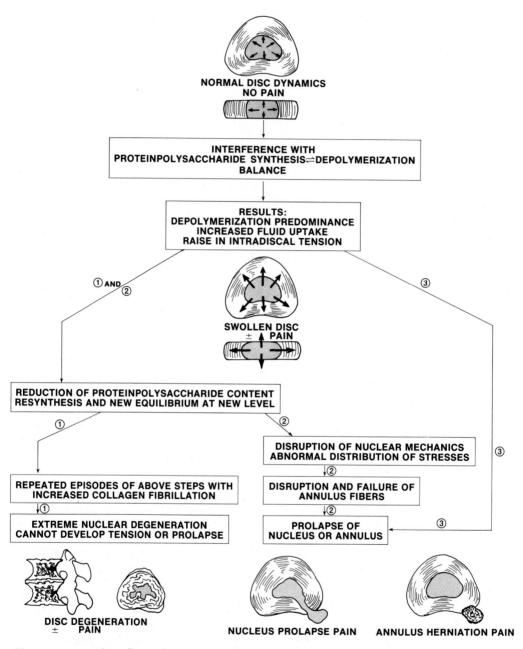

**NORMAL DISC DYNAMICS
NO PAIN**

**INTERFERENCE WITH
PROTEINPOLYSACCHARIDE SYNTHESIS⇌DEPOLYMERIZATION
BALANCE**

**RESULTS:
DEPOLYMERIZATION PREDOMINANCE
INCREASED FLUID UPTAKE
RAISE IN INTRADISCAL TENSION**

① AND ②

③

**SWOLLEN DISC
± ↑ PAIN**

**REDUCTION OF PROTEINPOLYSACCHARIDE CONTENT
RESYNTHESIS AND NEW EQUILIBRIUM AT NEW LEVEL**

① ②

**DISRUPTION OF NUCLEAR MECHANICS
ABNORMAL DISTRIBUTION OF STRESSES** ③

↓②

**REPEATED EPISODES OF ABOVE STEPS WITH
INCREASED COLLAGEN FIBRILLATION**

↓①

**DISRUPTION AND FAILURE OF
ANNULUS FIBERS**

↓②

**EXTREME NUCLEAR DEGENERATION
CANNOT DEVELOP TENSION OR PROLAPSE**

**PROLAPSE OF
NUCLEUS OR ANNULUS** ③

**DISC DEGENERATION
± PAIN**

**NUCLEUS PROLAPSE PAIN**

**ANNULUS HERNIATION PAIN**

**Figure 2.90.** This flow diagram explains the biochemical hypothesis of the basic mechanisms of spine pain, disc prolapse, and disc degeneration. A number of mechanical factors mentioned in this chapter probably play a large role in the clinical presentation and outcome of these various biochemical phenomena. (Reproduced with permission of A. A. White and M. M. Panjabi: *Clinical Biomechanics of the Spine.* Philadelphia, J. B. Lippincott, 1978, p. 291.)

spine are normally shared between the joints and discs. This load sharing can be influenced by the type of loading, the geometry of the motion segment, and the stiffness of the participating structures (61).

Miller et al. (62) have reported on the manner in which the intervertebral disc and the posterior elements share loads placed on the lumbar motion segment. For their report they made use of a two-dimensional biomechanical model to examine this load sharing. The model incorporated two rigid bodies to represent the vertebrae and six elastic springs to represent the tissues of the intervertebral disc and the posterior elements. Compression loads were resisted almost totally by the model intervertebral disc, but both the intervertebral disc and the posterior elements contributed substantially to resisting anteroposterior shear and flexion-extension loads. Motion segment morphology was a major determinant of load sharing in the model disc response to anteroposterior shear.

Both the intervertebral disc and the apophyseal (facet) joints of low lumbar motion segments are suspected sources of low back pain. When a low back disorder occurs, pain is aggravated by some physical activities but not by others. Different physical activities impose different loads on both the disc and the facets; perhaps pain aggravation is related to those loading patterns. Hence, it is important to know how much of a load imposed on a motion segment is distributed to the intervertebral disc, how much is distributed to the apophyseal joints, and what the determinants of that distribution are.

## Range of Internal Loads

Provided that facets were present, a shear force applied to the motion segment was resisted primarily by a combination of intervertebral disc shear and facet compression or tension. The portion of the overall shear resistance contributed by disc shear versus that contributed by facet tension compression depended little on how far posterior to the disc the facets were but depended very much on their superior-inferior location. When the

facets were low, almost all of that resistance was provided by shearing of the intervertebral disc. When the facets were high, each mechanism contributed substantially to the total resistance. Thus, in response to a large anteroposterior shear force, both the intervertebral disc and the facet joints can be loaded lightly to moderately or they can be loaded heavily. Which circumstance occurs seems to depend primarily on the location of the facets relative to the disc in the superior-inferior direction (62).

Facet inclination angle did not seem critical to motion segment response. When the facets were tilted 20° from the frontal plane, the facets were compressed 300 N at most in response to the 2,500-N compression force. when the facets were tilted only 5°, they were compressed 120 N at most. That is, *Facet inclination angle had only a modest effect on compression response.* In response to the 500-N shear force, changing the superior-inferior location of the facets by 2 cm caused about 3 times the change in load sharing between disc shear and facet inclination of 15° (62).

## CONCLUSIONS

The findings (62) suggest that when loads typical of those experienced in vivo are applied to a lumbar motion segment, the following occur:

1. The apophyseal joints are not loaded heavily by compression or flexion-extension loads but can be heavily loaded by anteroposterior shear loads.

2. Resistance developed by the apophyseal joints are not very effective in relieving loads on the intervertebral disc when the motion segment is compressed. They can be effective in relieving the disc, however, when the segment is flexed, extended, or anteroposteriorly sheared.

3. In response to anteroposterior shear loads, the location of the facet joints relative to that of the intervertebral disc in the superior-inferior direction is a major determinant of what loads each structure will bear.

Pathologic, experimental, and clinical studies indicate that excessive strain concentration may occur in the posterior elements of the spine and be increased by extension. These strains may cause small fractures in this region and can be responsible for episodes of back pain. The diagnosis of these fractures is usually missed.

Under compressive load, the highest compressive strains were recorded near the bases of the pedicles and deep surfaces of the pars interarticularis (63).

Experiments were carried out on cadaveric lumbar spines to determine the mechanical function of the apophyseal joints (64). It was found that in lordotic postures the apophyseal joints resist most of the intervertebral shear force and share in resisting the intervertebral compressive force. Apophyseal joints prevent excessive movement from damaging the discs. The posterior annulus is protected in torsion by the facet surfaces and in flexion by the capsular ligaments.

Recent experiments in our laboratory and elsewhere performed on cadaveric spines have determined the mechanical properties of the apophyseal joints when they are subjected to loading regimes calculated to simulate movements and postures in life. This experimental evidence has been collated to give a concise account of the mechanical function of the apophyseal joints and to indicate under what circumstances they might sustain damage.

## Resistance to Intervertebral Shear Forces

When an intervertebral joint is loaded in shear, the apophyseal joint surfaces resist about one third of the shear force, while the disc resists the remaining two thirds (64). This passive resistance to shear is complicated by two features, however. First, when an intervertebral disc alone is subjected to sustained shear, it readily creeps forward. In an intact joint, this readiness to creep would manifest itself as stress relaxation, thus placing an increasing burden on the apophyseal joint surfaces until they resist all of the intervertebral shear force. Second, the muscle slips attached to the posterior part of the neural arch brace it by pulling downward. This prevents any backward bending and brings the facets more firmly

together. This means that in the intact joint the intervertebral disc is subjected only to pure compression and that the intervertebral shear force is resisted by the apophyseal joints, producing a high interfacet force.

## Resistance to Intervertebral Compressive Force

The absence of a flattened articular surface in the transverse plane at the base of the articular facets clearly suggests that apophyseal joints are not designed to resist intervertebral compressive force. Experiments confirm that, provided the lumbar spine is slightly flattened (as occurs in erect sitting or heavy lifting), all the intervertebral compressive force is resisted by the disc. When lordotic postures such as erect standing are held for long periods, however, the facet tips do make contact with the laminae of the subadjacent vertebra and bear about one sixth of the compressive force (64).

This contact may well be of clinical significance, since it will result in high stresses on the tips of the facets, and possibly, nipping of the joint capsules. Perhaps this is the reason standing for long periods can produce a dull ache in the small of the back which is relieved by sitting or by using some device, such as a bar rail, to induce slight flexion of the lumbar spine. Disc narrowing results in as much as 70% of the intervertebral compressive force being transmitted across the apophyseal joints. Three such specimens tested exhibited gross degenerative changes in the apophyseal joints (64).

With increasing extension of an intervertebral joint, the compressive force transmitted across the apophyseal joints increases, and it is likely that the extension movements are limited by this bony contact. Thus, it is possible that hyperextension movements could cause backward bending of the neural arch, eventually resulting in spondylolysis, but again only as a fatigue fracture.

## Resistance to Torsion

Axial rotation of the lumbar spine takes place about a center of rotation in the posterior disc or neural canal. (If axial rotation of the lumbar spine were to occur about some axis posterior to the apophyseal joints, it would be most strongly resisted by the fibers of the anterior annulus fibrosus, since the posterior annulus would be nearer to the center of rotation.) The apophyseal joints are oriented to resist such rotations and protect the soft tissues from the effects of torsion.

Forced axial rotation could occur from a fall on one shoulder or from activities involving high angular momentum, such as discus throwing. Awkward bending (i.e., forward and to one side) is often mistakenly thought to involve significant axial rotation of the lumbar spine. Unlike axial rotation, awkward bending is limited by soft tissues and can lead to ligamentous damage and disc prolapse (64).

For normal intervertebral discs to fail completely, they must be rotated to angles of 22.6° on the average, although microscopic damage will occur at angles somewhat less than this. The margin of safety must be quite high in the lower lumbar spine, however, when we consider that because of the orientation of the facets the T12-L1 discs can be safely rotated about 5° to each side.

### Resistance to Flexion

The capsular ligaments of the apophyseal joints play the dominant role in resisting flexion of an intervertebral joint. In full flexion, as determined by the elastic limit of the supraspinous and interspinous ligaments, the capsular ligaments provide 39% of the joint's resistance. The balance is made up by the disc (29%) the supraspinous and interspinous ligaments (19%), and the ligamentum flavum (13%) (64).

In hyperflexion, the supraspinous and interspinous ligaments are damaged first, followed by the capsular ligaments and then the disc. Bending forward and to one side, however, could damage the capsular ligaments first because the component of lateral flexion would produce extra stretching of the capsule away from the side of bending while not affecting the supraspinous and interspinous ligaments which lie on the axis of lateral bending.

In flexion, as in torsion, the apophyseal joints protect the intervertebral disc.

Once the posterior spinal ligaments have been sprained in hyperflexion, the wedged disc is able to prolapse into the neural canal if subjected to a high compressive force.

### CONCLUSION

The function of the lumbar apophyseal joints is to allow limited movement between vertebrae and to protect the discs from shear forces, excessive flexion, and axial rotation. They are not well suited to resist intervertebral compressive forces and are usually protected by the discs. The ligaments of the apophyseal joints are most likely to be damaged in bending forward and to one side. The capsule could be a source of pain in sustained lordotic postures (64).

### References

1. Rees WS: Slipped disc syndrome. *Med J Aust* 2:948, 1973.
2. Rothman RH, Simeone FA: *The Spine*. Philadelphia, WB Saunders, 1975, vol II, p 444.
3. Feffer H: How to prevent back pain. *US News World Rep* 47–48, April 1975.
4. Cyriax J: *Textbook of Orthpedic Medicine*, ed 5, vol 1: *Diagnosis of Soft Tissue Lesions*. Baltimore, Williams & Wilkins, 1969, vol 1, pp 389–397.
5. Day PL: Early interim and long term observations on chemonucleolysis in 876 patients with special comments on the lateral approach. *Clin Orthop* 99:63–69, 1974.
6. Rothman RH, Simeone FA: *The Spine*. Philadelphia, WB Saunders, 1975, vol II, p 468.
7. Semmes RE: *Ruptures of the Lumbar Intervertebral Disc*. Springfield, IL, Charles C Thomas, 1964, pp 17–18.
8. Scoville WB, Corkill G: Lumbar spondylolisthesis with ruptured disc. *J Neurosurg* 40:530, 1974.
9. Abdullah AF, Ditto EW, Byrd EW, Williams R: Extreme lateral disc herniations, clinical syndrome and special problems of diagnosis. *J Neurosurg* 41:229–233, 1974.
10. Nachemson AL: The lumbar spine, an orthopaedic challenge. *Spine* 1(1):59–69, 1976.
11. Epstein BS: *The Spine, A Radiological Text and Atlas*, ed 3. Philadelphia, Lea & Febiger, 1969, pp 35, 38, 554.
12. Keele CA, Neil E: *Samson Wright's Applied Physiology*, ed 10. London, Oxford University Press, 1961, p 51.
13. Cailliet R: *Low Back Pain Syndrome*. Philadelphia, FA Davis, 1962, pp 4–5.
14. Puschel J: Der Wassergehalt Normaler und Degenerieter Zuracken Werbelscheben. *Beitr Pathol* 84:123, 1930.
15. DePukey P: The physiological oscillation of the length of the body. *Acta Orthop Scand.* 6:338d, 1935.
16. Hendry NGC: The hydration of the nucleus pul-

posus and its relation to intervertebral disc derangement. *J Bone Joint Surg* 40B:132, 1958.

17. Finneson BE: *Low Back Pain.* Philadelphia, JB Lippincott, 1973, p 27.
18. Morris JM, Lucas DB, Bresler B: Role of the trunk in stability of the spine. *J Bone Joint Surg* 43A:327, 1961.
19. Gresham JL, Miller R: Evaluation of the lumbar spine by diskography. *Orthop Clin* 67:29, 1969.
20. Finneson BE: *Low Back Pain.* Philadelphia, JB Lippincott, 1973, p 31.
21. Hoelein BF: *Canine Neurology: Diagnosis and Treatment.* Philadelphia, WB Saunders, 1965.
22. Finneson BE: *Low Back Pain.* Philadelphia, JB Lippincott, 1973, pp 264, 265.
23. Lecuire J, et al: 641 operations for sciatic neuralgia due to discal hernia, a computerized statistical study of the results. *Neurochirugie* 19:501–512, 1973.
24. Finneson BE: *Low Back Pain,* ed 2. Philadelphia, JB Lippincott, 1980, pp 33–37.
25. Panjabi MM, White A: Basic biomechanics of the spine. *Neurosurgery* 7(1): 76–77, 1980.
26. Gregerson GG, Lucas DB: An in vivo study of the axial rotation of the human thoraco-lumbar spine. *J Bone Joint Surg* 49A:247, 262, 1967.
27. Lumsden RM II, Morris JM: An in vivo study of axial rotation and immobilization at the lumbosacral joint. *J Bone Joint Surg* 50A:1591–1602, 1968.
28. White AA, Panjabi MM: *Clinical Biomechanics of the Spine.* Philadelphia, JB Lippincott, 1978, p 15.
28a. Bernini PM, Simeone FA: Reflex dystrophy. *Spine* 6(2):180–184, 1981.
28b. Farfan HF: *Mechanical Disorders of the Low Back.* Philadelphia, Lea & Febiger, 1973, p 24.
28c. Helfet AJ, Gruebel-Lee DM: *Disorders of the Lumbar Spine.* Philadelphia, JB Lippincott, 1978, p 46–47.
28d. Tsukada K: Histologische Studien über die Zwischenwirbelscheibe des Menschen. *Altersvanderugen Mitt Akad Kioto* 25:1–29, 207–209, 1932.
28e. Shinohara H: A study on lumbar disc lesions. *J Jpn Orthop Assoc* 44:553, 1970.
28f. Malinsky J: The ontogenetic development of nerve terminations in the intervertebral discs of man. *Acta Anat* 38:96, 1959.
28g. Hirsch C, Inglemark BG, Miller M: The anatomical basis for low back pain. Studies on the presence of sensory nerve endings in ligamentous, capsular and intervertebral disc structures in the human lumbar spine. *Acta Orthop Scand* 1:33, 1963–1964.
28h. Sunderland S: Anatomical paravertebral influence on the intervertebral foramen. In: *The Research Status of Spinal Manipulative Therapy.* Bethesda, MD, National Institute of Neurological and Communicative Disorders and Stroke, NINCDS Monograph No 15, DHEW No 76-998, 1975, p 135.
28i. Edgar MA, Ghadially JA: Innervation of the lumbar spine. *Clin Orthop* 115:35–41, 1976.
28j. Lazorthes G, Poulhes J, Espagno J: Etude. sur les nerfs sinu-vertebraux lumbaires le nerf de roofe existe-t-il? *CR Assoc Anat* 34:317, 1948.
28k. Yoshizawa H, O'Brien J, Smith WT, Trumper M: The neuropathology of intervertebral discs removed for low-back pain. *J Pathol* 132:95–104, 1980.
29. Bogduk N: The anatomy of the lumbar intervertebral disc syndrome. *Med J Aust* 1:878, 1976.
30. Vernon-Roberts B, Pirie CJ: Degenerative changes in the intevertebral discs of the lumbar spine and their sequelae. *J Rheumatol Rehabil* 16:13, 1977.
31. Farfan HF, Cossett B, Robertson GH, Wells RV, Kraus H: The effects of torsion on the lumbar intervertebral joints, the role of torsion in the production of disc degeneration. *J Bone Joint Surg* 52:3, 1970.
32. Farfan HF: *Mechanical Disorders of the Low Back.* Philadelphia, Lea & Febiger, 1973, pp 24, 44, 49.
33. Farfan HF: *Mechanical Disorders of the Low Back.* Philadelphia, Lea & Febiger, 1973, p 135.
34. Ritchie JH, Fahrni WJ: Age changes in the lumbar intervertebral disc. *Can J Surg* 13:65, 1970.
35. Hirsch C, Schajowicz F: Studies on the structural changes in the lumbar annulus fibrosus. *Acta Orthop Scand* 22:184, 1953.
36. Turek S: *Orthopaedics—Principles and Their Applications.* Philadelphia, JB Lippincott, 1956, chap 27, 748.
37. Keyes DC, Compere EL: The normal and pathological physiology of the nucleus pulposus of the intervertebral disc: an anatomical, clinical and experimental study. *J Bone Joint Surg* 14:897, 1961.
38. Yong-Hing K, Kirkaldy-Willis WH: The pathophysiology of degenerative disease of the lumbar spine. *Orthop Clin North Am* 14(13):501–503, 1983.
39. Lora J, Long D: So-called facet denervation in the management of intractable back pain. *Spine* 1(2):121–126, 1976.
40. Arns W, et al: Conservative therapy of lumbar intervertebral disc lesions. *Dtsch Med Wochenschr* 101:587–589, 1976.
41. Macnab I, et al: Chemonucleolysis. *Can J Surg* 14:280–289, 1971.
42. Macnab I: Negative disc exploration. *J Bone Joint Surg* 53A:891–903, 1971.
43. Maigne R: Low back pain of thoraco-lumbar origin. *Arch Phys Med Rehabil* 61:389–395, 1980.
44. Helfet AJ, Gruebel-Lee DM: *Disorders of the Lumbar Spine.* Philadelphia, JB Lippincott, 1978, p 72.
45. Deleted in proof.
46. Eagle R: A pain in the back. *New Scientist* 170–173, October 18, 1979.
47. Miller J: Empirical approaches to the validation of manipulation. Paper delivered at University of Michigan College of Osteopathic Medicine, April 30–May 1, 1983.
48. Lorenz M, Patwardhan A, Vanderby R: Load bearing characteristics of the lumbar spine in normal and surgically altered spinal segments. *Spine* 8(2):122–128, 1983.
49. Mooney V, Robertson JR: The facet syndrome. *Clin Orthop* 115:149, 1976.
50. Carrera CG: Lumbar facet injection in low back pain and sciatica. *Radiology* 737:665–667, 1980.
51. Dory M: Arthrography of the lumbar facet joints. *Radiology* 140:23–27, 1981.

52. Fahrni WH: Conservative treatment of lumbar disc degeneration: our primary responsibility. *Orthop Clin North Am* 6(1):93–103, 1975.

53. Fromelt K, Cox JM, Schreiner S: Activities causing injury to the lumbar spine: a computer study. *JACA* 17:3–16, 1983.

54. Hutton WC, Adam MA: Mechanical factors in the etiology of low back pain. *Orthopedics* 5(11):1461–1465, 1982.

55. Posner I, White AA, Edwards WT, Hayes WC: A biomechanical analysis of the clinical stability of the lumbosacral spine. *Spine*, 7(4):374–389, 1982.

55a. Ehni G, Weinstein P: *Lumbar Spondylosis*. Chicago, Year Book Medical Publishers, 1977, p 137.

55b. Dyck P, Pheasant HC, Doyle JB, Rieder JJ: Cauda equina compression. *Spine* 2(1):77, 1977.

55c. Raney F: The effects of flexion, extension, Valsalva maneuver, and abdominal compression on the myelographic column. International Society for the Study of the Lumbar Spine, San Francisco Meeting, June 5–8, 1978.

55d. Pilling JR: Water soluble radiculography in the erect position, a clinical radiological study. *Clin Radiol* 30:665–670, 1979.

55e. Matthews, Yates: *Lancet*, March 1974.

55f. Wilmink JT, Penning L: Influence of spinal posture on abnormalities demonstrated by lumbar myelography. *Am J Neuroradiol* 4:656–658, 1983.

55g. McNeil T, Warwick D, Andersson G, Schultz A: Trunk strengths in attempted flexion, extension, and lateral bending in healthy subjects and patients with low-back disorders. *Spine* 5(6):529–538, 1980.

55h. White AA, Panjabi MM: *Clinical Biomechanics of the Spine*. Philadelphia, JB Lippincott, 1978, p 55.

55i. Finneson BE: *Low Back Pain*. Philadelphia, JB Lippincott, 1973, p 96.

56. MacGibbon B, Farfan H: A radiologic survey of various configurations of the lumbar spine. *Spine* 4(3):258–266, 1976.

57. Naylor A, Happey F, Turner RL, Shentall RD, West RD, Richardson C: Enzymatic and immunological activity in the intervertebral disc. *Orthop Clin North Am* 6(1):51–58, 1975.

58. Elves MW, Bucknill T, Sullivan MF: In vitro inhibition of leucocyte migration in patients with intervertebral disc lesions. *Orthop Clin North Am* 6:1, 1975.

59. Gertzbein SD: Degenerative disc disease of the lumbar spine. *Clin Orthop* 129:68–71, 1977.

60. Eyre DR: Biochemistry of the intervertebral disc. *Int Rev Connect Tissue Res* 8:227–289, 1979.

61. Andersson GBJ: The biomechanics of the posterior elements of the lumbar spine. *Spine* 8(3):326, 1983.

62. Miller JAA, Haderspeck KA, Schultz AB: Posterior elements in lumbar motion segments. *Spine* 8(3):331–337, 1983.

63. Jayson MIV: Compression stresses in the posterior elements and pathologic consequences. *Spine* 8(3):338, 1983.

64. Adams MA, Hutton WC: The mechanical function of the lumbar apophyseal joints. *Spine* 8(3):327–329, 1983.

CHAPTER **3**

# Diagnosis

## DIAGNOSTIC BIOMECHANICS

The most important spinal component is the intervertebral disc. It is the key structure in the movable segment (or, as Schmorl calls it, the "motor segment"), and its lesions (tears, prolapses, and degeneration) affect the rest of the movable segment (1). The axis of sagittal movement of the spine passes through the middle to the posterior portion of the disc, and as the axis pivots around the nucleus pulposus which acts as a fulcrum, it may shift slightly. In horizontally rotatory movement, the annular fibers in the lumbar region undergo shearing stress leading to tears or rupture, even in younger people, since the vertical axis of rotation is posterior to the vertebral bodies.

Both rupture of annular fibers, or the dissecting prolapse of the nucleus pulposus through the annulus fibrosus, and fracture and destruction of the basal cartilaginous and bony apophyseal plate may allow prolapse of the nucleus pulposus. This happens especially in young people with high intradiscal pressures sustained on loading in flexion and on high shearing stress in rotation, either into the posterior lateral extradural space (with the middle being protected somewhat by the posterior longitudinal ligament in most instances) or vertically into the bone through gaps, weak places, or fractures of the bony cartilaginous plate (1).

Clinical and experimental observations suggest that the disc may be one of the sources of idiopathic low back pain (2). In patients who develop definite disc herniation, one or more episodes of back pain frequently precede the herniation. These episodes of pain may be very similar to the pain experienced by patients who do not develop disc herniation. Hirsch (2a) and Lindblom (2b) increased the intradiscal pressure in patients with a history of back pain by injecting saline into the discs. They found that increased intradiscal pressure reproduced the patient's pain. If the disc was injected with a local anesthetic prior to the increases in intradiscal pressure, pain did not develop. If Hypaque was injected into a disc and the dye extended into the annulus, severe pain was sometimes produced. If the dye remained in the nucleus, pain did not occur. Direct mechanical stimulation of the annulus and cartilage plate may also produce pain. These findings indicate that irritation or abnormalities of the disc may cause pain, but even if the disc is not the primary source of pain in some syndromes, alterations in the disc may produce symptoms by changing the loads on other structures, including facet joints, spinal ligaments, paraspinal muscles, and nerve roots.

### Discal Back Pain and Sciatica

Patients present with back pain and sciatica, with back pain and no sciatica, and with sciatica and no back pain. The most overlooked diagnosis of disc protrusion in clinical practice probably involves the patient with back pain without sciatica. Early nuclear protrusion into the annular fibers often involves the patient with acute back pain and perhaps an antalgic lean to one side. It is well documented that the annulus fibrosus is well innervated by the sinuvertebral nerve, becoming more so from the central portion to the peripheral portion of the disc (3). Radiating cracks in the annulus fibrosus develop in the most centrally situated lamellae and extend outward toward the periphery (4). Turek (5) states that this cracking and fissuring begins as early as the fifteenth year and may take place silently over many years. The annulus, under the pressure of nuclear protrusion, becomes progressively weaker and thinner. As this pathological state develops, the intensity of pain and the antalgic lean of the patient increase.

As the annular fibers progressively thin and the protruding nuclear material makes mild contact with the nerve root, the manifestations of sciatica are first observed. If the annular fibers completely tear and the protruding material bursts forth, the intensity of the sciatica proportionately increases.

The pressure on protruding nuclear material is greater in the young person with a turgid nucleus, which contains up to 80% water, than in the older person in whom the nucleus pulposus has become dehydrated and converted into a hardened mass. Therefore, a patient may have a nuclear bulge creating low back pain resulting from aggravation of the annular fibers, or he may have back pain and sciatica as the protruding disc material contacts the nerve root, or he may have only sciatica if the disc protrudes through the annulus and contacts only the nerve root, with no other structures innervated by the recurrent meningeal nerve being irritated.

Equally important is the fact that the nucleus which bulges through the annulus fibrosus and comes to lie free under the posterior longitudinal ligament may migrate cephalad and caudally along the posterior vertebral body. Nuclear material that breaks continuity with the remaining nucleus is called a free fragment or prolapsed disc.

White and Panjabi (6) prepared an update of Charnley's (7) hypothesis on low back pain.[1] The following are the classifications of back pain from White and Panjabi (6).

## ACUTE BACK SPRAIN (TYPE I)

Acute back sprain (type I) characteristically occurs when a laborer attempts to sustain a sudden additional load. There is immediate severe pain that may last for several weeks. The pain is primarily in the low back, without sciatica, and may be due to several factors. Charnley suggested the possibility of rupture of some of the deep layers of the annulus. We believe that, while this rupture is possible, the inner fibers are not innervated, and there is relatively less loading and deformation of the deeper fibers than of the periphery. There are other possibilities, however. One is that peripheral annular fibers may be injured or ruptured along with any of the other posterior ligaments or musculotendinous structures; another is that some of these injuries may involve rupture of muscle fibers or be associated with nondisplaced or minimally displaced vertebral end-plate fractures (Fig. 3.1). Whatever the cause, these conditions should respond to a period of rest, followed by a gradual resumption of normal activities.

## ORGANIC OR IDIOPATHIC FLUID INGESTION (TYPE II)

An attack of low back pain and muscle spasm may be produced by the sudden passage of fluid into the nucleus pulposus for some unknown reason (7, 8; and Footnote 2) (Fig. 3.2). Charnley suggested that this passage of fluid irritated the peripheral annular fibers, causing the characteristic pain. There is little to discredit the hypothesis 20 years later. Naylor (8) suggests that increased fluid uptake in the nucleus is a precipitating factor in the biochemical chain of events that can lead to disc disease. Very indirect evidence, however, suggests that increases in fluid

---

[1] Charnley's article (7) is a classic exposition on the topic. There is a clear theoretical presentation of the mechanism, diagnosis, and treatment of the various combinations of back pain and sciatica. It is highly recommended for both the primary care physician and the specialist.

[2] Naylor's article (8) provides a superb, comprehensive review of this hypothesis.

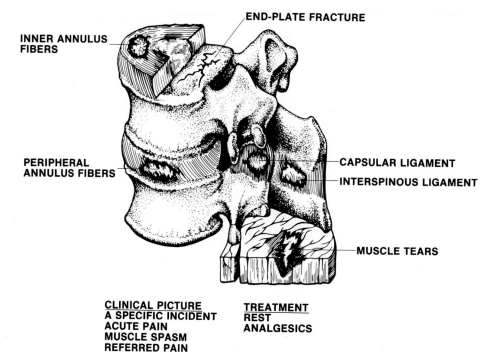

INNER ANNULUS
FIBERS

END-PLATE FRACTURE

PERIPHERAL
ANNULUS FIBERS

CAPSULAR LIGAMENT

INTERSPINOUS LIGAMENT

MUSCLE TEARS

CLINICAL PICTURE
A SPECIFIC INCIDENT
ACUTE PAIN
MUSCLE SPASM
REFERRED PAIN
NEGATIVE SLR

TREATMENT
REST
ANALGESICS

**Figure 3.1.** A clinical picture of acute back sprain (Type I) may involve damage to any number of ligamentous structures, the muscle, or even vertebral end-plate fracture. *SLR*, straight leg raising test. (Reproduced with permission from A. A. White and M. M. Panjabi: *Clinical Biomechanics of the Spine.* Philadelphia, J. B. Lippincott, 1978, p. 286 (6).)

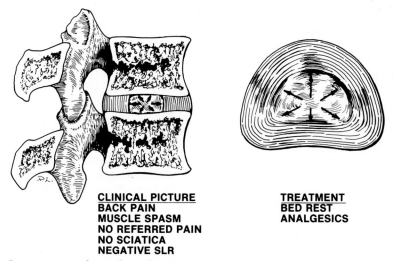

CLINICAL PICTURE
BACK PAIN
MUSCLE SPASM
NO REFERRED PAIN
NO SCIATICA
NEGATIVE SLR

TREATMENT
BED REST
ANALGESICS

**Figure 3.2.** Organic or idiopathic fluid ingestion (Type II). This mechanism may account for a large portion of back pain for which no distinct diagnosis nor etiology has been determined. (Reproduced with permission from A. A. White and M. M. Panjabi: *Clinical Biomechanics of the Spine.* Philadelphia, J. B. Lippincott, 1978, p. 286 (6).)

in the disc structure may not cause spine pain. This evidence is based on the observation that astronauts returning from outer space have heightened disc space but no back pain according to Kazarian (8a). On the other hand, there is evidence, although inconsistent, which suggests that fluid injection into the normal disc causes low back pain (9). This discrepancy may be partially explained by the differences in the rate of change in fluid pressure. The hypothesis of fluid ingestion is consistent with the clinical data because it is compatible with the characteristic clinical course of exacerbations and remissions, with or without progression to other clinical syndromes. In other words, movement of fluid in and out of the disc can explain the onset and resolution of the clinical symptoms. We suggest that this may be the explanation for spontaneous idiopathic organic spine pain (cervical, thoracic, or lumbar) unrelated to trauma, which accounts for a significant number of the many cases of spine pain.

## POSTEROLATERAL ANNULUS DISRUPTION (TYPE III)

If there is failure or disruption of some of the annular fibers, posterolateral irritation in this region may cause back pain with referral into the sacroiliac region, the buttock, or the back of the thigh (Fig. 3.3). This referred pain is due to stimulation of the sensory innervation by mechanical, chemical, or inflammatory irritants. Thus, "referred sciatica," as Charnley called it, is distinguished from true sciatica by a negative straight leg raising test and a lack of neuromuscular deficit. As suggested previously, this referred pain may be explained by the "gate" control theory. This referred sciatica may resolve itself through reabsorption or neutralization of the irritants and/or phagocytosis and painless healing of the disrupted annular fibers.

## BULGING DISC (TYPE IV)

Another proposed mechanism of low back pain and sciatica involves protrusion of the nucleus pulposus, which remains covered with some annular fibers and, possibly, the posterior longitudinal ligament (Fig. 3.4). There may be "true acute sciatica" with mechanical and, possibly, chemical and/or inflammatory irritation of the nerve roots. The pain may include the back, buttock, thigh, lower leg, and even the foot and may be increased with coughing and sneezing; the straight leg raising test is positive. In this situation, radiographs usually do not indicate narrowing. It is feasible that traction or spinal manipulation may alter the mechanics and possibly may be therapeutic. With rest, the irritation may subside and remain stable or may return spontaneously after mobilization.

## SEQUESTERED FRAGMENT (WANDERING DISC MATERIAL) (TYPE V)

A sequestered nucleus pulposus and/or annulus fibrosus (Fig. 3.5) associated with the normal degenerative processes of the disc and/or other presently unknown pathologic changes may develop with time. This sequestrum may move about in a random fashion in response to the directions and magnitude of forces produced at the motion segment by the activity of the individual. This movement may permit the sequestrum to irritate the annular fibers (by physical presence and/or chemical breakdown products) and to produce low back pain with or without sciatica. It may also produce a bulge in an area in which it can cause true sciatica. The sequestration may move about, so that it either may be asymptomatic or may cause some combination of spine pain, referred pain, and true radiculopathy. Because of the movement of the sequestered fragment in response to forces at the motion segment, it may be possible, through axial traction or spinal manipulation of the motion segment, to move the sequestrum temporarily or permanently from a location in which it stimulates a nerve to one in which it causes no irritation. Subsequent motion of the disc fragment into areas of pain insensitivity or subsequent scarring may result in no recurrence. On the other hand, if there is no scarring, the random movement of the sequestered portion of the disc may include positions of subsequent nerve root irritation.

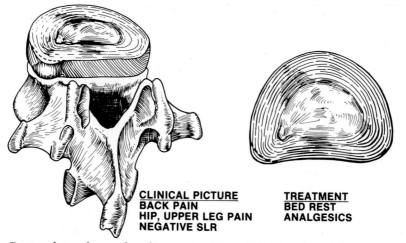

**CLINICAL PICTURE**          **TREATMENT**
**BACK PAIN**                 **BED REST**
**HIP, UPPER LEG PAIN**       **ANALGESICS**
**NEGATIVE SLR**

**Figure 3.3.** Posterolateral annulus disruption (Type III). The *dotted line* represents the original normal contour of the disc. Hip and thigh pain are referred pain rather than true sciatica. (Reproduced with permission from A. A. White and M. M. Panjabi: *Clinical Biomechanics of the Spine.* Philadelphia, J. B. Lippincott, 1978, p. 287 (6).)

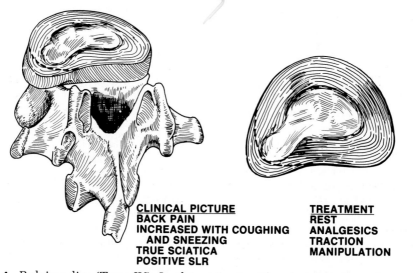

**CLINICAL PICTURE**              **TREATMENT**
**BACK PAIN**                     **REST**
**INCREASED WITH COUGHING**       **ANALGESICS**
**AND SNEEZING**                  **TRACTION**
**TRUE SCIATICA**                 **MANIPULATION**
**POSITIVE SLR**

**Figure 3.4.** Bulging disc (Type IV). In the patient with a bulging disc, the annulus is bulging to such an extent that nerve root irritation has caused sciatica. The *dotted line* shows the normal position of the annulus rim. (Reproduced with permission from A. A. White and M. M. Panjabi: *Clinical Biomechanics of the Spine.* Philadelphia, J. B. Lippincott, 1978, p. 287 (6).)

## DISPLACED SEQUESTERED FRAGMENT (ANCHORED) (TYPE VI)

Another clinical and mechanical cause of low back pain and sciatica is displacement of a sequestrum of the annulus and/or nucleus into the spinal canal or intervertebral foramen (Fig. 3.6). The fragment is to some degree fixed in position. The nerve root irritation results from inflammation due to mechanical pressure, chemical irritation, an autoimmune response, or some combination of the three. There is true sciatica with the positive straight leg raising sign. In association with a displaced portion of the intervertebral disc (sequestration), there may be narrowing of the interspace at the involved level. Axial traction, manipulation, and random movement are unlikely to help. Chymopapain injected into the disc space may never reach or affect the sequestrum, especially if there has been scarring or blockage of the hole in the disc structure. We hypothesize when this situation subsides spontaneously, it is the result of phagocytosis and/or some physiological adjustment of the neural structures to the irritation. Patients with a displaced sequestered fragment show the best results when treated with surgery, as suggested by Charnley and subsequently confirmed by Sprangfort (7, 10; and Footnote 3).

## DEGENERATIVE DISC (TYPE VII)

Disc degeneration (Fig. 3.7) involves a disruption of the normal annular fibers of the disc to such an extent that the disc is no longer able to serve an adequate mechanical function. This disruption may be associated with degenerative arthritic processes of the vertebral bodies and/or the intervertebral joints. There may be chronic pain, intermittent pain, or no pain.

## ORGANIC IDIOPATHIC SPINE PAIN

Organic idiopathic spine pain is the type of pain present in patients who are diagnosed clinically as having organic spine pain without sciatica for which there is no known etiology. Pain may emanate from the disc, or it may be caused by increased fluid uptake by the disc (Type II), any combination of the previously described etiologic factors, or some mechanism yet to be discovered.

## DIAGNOSIS OF THE DISC LESION

We classified the change within the nucleus pulposus when it escaped the confines of the annulus as a protrusion or prolapse. Protrusion of nuclear material

---

[3] Spangfort's article (10) is an excellent discussion of the significance of various physical findings in the evaluation and interpretation of low back pain and sciatica.

occurs when the protruding nucleus is contiguous with the remaining nucleus and the annulus fibrosus is stretched, thinned, and under pressure. The protrusion may cause only back pain if the outer nerve-innervated annulus is irritated, or it may cause both back and leg pain if the annulus bulge contacts the dural lined nerve root within the lateral recess of the vertebral column. Keep in mind that the pressure within the nucleus is 30 psi (11) and that Nachemson and Morris (11a) have found this pressure to be 30% less in the standing position than in the sitting position, with 50% less pressure in the reclining position than in the sitting position. The cerebrospinal fluid pressure is 100 mm of water in the recumbent posture and 400 mm in the sitting posture (12). This is important in treating the disc lesion, as sitting is to be avoided. An epidemiological study (13) conducted in Baltimore, Maryland, demonstrated that suburban dwellers who drive to work have twice the incidence of severe back pain than do those who do not drive and that those workers who drive during most of their working day, such as truck drivers, have three times the incidence. Fahrni (14) surveyed a jungle people in India who squat rather than sit and found that they had a zero incidence of back pain and a greatly diminished incidence of disc degeneration on x-ray.

Gresham and Miller (15) carried out postmortem discograms on 63 fresh autopsies; these patients who came to autopsy were between 14 and 80 years old and had had relatively asymptomatic backs. Gresham and Miller found that all of the specimens that came from patients between 46 and 59 years old revealed evidence of disc degeneration at L5-S1.

Prolapse exists when the extruded nucleus loses continuity with the remaining nuclear material and forms a free fragment, or what in Europe is termed a sequestered disc fragment, within the spinal canal. Arns et al. (16) state that the first stage of disc lesion is nuclear bulge which causes lumbago and symptoms of Déjérine's triad. The second stage is the onset of sciatica as the nuclear bulge contacts the nerve root, and the third and final stage is prolapse.

Opinions as to the efficacy of myelog-

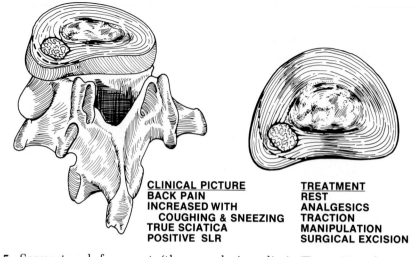

**CLINICAL PICTURE**
**BACK PAIN**
**INCREASED WITH**
    **COUGHING & SNEEZING**
**TRUE SCIATICA**
**POSITIVE SLR**

**TREATMENT**
**REST**
**ANALGESICS**
**TRACTION**
**MANIPULATION**
**SURGICAL EXCISION**

**Figure 3.5.** Sequestered fragment (the wandering disc) (Type V). The results of treatment with surgery are better in the Type V patient than in the Type I to Type IV patient, but they are probably not as good in the Type V patient as they are in the Type VI and Type VII patient. The wandering disc is a possible explanation for the clinical picture of exacerbations and remissions that are so frequently encountered. It may also be a partial explanation of why some patients show a good response to traction or manipulation. (Reproduced with permission of A. A. White and M. M. Panjabi: *Clinical Biomechanics of the Spine.* Philadelphia, J. B. Lippincott, 1978, p. 288 (6).)

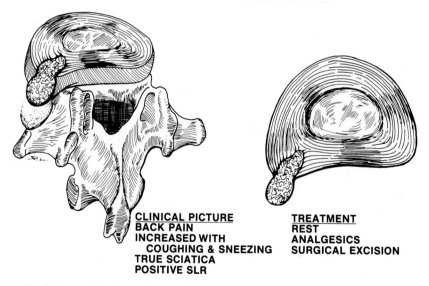

**CLINICAL PICTURE**
**BACK PAIN**
**INCREASED WITH**
    **COUGHING & SNEEZING**
**TRUE SCIATICA**
**POSITIVE SLR**

**TREATMENT**
**REST**
**ANALGESICS**
**SURGICAL EXCISION**

**Figure 3.6.** With Type VI, there is sequestration and displacement, but there is some anchoring of the ligament, so that it cannot move about. This is likely to be helped by traction or manipulation. (Reproduced with permission from A. A. White and M. M. Panjabi: *Clinical Biomechanics of the Spine.* Philadelphia, J. B. Lippincott, 1978, p. 289 (6).)

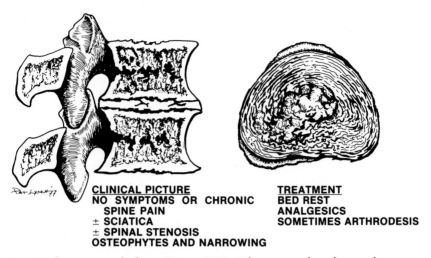

**CLINICAL PICTURE**
**NO SYMPTOMS OR CHRONIC**
   **SPINE PAIN**
**± SCIATICA**
**± SPINAL STENOSIS**
**OSTEOPHYTES AND NARROWING**

**TREATMENT**
**BED REST**
**ANALGESICS**
**SOMETIMES ARTHRODESIS**

**Figure 3.7.** A degenerated disc (Type VII) either may be the end process of the mechanical and biological effects of normal functioning or may be associated with considerable pain and disability. There may also be arthritis in the intervertebral joints. It is important to emphasize that these various stages are a continuum. A given disc may move or decelerate, stop or, in some instances, even reverse. (Reproduced with permission from A. A. White and M. M. Panjabi: *Clinical Biomechanics of the Spine.* Philadelphia, J. B. Lippincott, 1978, p. 290 (6).)

raphy, electromyography, and discography in the diagnosis of disc protrusions have varied. Semmes (17) states that because nearly one third of myelograms are not definitive or are misleading, the history and clinical findings have proved more reliable. He states that myelography is used too frequently for diagnosis and indication for surgery and that he has used it in less than 3% of his last 350 surgeries. In the Scandinavian countries, the use of oil-based media in myelography has been banned due to the risk of arachnoiditis (13).

Herlin states that myelography is not a sufficiently reliable method of investigation in the diagnosis of sciatica (18) and has utilized myelography in only 10% of his cases (19). A connection between lumbar disc degeneration and pelvic disease has been documented by Herlin who says that it has been suspected for years and that painful and chronic infectious conditions of the urogenital organs have been associated with compression of one or several of the lower sacral nerve roots. He further states that endometriosis sometimes is combined with sciatica and that

it seems justifiable to investigate the relationship between sacral nerve root compression and the development of endometriosis. He believes that in the man, lower sacral nerve root compression as a cause of chronic prostatovesiculitis ought to be considered (20). He has documented that in one patient, two miscarriages were due to sacral nerve root compression which caused most of the patient's sciatica later (21). In another patient, he believes that there is a probable connection between chronic urogenital infection due to disc compression of sacral nerve roots and rheumatoid arthritis (22). Herlin has also documented a connection between sacral nerve root compression and chronic prostatitis (23). He also believes that although there is no definite proof as yet, the possibility of sacral nerve root compression as a cause of sterility must be considered (23). He presents a case of pain originating bilaterally in the medial region of the gluteal muscles and radiating into the minor pudendal labiae and clitoris with a decrease to loss of the duration of intensity of orgasm. Following surgery for the removal of a medial 5th lumbar disc lesion, the patient's sexual function normalized within 2 months (24).

Emmett and Love (25) and Ross and Jackson (26) believe that disc disease should be ruled out in young and middle-aged patients who develop problems of urinary retention, vesicle irritability, or incontinence. Amelar and Dubin (27), however, link lumbar disc disorders with sexual impotence and bladder function disturbances through organic parasympathetic involvement rather than to psychological causes.

## Pudendal Plexus

Understanding the neurovisceral connection between the disc lesion and disease of the pelvic organs requires understanding of the pudendal plexus. The pudendal plexus is formed from the 2nd, 3rd, and 4th sacral nerves and is the innervation of certain pelvic organs (28). Parasympathetic fibers innervate the urinary bladder, prostate gland, and seminal vesicles. The uterus and external genitalia also are innervated by nerve fibers from this plexus, and the alimentary tract is controlled by the pudendal plexus as well. The pudendal nerve, a branch of the pudendal plexus, gives rise to the inferior hemorrhoidal nerve, the perineal nerve to the transversus perinei profundus, the sphincter urethrae membranacea, bulbocavernosus, ischiocavernosus, transversus perinei superficialis, the corpus cavernosum urethrae, the urethra, the mucous membrane of the urethra, the urogenital diaphragm, and a scrotal branch to the scrotum and labiae. Another branch of the pudendal nerve, the dorsal nerve of the penis, innervates the urogenital diaphragm, the corpus cavernosum penis, and dorsum of the penis ending in the glans. The clitoris is innervated similarly in the female.

Neuroanatomically, the pressure on the sacral nerve roots by disc lesion can create aberrant nerve supply to the organs described and resultant disease. On this neurological basis one can see the reason many authorities state that disc lesion should be considered in the etiology of any condition of the urogenital system or reproductive system.

## Occurrence and Onset of Back and Leg Pain

The onset of sciatica or back pain represents a starting point for diagnosis. It is possible for a disc to protrude and contact a nerve root, resulting in the sudden onset of sciatica without accompanying back pain. This protrusion may result in isolated pain in an area of specific nerve innervation such as the heel, calf, great toe, or posterior thigh. Back pain preceding sciatica indicates irritation of the annulus fibrosus, ligaments, and dura mater innervated by the recurrent meningeal nerve prior to contact with the involved nerve root. The sudden onset of leg pain without back pain indicates extrusion (prolapse) of the disc (29).

A differential diagnosis between protrusion and prolapse may include the findings shown in Table 3.1.

The cauda equina symptoms caused by large midline disc protrusions contacting several roots of the cauda equina present a particular problem in diagnosis. Difficulty with urination, incontinence, rectal difficulties, difficulty in walking, or symptoms of abdominal viscera are indicative of the diagnosis of a large midline disc protrusion. These represent true surgical emergencies and must be handled as such.

The delay in the onset of pain in disc injuries can be the key to diagnosis. The cartilage of the spine has a poor blood supply and reacts to injuries slowly.

**Table 3.1.**
**Clinical Differentiation Findings in Protrusion and Prolapse**

| Differential Diagnosis | Protrusion | Prolapse |
|---|---|---|
| Pain on compression and distraction | Yes, usually | Not as frequently |
| Flexion and extension | Yes | Only on flexion |
| Cough, sneeze, and strain | Yes | Not always |
| Onset of pain | Gradual | Sudden, intense |

Therefore, it may be 2 or 3 days after the oozing of the nuclear material and the slow swelling of the disc result in the pain that follows an injury and protrusion of a disc (30).

## Summary of Diagnosis of the Disc Lesion

1. Note the specific distribution of pain into the lower extremity and whether it involves the L4, L5, or S1 nerve root.

2. Note whether there is any lean of the lumbar spine.

3. Do x-rays reveal any right or left lateral flexion of the vertebrae at the level of disc involvement ascertained from dermatome evaluation? That is, if an L5 dermatome sensitivity is found, does the L4 vertebra have a right or left lateral flexion subluxation? If it is the S1 dermatome, does the L5 vertebra have a left or right lateral flexion?

4. Correlate the findings from above to differentiate protrusion from prolapse. Statistically, prolapses are much more difficult to treat than are protrusions.

5. Correlate the straight leg raising sign with a medial or lateral disc. That is, is it positive on the side of sciatica, indicating lateral disc or medial disc, or is it positive on the well leg raising sign, indicating a medial disc on the side of sciatica?

6. Investigate the site of original pain; i.e., whether it was back or leg, to rule out tumor, infection, or other organic disease as a probable etiology. Refer to Table 3.2 to aid in the differential diagnosis between a tumor and a disc lesion.

7. If a disc involvement truly seems probable, after the site has been determined to be either medial or lateral, explain to the patient that manipulative therapy may not be adequate and that surgical intervention may be necessary.

Rothman and Simeone (29) state that radiating cracks in the annulus fibrosus develop in the most centrally situated lamellae and extend outward to the periphery. These radiating clefts in the annulus weaken its resistance to nuclear herniation. Herniation is a greater threat to a younger individual between the ages of 30 and 50 having good nuclear turgor than it is to the elderly in whom the nucleus is

**Table 3.2.**
**Differential Diagnostic Findings of Discal versus Tumor Etiology**

| Differential Diagnosis | Neoplasm | Protrusion |
|---|---|---|
| Sitting and standing | No change | Aggravates |
| Bilateral | Often | Seldom |
| Night pain | Yes | Less |
| Character of pain | Unrelenting | Intermittent |
| Cauda equina symptoms | More | Less |
| Onset first leg or back pain | Back usually | Either |

fibrotic. Falconer (31) states that myelographic defects are seen unchanged after successful conservative treatment of sciatica and that this is due not to mechanical factors but to clinical nerve root symptoms created by the biochemical irritation of the nerve root degeneration and its resultant irritants on the nerve root. Rothman and Simeone (29) discuss variations of the spinal canal in detail. The trefoil canal, which Finneson (32) discussed also, is common at the L4- and L5 level. The trefoil canal has lateral recesses which render the canal narrower and thereby more vulnerable to compression by extruded disc material. We discuss the finding on x-ray of underdeveloped pedicles which would result in a decreased anteroposterior measurement of the vertebral canal and thus create a stenotic vertebral canal. This would result in more pronounced symptoms of disc protrusion. Imagine the combination of a trefoil canal with lateral recesses, underdeveloped pedicles, and articular facet degenerative arthrosis, all of which are narrowing the vertebral canal and, when coupled with disc protrusion, result in an exceptionally painful condition. It is well to remember that the lumbar nerve roots lie in the superior part of the intervertebral foramen in a relatively protected position and that it is only in disc narrowing that the superior articular facet of the vertebra below might subluxate in a position to create nerve root pressure. Rothman and Simeone (29) also state that a small nuclear herniation of only 1 to 2 mm in height can cause marked nerve root compression in a patient with a small lumbar spinal canal and particularly with a narrow lateral recess which makes the patient susceptible to degenerative changes of the intervertebral disc (29).

## EXAMINATION

### History

Table 3.3 shows the low back pain examination form which we use. A history of the patient usually is compiled by an assistant. The patient's chief complaint should be recorded as exactly as possible; e.g., pain in the low back radiating into the calf of the right leg or pain in the side of the leg with numbness of the great toe. The history of the complaint should include specific details as to how the pain began; i.e., whether the pain in the back started with or without leg pain or whether the leg pain started sometime after the pain in the back. *A chronological sequence of back or leg pain from its first incidence in life to the present should be recorded by month and year and should include the present symptoms.* Note that on this form the date of pain onset and the date of first examination are requested. These dates allow the doctor to notice the time lapse between the onset of symptoms and the consultation. If this lapse has been long, the patient may have sought other care, and a careful screening of past procedures and diagnosis is necessary.

The history of the patient should include any surgical interventions. Be particularly alert to any disease that could metastasize to the spine and mimic a disc lesion. Any symptoms of gastrointestinal, genitourinary, and menstrual problems should be listed. These allow for documentation of any pudendal plexus symptoms for evaluation following the mechanical relief of back pain. Thus, it is possible to evaluate the effects of chiropractic treatment not only on biomechanical faults but also on organic disease.

The family incidence of back pain also is recorded. This record should include whether the father, mother, or siblings have had low back pain, leg pain, or surgery, whether the back pain or leg pain started first or both began simultaneously, whether the pain is aggravated by coughing, sneezing, straining at the stool, bending and lifting, or sitting, and how far down the lower extremity the pain radiates.

### Physical Examination

As you proceed through the examination, mark the proper answer on the examination form and keep in mind the findings indicative of intervertebral disc protrusion and prolapse as shown in Table 3.4.

EXAMINATION WITH THE PATIENT SITTING

*Minor's Sign (Fig. 3.8).* Minor's sign is manifest when the patient, in rising from sitting, lifts his body weight with his arms and places his body weight on the unaffected leg. He may place his hand on his low back. The painful lower extremity is spared of weight bearing.

*Bechterew's Sign (Fig. 3.9).* The test for Bechterew's sign is performed by having the patient extend the knee while in a sitting position. This sitting straight leg raise again stretches the sciatica nerve root and creates either back or leg pain or both if there is a disc lesion.

Please note that, according to Finneson, the straight leg raising sign is a more positive sign of disc lesion in younger people; i.e., under age 40, than it is in older people. This is because as the intradiscal pressure decreases with age, the turgor of the nucleus becomes less and the nucleus is less likely to compress severely against the nerve root during such maneuvers as straight leg raising, Valsalva, or Bechterew's.

*Valsalva Maneuver and Lindner's Sign (Fig. 3.10).* For the Valsalva maneuver, the patient attempts to expel air against a closed glottis. This movement can be described to the patient as straining to move the bowel. During this maneuver, the intradiscal pressure increases and the increased force against the anterior dura lining of the nerve root accentuates the patient's back and/or leg pain.

**Table 3.3.**
**Low Back Examination Form**

### LOW BACK EXAMINATION FORM FOR CLINICAL EVALUATION
### AND STATISTICAL RESEARCH OF LOW BACK AND DISC DISORDERS

Name _____ Age _____ Sex _____ S.M.W.D.

Occupation  _____

Date of Pain Onset _____ Date of First Examination  _____

Chief Complaint:

History of Complaint:

**PHYSICAL EXAMINATION**

Surgical History:

Bowel Habits:

Urinary Habits:

Menstrual Periods:

Digestion:
Drugs:
Past Illnesses:
B/P:            Heart Rate:            Rhythm:            Sounds:            Lung:

Abdomen:                                                        Prostate:
Testicle Pain:                                                  Impotency:

**FAMILY HISTORY OF BACK PROBLEMS:**

| Sciatica | Low Back Pain | Surgery for Disc |
|---|---|---|
| ____ None | ____ None | ____ None |
| ____ Father | ____ Father | ____ Father |
| ____ Mother | ____ Mother | ____ Mother |
| ____ Brother | ____ Brother | ____ Brother |
| ____ Sister | ____ Sister | ____ Sister |
| ____ Other | ____ Other | ____ Other |
| ____ Unknown | ____ Unknown | ____ Unknown |

| Location of Pain | Pain Aggravated by | Extent of Pain |
|---|---|---|
| ____ Right Leg | | ____ Buttock |
| ____ Left Leg | | ____ Thigh |
| ____ Both Legs | ____ Coughing | ____ Knee |
| ____ Alternating | ____ Sneezing | ____ Calf |
| ____ Leg Pain Came | ____ Straining at stool | ____ Ankle |
| ____ Before Back Pain | ____ Bending & Lifting | ____ Foot |
| ____ Simultaneous with | ____ Sitting | ____ Toes |
| back pain | | ____ Unknown |
| ____ After Back Pain | | |

## Table 3.3—*Continued*

### Examination · Sitting

| Minor's Sign | Bechterew's Sign | Valsalva | Valsalva with Bechterew's |
|---|---|---|---|
| ___ Positive<br>___ Negative | ___ Positive<br>    ___ L.B.P.<br>    ___ L.P.<br>___ Negative | ___ Positive<br>    ___ L.B.P.<br>    ___ L.P.<br>___ Negative | ___ Positive<br>    ___ L.B.P.<br>    ___ L.P.<br>___ Negative |

### Examination · Standing

| Neri's Bow | Lewin's Standing |
|---|---|
| ___ Negative<br>___ Positive<br>    ___ Rt.<br>    ___ Lt | ___ Positive<br>    ___ L.B.P<br>    ___ S.I.<br>___ Negative |

### Examination · Standing Cont.

| Gait | Spine Tilt | Pain on Palpation | Percussion | Kemp's | Motion | Toe Walk | Heel Walk |
|---|---|---|---|---|---|---|---|
| ___ Normal<br>___ Rt Limp<br>___ Lt Limp<br>___ Other | ___ None<br>___ Right<br>___ Left<br>**Lordosis**<br>___ Normal<br>___ Loss<br>___ Increased | ___ Negative<br>**Paravertebral**<br>Rt.    Lt<br>___ L1 ___ L1<br>___ L2 ___ L2<br>___ L3 ___ L3<br>___ L4 ___ L4<br>___ L5 ___ L5<br>___ S1 ___ S1 | ___ Negative<br>___ L1<br>___ L2<br>___ L3<br>___ L4<br>___ L5<br>___ S1 | Right<br>___ Negative<br>___ Positive<br>Left<br>___ Negative<br>___ Positive | Pain Present<br>Flexion ____/90 ____<br>Extension ____/30 ____<br>Lateral Flexion<br>Rt ____/20 ____<br>Left ____/20 ____<br>Rotation<br>Rt ____/30 ____<br>Lt ____/30 ____ | ___ Positive<br>    ___ Rt<br>    ___ Lt<br>___ Negative | ___ Positive<br>    ___ Rt<br>    ___ Lt<br>___ Negative |

### Examination · Supine

| Lindner's | Straight Leg Raise | | | Patrick's | Gaenslen's |
|---|---|---|---|---|---|
| ___ Positive<br>    ___ L.B.P.<br>    ___ L.P.<br>___ Negative | Right<br>___ Negative   o<br>___ Positive at     ___ L.B.P.<br>    ___ L.P.<br>    ___ Both<br><br>Left<br>___ Negative   o<br>___ Positive at     ___ L.B.P.<br>    ___ L.P.<br>    ___ Both | **Braggard's**<br>___ Negative<br>___ Positive<br><br>**Braggard's**<br>___ Negative<br>___ Positive | **Well Leg Raising**<br>___ Positive<br>___ Negative<br><br>**Medial Hip Rotation**<br>___ L.B.P.<br>___ L.P.<br>___ Negative | Right<br>___ Negative<br>___ Positive<br><br>Left<br>___ Negative<br>___ Positive | Right<br>___ Negative<br>___ Positive<br><br>Left<br>___ Negative<br>___ Positive |

| Cox's Sign | Amoss' | MUSCLE STRENGTH | | | | | | | | | |
|---|---|---|---|---|---|---|---|---|---|---|---|
| | | | Dorsi-Flexion | | Plantar-Flexion | | Great Toe Flexion | | Great Toe Extension | | Foot Eversion |
| | | | Rt. | Lt. | Rt. | Lt. | Rt. | Lt. | Rt. | Lt. | Rt.   Lt. |
| ___ Positive<br>___ Negative | ___ Positive<br>___ Negative | Normal | | | | | | | | | |
| | | Weakness | | | | | | | | | |

| Thigh & Calf Circumference | Milgram's | Tendon Relexes | | | Sensory Examination | | | |
|---|---|---|---|---|---|---|---|---|
| | | | | | Hyperesthesia | | Hypoesthesia | |
| Rt Thigh _____<br>Lt Thigh _____<br>Rt Calf _____<br>Lt Calf _____ | Positive<br>    ___ Rt<br>    ___ Lt<br>Negative | 0 Active & Equal<br>1 Increased<br>2 Decreased<br>3 Absent<br>4 Unknown | Ankle<br>Rt.    Lt. | Knee<br>Rt.    Lt. | Rt        Lt<br>___ None ___ None<br>Dermatome<br>___ L3 ___ L3<br>___ L4 ___ L4<br>___ L5 ___ L5<br>___ S1 ___ S1<br>___ S2 ___ S2<br>___ Other ___ Other | | Rt.        Lt.<br>___ None ___ None<br>Dermatome<br>___ L3 ___ L3<br>___ L4 ___ L4<br>___ L5 ___ L5<br>___ S1 ___ S1<br>___ S2 ___ S2<br>___ Other ___ Other | |

| Circulation | Normal | Diminished | Moses' |
|---|---|---|---|
| Femoral Artery | | | Positive |
| Popliteal Artery | | | Rt. |
| Post. Tibial Artery | | | Lt. |
| Dorsalis Pedis Artery | | | Negative |

## Table 3.3—*Continued*

### Prone Examination

| Nachlas' | Yeoman's | Ely's | Prone Lumbar Flexion | Popliteal Fossa Pain |
|---|---|---|---|---|
| ___ Positive<br>___ Rt<br>___ Lt<br>___ Negative | ___ Positive<br>___ Rt<br>___ Lt<br>___ Negative | ___ Positive<br>___ Rt<br>___ Lt<br>___ Negative | ___ No Change<br>___ Change | ___ Positive<br>___ Rt.<br>___ Lt.<br>___ Negative |

### NONORGANIC PHYSICAL SIGNS

| Libman's | Tenderness to Skin Pinch | Mannkopf's | Burns' Bench | Flip Test | Plantar Flexion | Flexed Hip Test |
|---|---|---|---|---|---|---|
| ___ Positive<br>___ Negative | ___ Specific<br>___ Nonanatomic | ___ Positive<br>___ Negative | ___ Positive<br>___ Negative | ___ Positive<br>___ Negative | ___ Positive<br>___ Negative | ___ Positive<br>___ Negative |

| Axial Loading | Rotation of Shoulders & Pelvis |
|---|---|
| ___ L.B.P.<br>___ Negative | ___ L.B.P.<br>___ Negative |

### X-RAYS STANDING OR RECUMBENT

| | | | SPINAL MECHANICS | | |
|---|---|---|---|---|---|
| Spinal Tilt | Scoliosis | Sacral Angle | Facet Asymmetry | Facet Syndrome | Van Ankerveeken Stability |
| ___ No<br>___ Rt<br>___ Lt<br>___ L1<br>___ L2<br>___ L3<br>___ L4<br>___ L5 | ___ No<br>___ Rt<br>___ Lt<br>___ L1<br>___ L2<br>___ L3<br>___ L4<br>___ L5<br>___ Mild<br>___ Moderate<br>___ Severe | Lumbar Lordosis Angle | S Sagittal<br>C Coronal<br>Lt    Rt<br>L1-L2<br>L2-L3<br>L3-L4<br>L4-L5<br>L5-S1 | ___ Present<br>___ L5-S1<br>___ L4-L5<br>___ Not Present | ___ Stable<br>___ Unstable |

### CONGENITAL ABNORMALITIES

| Spina Bifida | Spondylolysis | Spondylolisthesis | Transitional Vertebra | Stenosis | | Intercrestal Line Cuts | L5 Transverse Processes |
|---|---|---|---|---|---|---|---|
| ___ None<br>___ L1<br>___ L2<br>___ L3<br>___ L4<br>___ L5<br>___ S1<br>___ S2<br>___ S3 | ___ None<br>___ L1<br>___ L2<br>___ L3<br>___ L4<br>___ L5<br>___ S1 | ___ No<br>___ L1<br>___ L3<br>___ L4<br>___ L5<br><br>Per Cent | Sacralization<br>___ Right<br>___ Left<br>Lumbarization<br>___ Right<br>___ Left<br>___ True<br>___ False | Sagittal Diameter Spinal Canal<br>L1-L2<br>L2-L3<br>L3-L4<br>L4-L5<br>L5-S1 | Sagittal Diameter Vertebral Body<br>L1-L2<br>L2-L3<br>L3-L4<br>L4-L5<br>L5-S1 | ___ L4 Body<br>___ L5 Body | ___ Less<br>___ Greater Than L3 |

| Other |
|---|
| |

### ACQUIRED ABNORMALITIES

| Schmorl's Nodes | Narrowed Disc Space | Spondylosis | Articular Facet Arthrosis | Retrolisthesis | Other |
|---|---|---|---|---|---|
| ___ No<br>___ L1<br>___ L2<br>___ L3<br>___ L4<br>___ L5 | ___ No<br>___ L1-L2<br>___ L2-L3<br>___ L3-L4<br>___ L4-L5<br>___ L5-S1 | ___ None or Slight BODY<br>L1-L2<br>L2-L3<br>L3-L4<br>L4-L5<br>L5-S1 | ___ None or Slight<br>Rt        Lt<br>___ L1-L2   ___ L1-L2<br>___ L2-L3   ___ L2-L3<br>___ L3-L4   ___ L3-L4<br>___ L4-L5   ___ L4-L5<br>___ L5-S1   ___ L5-S1 | ___ None<br>___ L1<br>___ L2<br>___ L3<br>___ L4<br>___ L5 | |

**Table 3.3—*Continued***

**CORRELATIVE DIAGNOSIS OF LOW BACK PAIN**

**Disc**

| L3 | | ___ Medial | ___ Annular Tear (Cat. I) | ___ Lumbar Spine Stenosis (Cat. VIII) |
|----|----|----|----|----|
| L4 | Rt. | ___ Lateral | ___ Nuclear Bulge (Cat. II) | ___ Iatrogenic Back Pain (Cat. IX) |
| L5 | Lt. | ___ Subrhizal | ___ Nuclear Protrusion (Cat. III) | ___ Functional Low Back Pain (Cat. X) |
| | | | ___ Nuclear Prolapse (Cat. IV) | ___ Lumbar Spine Sprain and Strain |
| | | | ___ Discogenic Spondyloarthrosis (Cat. V) | (Cat. XI) |
| | | | ___ Facet Syndrome (Cat. VI) | ___ Subluxation (Cat. XII) |
| | | | ___ Spondylolisthesis (Cat. VII) | ___ Tropism (Cat. XIII) |
| | | | | ___ Transitional Segment (Cat. XIV) |
| | | | | ___ Other Pathologies (Cat. XV) |

**OTHER**

---

**Table 3.4.**
**Criteria for Diagnosis of Sciatica due to a Herniated Intervertebral Disc (55)**

1. Leg pain is the dominant symptom when compared with back pain. It affects one leg only and follows a typical sciatic (or femoral) nerve distribution.
2. Paresthesiae are localized to a dermatomal distribution.
3. Straight leg raising is reduced by 50% of normal, and/or pain crosses over to the symptomatic leg when the unaffected leg is elevated, and/or pain radiates proximally or distally with digital pressure on the tibial nerve in the popliteal fossa.
4. Two of 4 neurologic signs (wasting, motor weakness, diminished sensory appreciation, and diminution of reflex activity) are present.
5. A contrast study is positive and corresponds to the clinical level.

Note also that the patient is asked to flex the head upon the chest, which increases the traction of the nerve root against the disc bulge (Lindner's sign).

Rainey (33) has stated that with a contained disc; i.e., the posterior annulus is not ruptured, flexion or maintenance of the flexed position obliterates the disc bulge and, assuming that motion of an irritated nerve root over a bulging disc is often the source of the patient's back and leg pain, thus could be the explanation for relief of pain with flexion treatment. We have also demonstrated that both the

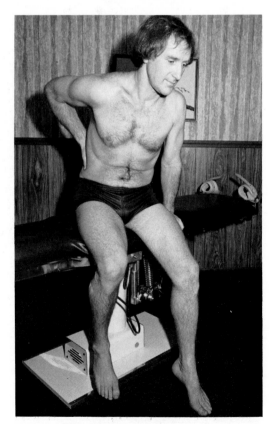

**Figure 3.8.** Minor's sign.

Valsalva maneuver and abdominal compression obliterate the myelographic defect. Again if it is assumed that motion of an irritated nerve root over a disc bulge is one of the causes of pain, the findings

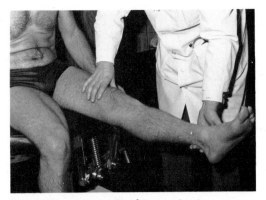

**Figure 3.9.** Bechterew's sign.

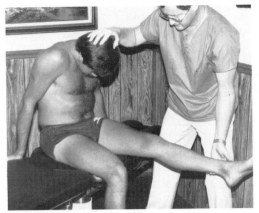

**Figure 3.11.** Bechterew's test, Lindner's sign, and the Valsalva maneuver.

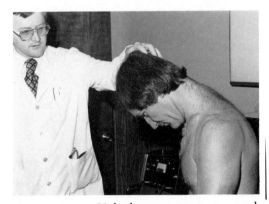

**Figure 3.10.** Valsalva maneuver and Lindner's sign.

here could explain how abdominal compression or Valsalva maneuver done abruptly increases the patient's pain as the defect appears and disappears and thereby moves the nerve root over the disc.

***Bechterew's Test, Lindner's Sign, and Valsalva Maneuver (Fig. 3.11).*** If Bechterew's test is added to the Valsalva maneuver, further stretching the nerve roots behind the intervertebral disc space, this increased stretching accentuates the patient's pain in nuclear escape. The combination of the Valsalva maneuver, Bechterew's test, and Lindner's sign indicates the presence of a disc lesion. One test alone might not be positive.

## EXAMINATION WITH THE PATIENT STANDING

***Néri's Bowing Sign (Fig. 3.12).*** With Néri's sign, as the patient bows forward,

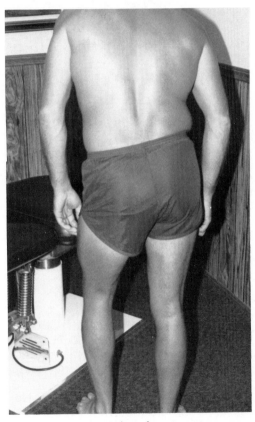

**Figure 3.12.** Néri's bowing sign.

the affected leg flexes, as in a curtsey, as the sciatic nerve is irritated.

***Lewin's Standing Sign (Fig. 3.13).*** Lewin's standing sign is manifested with the patient's knees placed in extension. Increased pain in the low back or leg can

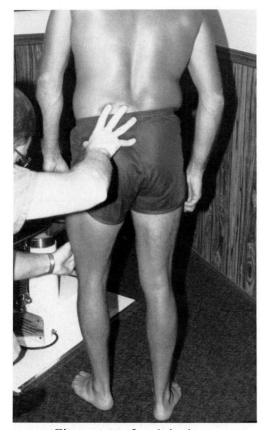

**Figure 3.13.** Lewin's sign.

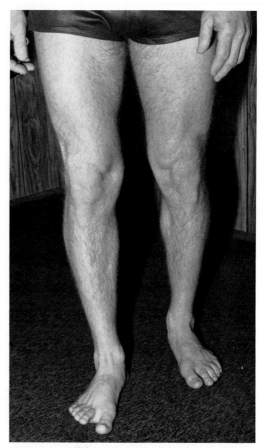

**Figure 3.14.** Gait.

cause the knee to snap back into flexion. If this is observed, a disc, gluteal, or sacroiliac disturbance is indicated.

*Gait (Fig. 3.14).* Note whether the patient limps while walking and the extremity affected.

*Patient Lean (Fig. 3.15).* Note whether the patient leans to the right or the left. Later, correlation of this antalgia with the side of pain will aid in determining whether the nuclear bulge is medial, lateral, or subrhizal. - *under root*

*Lumbar Lordosis (Fig. 3.16).* Note whether the patient while standing reveals increased, decreased, or normal lumbar lordosis. The typical disc patient will have a loss of lumbar lordosis because this posture opens the dorsal intervertebral disc space, thus relieving the pressure of nuclear bulge on the involved nerve root and/or cauda equina.

*Pain on Palpation (Fig. 3.17).* Note the levels of pain that the patient experiences upon deep digital pressure. Sometimes, not only the back pain but also a radiating sciatic discomfort can be elicited.

*Percussion (Fig. 3.18).* Tapping over the involved paraspinal and spinous process levels creates pain if there are inflammatory changes around the involved nerve roots.

*Kemp's Sign (Fig. 3.19).* The test for Kemp's sign can be performed with the patient in either the standing or the sitting position. Sitting increases intradiscal pressure and, therefore, maximizes stress to the disc, whereas standing increases weight bearing and maximizes stress to the facets. The test for Kemp's sign should be performed in both positions. Kemp's sign can be positive for facet irritation or compression of a bulging nucleus against a nerve root. If both are present, low back

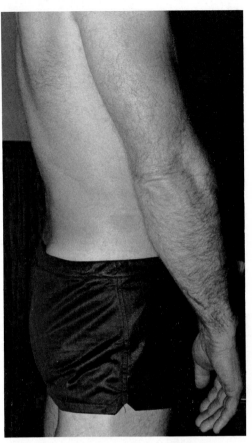

**Figure 3.16.** Lumbar lordosis.

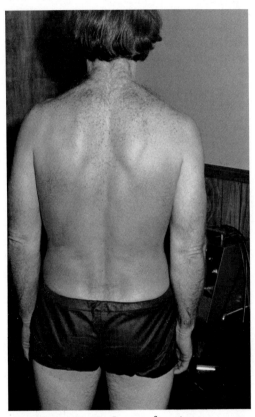

**Figure 3.15.** Lean of patient.

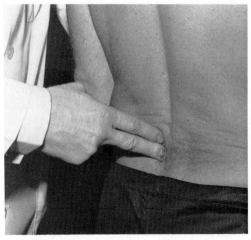

**Figure 3.17.** Pain on palpation.

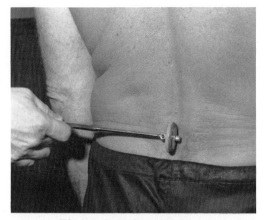

**Figure 3.18.** Percussion.

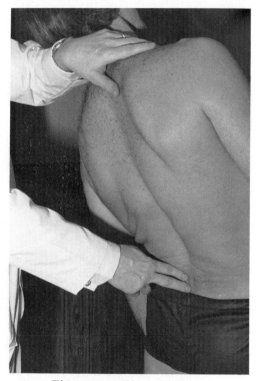

**Figure 3.19.** Kemp's sign.

less of the direction in which the patient is posteriorly and laterally flexed. It is to be expected that in medial disc protrusion, the patient will experience greater pain when flexed away from the side of pain or disc lesion whereas in lateral disc protrusion, the patient will experience greater pain when flexed into the side of low back and lower extremity pain.

***Goniometric Measurements (Figs. 3.20 to 3.23).*** Goniometric measurements should be taken with the patient in flexion, extension, lateral bending, and rotation of the lumbar spine. These measurements provide a record of the ranges of motion for comparison with future measurements and for verification of patient response or failure to treatment.

***Toe Walk (Fig. 3.24).*** The inability to walk on the toes indicates an L5-S1 disc problem due to weakness of the calf muscles supplied by the tibial nerve.

***Heel Walk (Fig. 3.25).*** The inability to walk on the heels indicates an L4-L5 disc problem due to weakness of the anterior leg muscles supplied by the common peroneal nerve.

pain is elicited. With a disc bulge, accentuation of the lower extremity radiculopathy is increased. Some patients with disc lesion experience only back pain with Kemp's sign. With a medial disc, Kemp's sign is usually positive when the patient is flexed either to the right or to the left in extension. Pain occurs because a medial disc can irritate a nerve root regard-

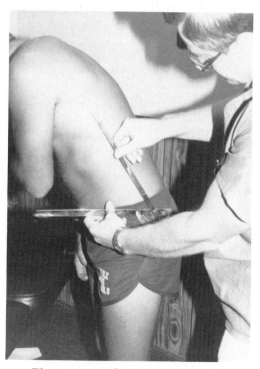

**Figure 3.20.** Flexion measured.

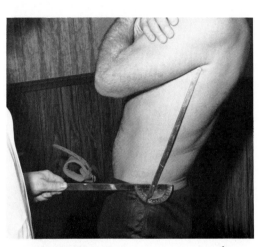

**Figure 3.21.** Extension measured.

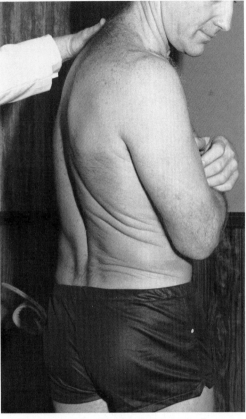

**Figure 3.23.** Rotation measured.

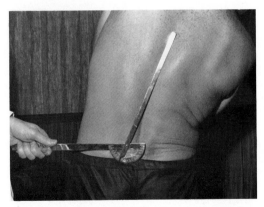

**Figure 3.22.** Lateral flexion measured.

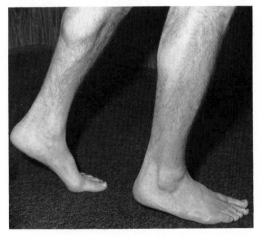

**Figure 3.24.** Toe walk.

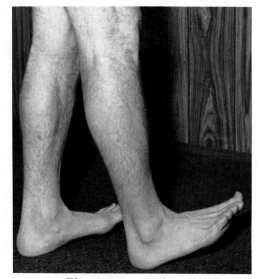

**Figure 3.25.** Heel walk.

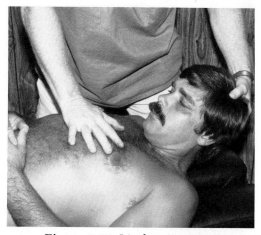

**Figure 3.26.** Lindner's sign.

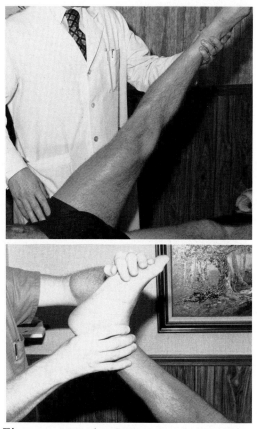

**Figures 3.27 (top) and 3.28 (bottom).** Straight leg raising sign, medial hip rotation, and Braggard's sign.

## EXAMINATION WITH THE PATIENT IN THE SUPINE POSITION

Some of these tests may be done with the patient in the prone position, depending on which position is more comfortable for the doctor and/or patient.

***Lindner's Sign (Fig. 3.26).*** The test for Lindner's sign (also known as the Brudzinski or Soto-Hall sign) is often performed in conjunction with the straight leg raising test or the Valsalva maneuver for maximum effect. Lindner's sign refers to stretching of the dural linings of the nerve roots behind the bulging disc material, which causes pain when performed.

***Straight Leg Raising Sign (Figs. 3.27 and 3.28).*** Lasègue (34) described the painful effect in patients with sciatica of stretching the sciatic nerve by extending the knee with the hip flexed and also the relief from pain when the knee was then flexed. This is the classic leg raising sign. Variations of this sign along with interpretations of its meaning lend much more knowledge to the examining physician than merely noting that at a certain degree of leg raise the patient experiences either back or leg pain or both back and leg pain. On the examination form, record whether the leg raising sign is positive and, if so, at what degree of elevation.

Breig and Troup (35) add a degree of sophistication to this test. After noting the level of pain on straight leg raising, lower the extremity a few degrees to relieve the pain and then dorsiflex the ankle while medially rotating the hip. Medial hip rotation places greater stretch upon the lumbar and sacral nerve roots and accentuates the straight leg raising sign. These authors state that if the pain which limits straight leg raising is elicited by such dorsiflexion and medial hip rotation, increased root tension is indicated and the site of pain may help in locating the level of the disc causing the pain. Figure 3.27 shows medial hip rotation and Figure 3.28 shows dorsiflexion of the foot (Braggard's sign).

By stretching the lumbosacral nerve roots, the straight leg raising sign proves that the 1st sacral nerve root allows the greatest movement.

In theory, the straight leg raise (SLR) should identify not only the presence of increased root tension but also, possibly, the site of such irritation. The production of pain on passive dorsiflexion of the ankle near the limit of the pain-free range of straight leg raising confirms that the root is mechanically compromised. Pain on pressure in the popliteal fossa after flexion of the knee at the limit of straight leg raising has a similar significance, and when the well leg raising test is positive, this pain is a strong confirmation of root involvement.

The angulatory stress exerted on the lumbar nerve roots during straight leg raising was measured on cadavers within 4 hours of death (36). A short length of rubber tube was inserted between the disc and nerve root and the tension was monitored by use of semiconductor pressure transducers. Results of this testing were:

1. With the straight leg raising sign, the pressure between the nerve root and the disc does not change until the leg is raised to about 30°, with a progressive rise occurring as the angle of the leg increases.

The pressure increase is highest at the L5-S1 disc level and half as high at the L4-L5 level. The pressure increase on SLR at L3-L4 was $\frac{1}{10}$ of that at L5-S1.

It can be concluded that:

a.) SLR that is positive under 30° reveals a large disc protrusion. The nerve root is stretched here long before it normally would be.

b.) SLR is most useful for identifying L5-S1 disc lesions, since the pressures are highest at this level. On SLR, L4-L5 is not as apt to give as much pain as is L5-S1, since the pressure between the disc and the nerve root is half that at L5-S1. Therefore, the L5-S1 disc lesion gives more pain in the low back and leg than does the L4-L5 disc lesion.

c.) No movement on the nerve root occurs until SLR reaches 30°.

d.) No movement of the L4 nerve root occurs during SLR (37).

2. Adduction of the hip on SLR increases the pressure on the nerve root.

3. O'Connell (38) reported that the 2nd, 3rd, and 4th lumbar nerve roots did not show an increase in tension during SLR but did show an increase during the femoral stretch test.

***Straight Leg Raising and Lindner's Signs (Fig. 3.29).*** Whenever the straight leg raising test produces a questionable result for pain, combine it with flexion of the cervical spine (Lindner's sign). This combination places the greatest pull and stretch on the nerve roots behind the intervertebral disc and often elicits pain. Along with this combination, dorsiflex the foot, have the patient cough, or perform the Valsalva maneuver. These maneuvers further accentuate intradiscal pressure and elicit pain that otherwise might be missed.

Interpretation of the Well Leg Raising Sign

***Well Leg Raising (Fajersztajn) Sign (Figs. 3.30 and 3.31).*** The well leg raising

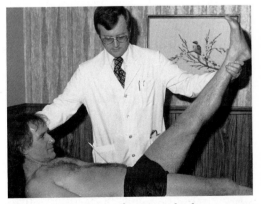

**Figure 3.29.** Tests for straight leg raising and Lindner's signs, performed together.

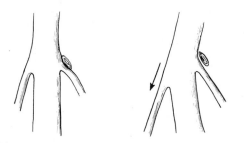

**Figure 3.30.** Interpretation of the well leg raising sign in lateral disc bulge.

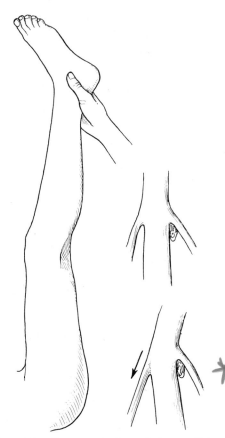

**Figure 3.31.** Interpretation of the well leg raising sign in medial disc bulge.

sign (Fajersztajn sign) is exacerbation of pain down the involved or painful lower extremity when the opposite or noninvolved extremity is placed in straight leg raise. Hudgins (39) states that increased sciatica on raising the opposite or well leg, the crossed straight leg raising sign, is associated with a herniated lumbar disc in 97% of patients. Myelography is unnec-

essary for the diagnosis of disc hernia in patients with this sign. Although it is possible for patients with this sign to have a normal myelogram, nevertheless, 90% prove to have a herniated disc.

When the disc protrusion is displaced lateral to the nerve root (Fig. 3.30), raising the uninvolved leg actually pulls the nerve root away from the disc and can relieve back or leg pain.

When the disc protrusion is displaced medial to the nerve root (Fig. 3.31), raising the uninvolved leg pulls the nerve root into the disc bulge and causes radiculopathy down the involved leg.

Interpretation of the Straight Leg Raising Sign

In a study of 50 patients in a 2-year period, Edgar and Park (40) found that the pattern of pain on straight leg raising was closely related to the central or lateral position of the disc protrusion. In addition to its use in the diagnosis and assessment of progress, the straight leg raising sign may be helpful in localizing the protrusion by analysis of the distribution of the pain so induced. Clinically, myelographic and operative observations were carried out prospectively on 50 such patients to investigate the relation between the the the pattern of pain in straight leg raising and the site of the protrusion. In 80% of the patients the following correlation was found:

| Location of Protrusion | Back Pain | Leg Pain |
|---|---|---|
| Lateral protrusion | | + |
| Medial protrusion | + | |
| Intermediate protrusion (Subrhizal) | + | + |

Therefore, a lateral protrusion causes a patient to experience leg pain; a medial protrusion, back pain; and a subrhizal protrusion, both back and leg pain.

The straight leg raising sign can provide a wealth of information: the level of pain can indicate the disc at fault, the presence of back pain, leg pain, or both can indicate the type of protrusion, and various combinations of Valsalva, cervical flexion, dorsiflexion of the foot, and medial hip rotation can aid significantly in diagnosis.

***Patrick's Sign (Fig. 3.32).*** Patrick's sign refers to pain in the groin and hip area, which is common with disc lesion because of the irritation of nerve supply to these structures. Evaluation of the hip by x-ray will rule out any hip disease.

***Gaenslen's Sign (Fig. 3.33).*** The test for Gaenslen's sign is performed by flexion of one knee upon the chest while the other is placed in extension over the side of the table. This is a differential sign between sacroiliac and lumbar spine pain. When the test is performed, the pain will appear at the location of the lesion, whether it be in the sacroiliac or lumbar spine.

***Cox's Sign (Fig. 3.34).*** Cox's sign occurs when, during SLR, the pelvis rises from the table rather than the hip flexing. The author has noticed this occurrence in 2 patients with prolapse into the intervertebral foramen—a grave condition.

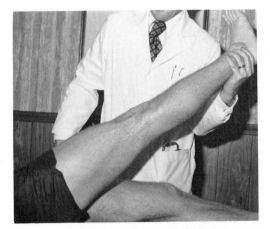

**Figure 3.34.** Cox's sign.

***Amoss' Sign (Fig. 3.35).*** Amoss' sign is manifested by difficulty rising from the supine position. The patient must use his arms to lift himself and prevent flexion or motion of the lumbar spine.

***Dorsiflexion of the Foot (Ankle Extension) (Fig. 3.36).*** The sciatic nerve is made up of tibial and common peroneal nerves. The common peroneal nerve divides into the superficial and the deep peroneal branch. Dorsiflexion as shown in Figure 3.36 depends upon nerve supply via the deep branch of the peroneal nerve to the anterior tibialis muscle, the extensor hallucis longus muscle to the great toe, and the extensor digitorum longus muscle to the toes. The superficial peroneal nerve supplies the peroneal muscles that allow the foot to flex laterally at the ankle as well as flex upward (dorsiflexion). Weakness of dorsiflexion of the foot at the ankle is indicative of 5th lumbar nerve root compression by an L4-L5 disc level lesion.

The inability of the patient to walk on his heels is also indicative of the same finding, but testing the patient's strengths as shown in Figure 3.36 is a much more intricate evaluation. The patient may be able to walk on his heels, yet demonstrate weakness of the muscle on dorsiflexion.

***Dorsiflexion of the Great Toe (Fig. 3.37).*** Dorsiflexion strength of the great toe is determined by testing the strength of the extensor hallucis longus muscle. Weakness of dorsiflexion of the great toe is indicative of L5 nerve root irritation by an L4-L5 disc lesion.

***Plantar Flexion or Ankle Flexion of***

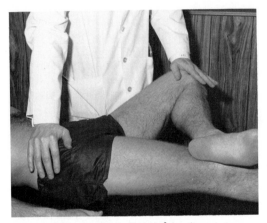

**Figure 3.32.** Patrick's sign.

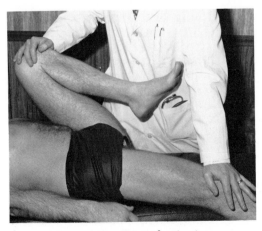

**Figure 3.33.** Gaenslen's sign.

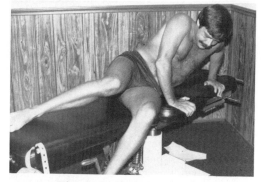

**Figure 3.35.** Amoss' sign.

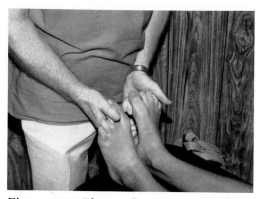

**Figure 3.38.** Plantar flexion of the ankle.

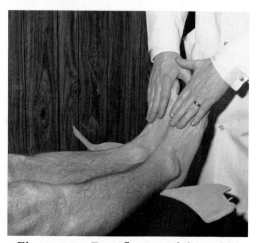

**Figure 3.36.** Dorsiflexion of the ankle.

A variation of this test is to ask the patient to walk on his toes. The inability to do so indicates the same finding as that of the plantar flexion sign. As in testing in dorsiflexion, testing the strength of one foot against the other is a much more reliable sign, since a patient may be able to walk on his toes and still have a weakness of calf muscles on one side.

The peroneal muscles are the evertors of the ankle and foot and receive supply from the 1st sacral nerve root. Test them by asking the patient to walk on the medial borders of his feet; or have him sit on the edge of the table, secure the ankle by stabilizing the calcaneus while placing your other hand in a position that forces him to plantar flex and evert his foot to reach it with his small toe. Oppose his plantar flexion and eversion by pushing against the head and shaft of the 5th metatarsal bone with the palm of your hand.

***Plantar Flexion of the Great Toe (Fig. 3.39).*** The flexor hallucis longus tendon is tested for strength in plantar flexion of the great toe. Weakness here is indicative of a 1st sacral nerve root compression by an L5-S1 disc lesion.

***Thigh Measurements (Fig. 3.40).*** Both thighs are measured at the same distance above the superior patellar pole. Differing sizes indicate atrophy.

***Calf Measurement (Fig. 3.41).*** Both calves are measured at the same distance below the inferior patellar pole. Differing sizes indicate atrophy.

***Milgram's Sign (Fig. 3.42).*** The inability to hold the feet 6 inches off the floor while in the supine position indicates ex-

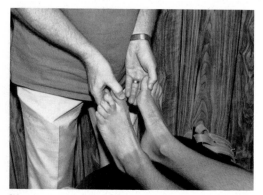

**Figure 3.37.** Dorsiflexion of the great toe.

***the Foot (Fig. 3.38).*** The tibial branch of the sciatic nerve supplies the posterior tibialis, gastrocsoleus, flexor digitorum longus, and hallucis longus muscles. Weakness of plantar flexion of the foot is indicative of compression of the 1st sacral nerve root by an L5-S1 disc lesion.

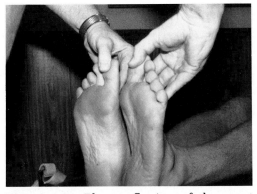

**Figure 3.39.** Plantar flexion of the great toe.

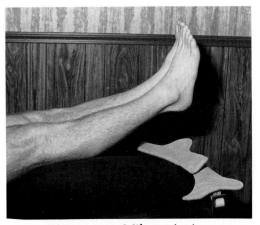

**Figure 3.42.** Milgram's sign.

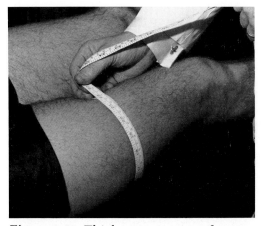

**Figure 3.40.** Thigh measurement for atrophy.

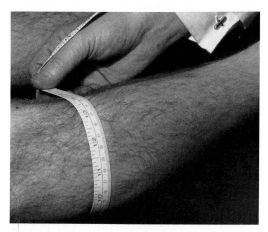

**Figure 3.41.** Calf measurement for atrophy.

treme nerve root irritation and is believed to be a sign of arachnoiditis due to Pantopaque dye as well as disc lesion.

*Ankle Jerk Reflex (Fig. 3.43).* The deep reflex of the ankle known as the Achilles reflex is diminished or absent in the presence of an L5-S1 disc irritation of the 1st sacral nerve root and, therefore, is of extreme importance for evaluating lower disc involvement. Note that the patient's foot is held in dorsiflexion while the ankle jerk reflex is elicited. Thus, not only the reflex but also the strength of the muscular contraction of the calf muscles is observed. This test can be performed with the patient prone or supine.

*Patellar Reflex (Knee Jerk) (Fig. 3.44).* The patellar reflex sign indicates involvement of the L3 disc, which would effect the 4th lumbar dermatomes. Since discs other than the L4 or L5 discs are seldom involved, this is relatively useless in evaluating disc lesions in the lower extremity.

*Pinwheel Examination (Figs. 3.45 to 3.48).* Pinwheel examination of the lower extremities is shown in Figures 3.45 to 3.48. The weight of the pinwheel is the only downward force applied so as to equalize the pressure of each leg. The same dermatome of each leg is stimulated, and the patient is asked which feels less sharp. Figure 3.45 shows testing of the 5th lumbar dermatome above the knee. Figure 3.46 shows testing of the L5 dermatome below the knee. Figure 3.47 shows testing of the dermatomes at the 1st sacral level of the thigh. Figure 3.48 shows testing of the dermatomes at the 1st sacral

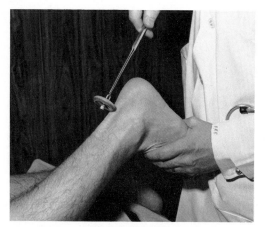

**Figure 3.43.** Ankle jerk reflex.

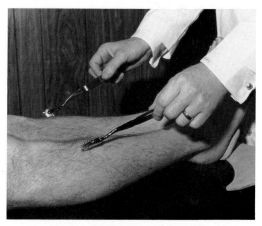

**Figure 3.46.** L5 dermatome.

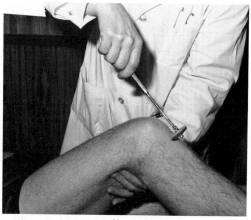

**Figure 3.44.** Patellar reflex (knee jerk).

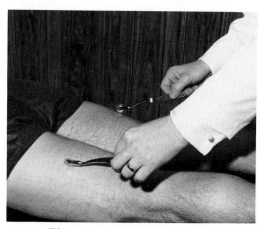

**Figure 3.47.** S1 dermatome.

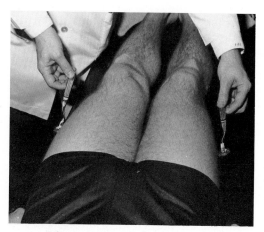

**Figure 3.45.** L5 dermatome.

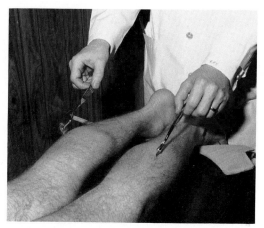

**Figure 3.48.** S1 dermatome.

level below the knee. The 1st sacral dermatome is tested with the patient prone.

Measurement of Lower Limb Circulation

*Femoral Artery (Fig. 3.49).* Draw a line between the anterior superior iliac spine (ASIS) and the symphysis pubes and midway between this point drop down 1 inch and that will be the femoral artery. Palpate the pulse and compare right to left for strength of pulse.

*Popliteal Artery (Fig. 3.50).* By Doppler or palpation determine the patency of the popliteal artery.

*Posterior Tibialis Artery (Fig. 3.51).* By Doppler or palpation compare the two pulses of the posterior tibialis arteries.

*Dorsalis Pedis Artery (Fig. 3.52).* By

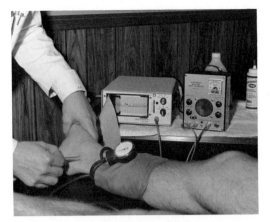

**Figure 3.51.** Posterior tibialis artery.

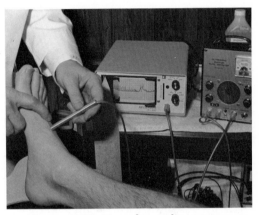

**Figure 3.52.** Dorsalis pedis artery.

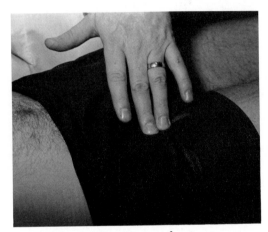

**Figure 3.49.** Femoral artery.

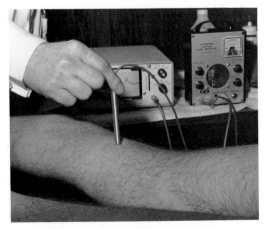

**Figure 3.50.** Popliteal artery.

Doppler or palpation compare the pulse of the dorsalis pedis artery and its strength in the two extremities. This artery is located between the 1st and 2nd metatarsal bones on the dorsum of the foot.

These pulses are important in differentiating intermittent claudication of ischemic etiology from that of neurogenic etiology. When these pulses are present and the patient has the cramp-like pains of claudication, the origin of pain is not vascular but neural. Look for discal lesion, ligamentous hypertrophy, stenosis, or peripheral neuropathy.

*Moses' Sign (Fig. 3.53).* The test for Moses' sign is performed by grasping the calf of the patient's leg, which creates pain if phlebitis or vascular occlusion is present.

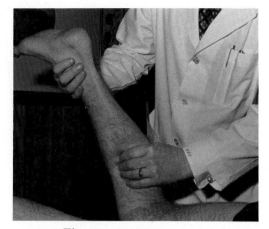

**Figure 3.53.** Moses' sign.

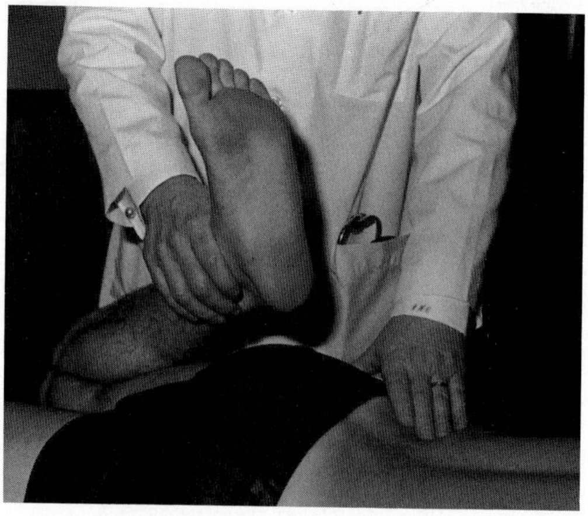

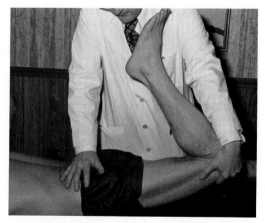

**Figure 3.54.** Nachlas' sign.

## EXAMINATION WITH THE PATIENT IN THE PRONE POSITION

***Nachlas' Knee Flexion Sign (Fig. 3.54).***
On passive flexion of the knee, the patient
lying in the prone position will experience pain in the low back or lower extremity. This sign is positive for sacroiliac,
lumbosacral, and disc lesions.

***Yeoman's Sign (Fig. 3.55).*** The test for
Yeoman's sign is performed by applying
pressure over the suspected sacroiliac
joint to fix the pelvis to the table. The
patient's leg, flexed at the knee, is hyper-
extended by lifting the thigh from the
table. Increased pain in the sacroiliac is
indicative of a lesion at that level.

***Ely's Heel-to-Buttock Sign (Fig. 3.56).***
The test for Ely's sign is performed by
bringing the patient's heel to the opposite
buttock by flexing the knee. Ely's sign
identifies any irritation of the psoas muscle or a lumbosacral lesion.

***Prone Knee Flexion Test (Fig. 3.57).***
Prone knee flexion provides provocative
testing for lumbar disc protrusion (41).
The pathophysiology of this test depends
upon compression of spinal nerves during
hyperextension of the lumbar spine,
which intensifies intervertebral disc protrusion into the spinal canal. Also, the
lumbar intervertebral foramina are narrowed and the spinal canal cross-sectional
area is decreased by lumbar extension.
Compression of a spinal nerve by lumbar
disc protrusion may be intensified; therefore, a protruded disc that has not pro-

**Figure 3.55.** Yeoman's sign.

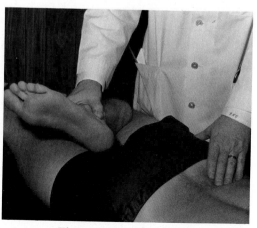

**Figure 3.56.** Ely's sign.

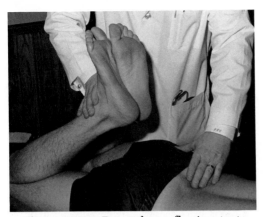

**Figure 3.57.** Prone knee flexion test.

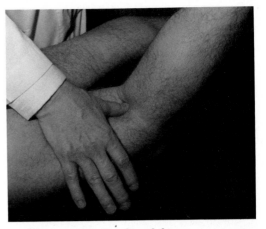

**Figure 3.58.** Popliteal fossa pressure.

duced sufficient neurocompression to cause weakness or reflex changes on testing with the spine normally aligned may be provoked by this test to produce changes which the examiner may elicit by testing in the prone knee flexion position.

The patient lies prone and the knees are hyperflexed, producing lumbar extension. The patient remains in the posture for approximately 45 to 60 seconds, and then the deep reflexes and muscle strength of the lower extremity are again evaluated. Weaknesses not observed prior to this manuever may well be evident following it.

***Popliteal Fossa Pressure (Fig. 3.58).*** In sciatica, the tibial branch of the sciatic nerve will be very tender in the popliteal space on deep pressure; this is known as the bowstring sign and, according to Macnab (42), is probably the single most important sign in the diagnosis of a ruptured intervertebral disc. The test for this sign can be performed with the patient in either the prone position, as shown in Figure 3.58, or the supine position. With the patient in the supine position, the straight leg raise is performed until the patient experiences some discomfort. At this level, the knee is allowed to flex and the examiner allows the patient's foot to rest on his shoulder. The test demands sudden firm pressure applied to the popliteal nerve. This action may startle the patient enough to make him jump. Reproduction of pain in the leg or in the back

is irrefutable evidence of nerve root compression.

## NONORGANIC PHYSICAL SIGNS (MALINGERING)

*A patient with three or more of the following signs should be suspected of malingering.* For more information on psychological screening of patients, see the article by Waddell et al (43).

***Libman's Sign (Fig. 3.59).*** Deep palpation of the mastoid processes indicates the patient's pain threshold. Compare the patient's pain response to palpation of the mastoid processes to his pain response to examination of the low back. The two of these pain sensitivities should be the same.

***Tenderness to Skin Pinch (Fig. 3.60).*** With a pen lay out specific spinal segments on the patient's back. Then pinch the skin segment by segment, which should elicit pain in the pathway of the appropriate segment. If the patient complains of a generalized pain over many segments of the spinal nerve, he is probably exaggerating his symptoms.

***Mannkopf's Sign (Fig. 3.61).*** Take the patient's pulse prior to deep palpation of a painful area. Such deep palpation should increase the pulse approximately 10 bpm if it is a true marked pain. If palpation does not accentuate the pulse, the patient may be exaggerating his symptoms.

***Burns' Bench Sign (Fig. 3.62).*** Have the

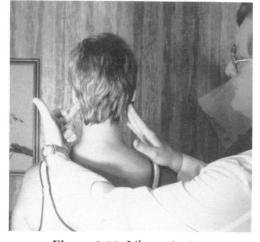

**Figure 3.59.** Libman's sign.

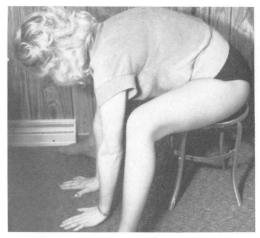

**Figure 3.62.** Burns' bench sign.

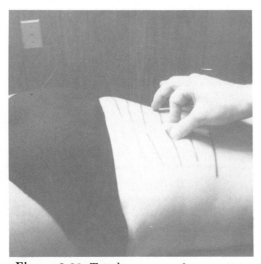

**Figure 3.60.** Tenderness to skin pinch.

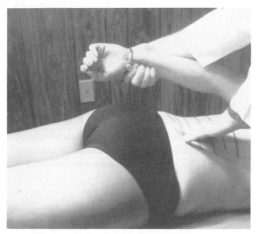

**Figure 3.61.** Mannkopf's sign.

patient sit on a low stool and bend forward and touch the floor with the palms of his hands. If he says he cannot do this because of low back pain, suspect malingering, since flexion in this particular posture will not effect the low back specifically. Primary motion occurs at the hip joints and not the lumbosacral spine.

*Flip Test (Fig. 3.63).* Have the patient sit on the examination table with his back straight and his legs extended. If he truly suffers from a disc lesion compressing the sciatic nerve, he cannot perform this test and will have to flex the knee or raise the hip from the table in order to relieve the sciatic stretch. If he can perform this test, he probably has no true sciatica or disc lesion and is malingering.

*Plantar Flexion Test (Fig. 3.64).* Ask the patient to raise his legs one at a time until he feels low back or leg pain. Note the angle at which the pain is elicited and ask the patient to lower the leg. Then place one hand under the patient's knee and one under the patient's foot and raise the lower extremity, keeping the knee slightly flexed. Raise the leg to one half of the height at which pain was originally elicited and plantar flex the foot. If the patient says that this causes pain, suspect malingering.

*Flexed Hip Test (Fig. 3.65).* Place one hand under the patient's lumbar spine and the other under the patient's knee. Lift the knee, and if the patient says he feels pain in his low back before the lumbar spine moves, suspect malingering.

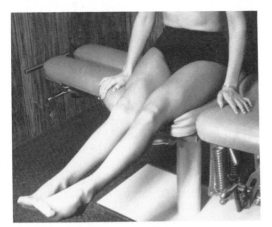

**Figure 3.63.** Flip test.

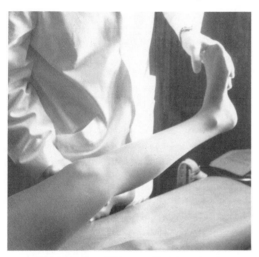

**Figure 3.64.** Plantar flexion test.

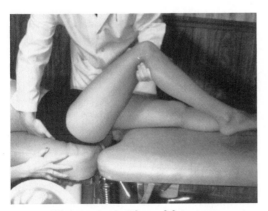

**Figure 3.65.** Flexed hip test.

*Axial Loading Test (Fig. 3.66).* Press the patient's cranium in a downward position. The axial loading may elicit pain in the neck but should not elicit pain in the low back. Suspect malingering if the patient says he feels pain in the low back.

*Rotation Test of the Shoulders and Pelvis (Fig. 3.67).* Have the patient turn his shoulders to rotate his entire spine. If he complains of low back pain, suspect malingering, since he is not truly moving his lumbar spine but rather is moving his spine from the thighs upward.

## Correlative Diagnosis of Low Back Pain

With the history and physical examination of the patient completed, including the x-ray examination, we can now correlate our findings. The Cox Clinical Classification of Low Back Pain Progression is therefore, presented as an aid to understanding the clinical findings, as a means of standardizing terminology about low

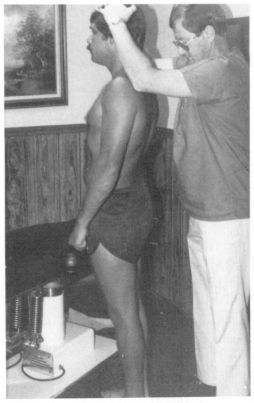

**Figure 3.66.** Axial loading test.

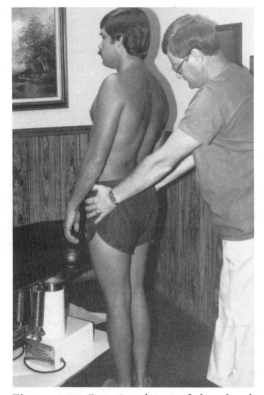

**Figure 3.67.** Rotational test of the shoulders and pelvis.

back pain, and as a tool to be used in its diagnosis and treatment.

## COX CLINICAL CLASSIFICATION OF LOW BACK PAIN PROGRESSION

The Cox system classifies back pain into 15 categories. Low back pain, in both its etiology and progression, is well suited to placement in one of or a combination of these categories. Description of each of these categories follows.

### Category I—Annulus Fibrosus Injury

The patient with annulus fibrosus injury presents with the typical low back pain syndrome; i.e., the patient is young and usually on the first visit complains of low back pain following some flexion, twisting, or combined movement. No leg pain is usually noted, and relief is usually obtained within a few days. This type of pain may recur with progressive worsening of symptoms.

Clinically, the patient may present with muscle spasm, a loss of lordosis, and a positive Kemp's sign, but with no findings on the straight leg raising test and no altered motor or sensory changes of the lower extremity. Any leg pain is transient and not subjectively severe.

X-ray may reveal no change of discal space nor signs of discogenic spondylosis.

This patient responds well to distraction manipulation and is usually satisfied with the clinical results.

The patient in Category I has undergone tearing, cracking, or severe sprain of the annular fibers, causing irritation of the sinuvertebral nerve and resultant back pain. This patient is similar to the Type I or Type II patient of Charnley, White and Panjabi's classification (6, 7).

### Category II—Nuclear Bulge

The patient with nuclear bulge presents with a worsening of low back pain and minimal leg pain.

Clinically, the patient may have paresthesias of the lower extremities but has no frank altered deep reflexes. There is minimal irritation of the root of the nerve into the lower extremity, and a more positive straight leg raising sign, Kemp's sign, and other orthopedic tests for early disc protrusion are demonstrated. Déjérine's triad may increase the pain.

X-rays may show some early thinning of the disc space and discogenic spondylotic change, which may be minimal.

With prolonged exacerbation of low back and leg symptoms, the patient in Category II requires a longer treatment period than does the patient in Category I. At this stage, it is important that the patient wear a lumbosacral support in order to stabilize the low back for healing. Sitting must be strictly avoided in order to reduce the intradiscal pressure and allow the annulus to heal. The use of the Cox exercises to open the dorsal intervertebral disc space are most helpful at this time, and nutrition with Discat may be incorporated into the treatment regimen.

The patient in Category II shows progression of the tears and cracks of the annulus found in the Category I patient, with the nucleus pulposus bulging into these annular fibers and causing further irritation of the sinuvertebral nerve and early and minimal irritation of the nerve roots that exit from the cauda equina within the vertebral canal.

The articular facets also become pain-producing entities because of disruption of the articular cartilage and fibrous capsule and because of the subluxation resulting from the loss of normal mobility of the motion segment. With increased intradiscal pressure or annular disruption, this patient is analogous to the Type II or Type III patient of Charnley's classification (7).

### Category III—Nuclear Protrusion

The patient with frank nuclear protrusion has severe antalgia, marked lower extremity pain, and altered deep motor and sensory abnormalities.

Clinically, the patient demonstrates difficulty in straightening from a flexed position and marked loss of lumbar lordosis.

X-rays show antalgia and possible discal change.

Depending upon medial or lateral relationship of the disc bulge to the nerve root, the range of motion in the low back is markedly limited and Kemp's sign is definitely positive.

The patient in Category III requires prolonged treatment, and ambulation will be limited because of pain on weight bearing. It is mandatory that the patient wear a lumbosacral support and remain recumbent. At the outset of treatment, two or three visits/day may be necessary for maximum relief from pain. This patient is similar to the Type IV patient of Charnley's (7).

### Category IV—Nuclear Prolapse

The patient with nuclear prolapse has primarily lower extremity pain with minimal or absent low back pain. Nuclear material has completely torn through the annulus and lies within the canal as a free fragment severely irritating the nerve root and perhaps the cauda equina. The patient may have bowel and bladder problems. The decision to use surgery is based on the clinical differential diagnosis. If the patient does not show a 50% improvement within 3 weeks, surgery becomes imminent. This patient is analogous to the Type V or Type VI patient of Charnley's (7).

### Category V—Discogenic Spondyloarthrosis

The patient with discogenic spondyloarthrosis (chronic advanced degenerative disc diseases) has a history of intermittent low back pain; i.e., the patient is relatively free of pain except for acute exacerbations. The straight leg raising test is negative except for low back pain. Repeated motion of the spine, especially rotatory movements, causes low back pain. The patient must exercise care when bending and lifting and is analogous to the Type VII patient of Charnley's (7).

### Category VI—Facet Syndrome

The patient with facet syndrome presents with hyperextension of the lumbar spine, which usually produces pain. X-rays may well reveal a degenerative change of the facets, which follows degenerative disc disease. Macnab's line is positive, and the work of Van Akkerveeken is important here to determine the stability of the facet syndrome.

### Category VII—Spondylolisthesis

X-ray is diagnostic in the patient with spondylolisthesis.

### Category VIII—Lumbar Spine Stenosis

The patient with lumbar spine stenosis may present with symptoms of neurogenic intermittent claudication. For a full explanation of lumbar spine stenosis, see Chapter 7.

### Category IX—Iatrogenic Back Pain

The patient with iatrogenic back pain, due to either myelograms or surgery, suffers from irritation to the neural contents of the vertebral canal, which is perhaps severe enough to cause cauda equina symptoms. These patients are the most challenging to treat due to the difficulty in pinpointing the diagnosis and the consequent difficulty in arranging proper treatment. Many of these patients are failed back surgery syndrome (FBSS) patients whose biomechanics are so altered as to make relief from pain difficult, if not impossible, to attain.

## Category X—Functional Low Back Pain

The patient with functional low back pain often has personality aberrations and does not understand or will not understand the cause and treament of low back pain. Sometimes emotional upset manifests itself through low back pain symptoms. This type of patient represents a challenge to both the surgeon and the nonsurgeon in management.

## Category XI—Sprain and Strain

The patient with sprain or strain presents with an innocuous injury of nonrecurring frequency that seems to involve muscle and ligament damage rather than discal or facetal damage. No nerve damage can be found. The pain may be present for several weeks following an athletic injury or automobile accident, but it is not chronic unless facet or disc damage has occurred.

Treatment consists of maintaining normal range of facet motion, restriction of motion in the early stages of injury, and rehabilitative exercises later.

## Category XII—Subluxation

When a patient with subluxation presents with back pain, note the level and type of subluxation, e.g., a right lateral flexion subluxation of L5 on S1.

## Category XIII—Tropism

In the patient with tropism, the level of asymmetry of the facet facings is marked. For a full explanation, see Chapter 11.

## Category XIV—Transitional Segment

When a patient with transitional segment presents with back pain, decide whether there are 23 or 25 spinal segments, so as to determine whether the patient has lumbarization or sacralization.

## Category XV—Pathologies

Category XV is a catchall for patients with any other pathology.

Following this examination procedure, a correlative diagnosis can be made as to the level of disc involvement and its position, i.e., medial or lateral, in relation to the compressed nerve root. Also, other causes of back pain and the disc lesion can be noted from the examination and x-rays. Such things as facet syndrome, discogenic spondylosis and spondyloarthrosis, congenital defects as well as acquired pathologies can be identified at this time.

## SPECIAL DIAGNOSTIC CONSIDERATIONS

1. Finneson (44) states that transitional lumbosacral vertebra, namely, 6th lumbar segments, normally react as a protrusion at the L5-S1 disc level but that this is not an infallible rule and root localization may be uncertain.

2. Nashold and Hrubec (45) state (and we completely concur) that transitional vertebra is not increasingly found in association with disc compression.

3. Spondylolisthesis in conjunction with disc protrusion is an exception to the rule, since we have learned of one patient whose 4th lumbar disc after surgical removal showed bilateral pars interarticularis defects. No fusion was performed on this patient, and subsequent hypermobility of L4 resulted. The patient actually had worse pain following the surgery than before. Fusion seems necessary when disc removal is performed on patients with spondylolisthesis.

4. Hanrats (46) states that the occurrence of herniated nucleus pulposus in male members of the same family seems to point to a possible hereditary or congenital association, but he has not found a tendency for disc protrusions to occur in the presence of congenital vertebral anomalies.

5. White and Panjabi (6) state that a narrowed disc space without spondylosis is a sign of instability. Clinical instability is defined as the loss of ability of the spine, under physiological loads, to maintain normal relationships between vertebrae so that there is no damage and no subsequent limitation to the spinal cord or nerve roots and no development of incapacitating deformity or pain due to structural change.

6. When a disc lesion is present, a differential diagnosis between protrusion

and prolapse is necessary. Remember that sudden onset of leg pain and absence of low back pain indicates prolapse [Category IV] whereas low back pain followed later by leg pain indicates protrusion [Category III].

7. Relief of aggravation of pain on lateral flexion may indicate whether the disc protrusion is lateral or medial to the nerve root (47) (Fig. 3.68).

## RE-EVALUATION OF PATIENT RESPONSE TO CARE

The reliability of tests for re-evaluation of patient response to care is not good. Straight leg raising and range of motion tests are the most reliable, as the following facts substantiate.

The epineurium of the spinal nerve root is supplied with direct fibers from the spinal ganglion cells, whereas the epineurium in the anterior spinal roots is sup-

plied by the sinuvertebral nerve. Numerous free nerve endings associated with pain sensation are found in the spinal nerve roots.

The venous plexus of the vertebral column is enmeshed by an adventitial plexus of unmyelinated nerve fibers and is a vast source of pain sensation.

In SLR, tension and movement develop first in the sciatic notch, then in the ala of the sacrum as the nerve passes over the pedicle, and finally at the intervertebral foramen itself. Movement of the nerve root through the intervertebral foramen has been given by Falconer (31) as 2 to 6 mm, by Charnley (31a) as 4 to 8 mm, and by Inman and Saunders (48) as to 2 to 5 mm.

It is important to remember that compressing or stretching a normal nerve is not painful. The SLR pain is a reflex or sensory input mechanism to protect us from injury. The reason for SLR pain is

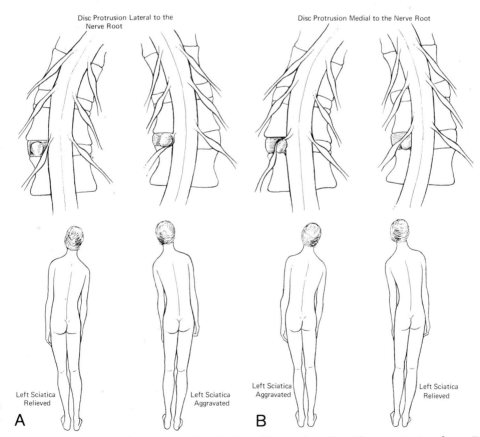

**Figure 3.68.** Sciatic scoliosis in a disc lesion. (Reproduced with permission from B. E. Finneson: *Low Back Pain*, edition 2. Philadelphia, J. B. Lippincott, 1980, p. 302.)

explained as sensitivity of the dorsal roots due to mechanical pressure. Perl (49) believes, however, that SLR pain is caused by a chemical noxious irritation by substances liberated by mechanical pressure.

Charnley (31a) found SLR to be the best clinical or radiological sign for diagnosing disc protrusion. Hakelius and Hindmarsh (50) state that they found an inverse proportion to the degree of limitation of SLR and the percentage of positive disc herniation at surgery. Sprangfort (51) states that in young people the sign has no specific value for diagnosing disc herniation and that a negative SLR excludes a disc herniation. After age 30, however, positive SLR is seen less often but its diagnostic value increases, and a negative SLR no longer excludes the diagnosis of disc herniation (51).

Objective assessment of spinal motion and straight leg raising and a global objective index show a high degree of intraobserver reproducibility. Million et al. (52) conclude that the emphasis in assessing the progress of the back pain patient must be on the subjective parameters, and the technique for this assessment developed.

Nineteen low back pain patients and 8 patients not suffering from low back pain were given several tests of flexibility and asymmetry by two different examiners. Three criteria of reliability and validity were used: (a) significant agreement between independent observers, (b) significantly different scores in the groups with and without low back pain, and (c) significant improvement following a successful spinal manipulation.

Tests of anterior flexion and asymmetry of foot eversion met only the first and second criteria, whereas tests of hamstring tightness and asymmetry of voluntary straight leg raising met only the first and third criteria. Passive and voluntary straight leg raising met only the first three criteria. Therefore, of the objective tests investigated here, only passive or voluntary straight leg raising can be strongly recommended for use in the evaluation of spinal manipulative therapy for low back pain (53).

*We utilize four tests in determining patient response to manipulative care—Kemp's, Déjérine's triad, range of motion, and the straight leg raise. Only the latter two have proven clinically reliable.*

## Motor Changes in Discal Lesions

Special mention of motor changes in these radicular compressions is needed, since they represent perhaps the most serious side effects of disc protrusion. Disc lesions can cripple and motor changes are the most serious side effects for the patient and the most serious potential medicolegal problems for the physician, whether the approach be conservative or surgical.

Occasionally, muscle weakness due to neurapraxia or degeneration may be present with little or no pain. Of course, muscle weakness usually follows sensory changes of the lower extremity. Nevertheless, regardless of the pain in a patient complaining of low back pain, leg pain, or an inability to walk on the toes or heels the clinician must always do kinesiological muscle testing.

Depending on the muscle involved, patients may complain of falling, having equilibrium problems (which really means they tend to limp due to weak muscles), or having the knee "give out" under them. Gait changes, such as limping due to calf muscle weakness and inability to lift the heel, or "stubbing" the great toe on carpet or steps due to weak anterior tibialis muscles or peroneal muscles, may be present. Patients may walk with the knee flexed so as to prevent "stretching" of the swollen or inflamed sciatic nerve. This would be a "walking" Néri bowing sign.

## Specific Diagnostic Criteria of Disc Lesions

---

L3-L4 DISC PROTRUSION (L4 NERVE ROOT COMPRESSION) FINDINGS

Weakness of the quadriceps muscle (Fig. 3.69). Diminished or absent patellar reflex (Fig. 3.70).

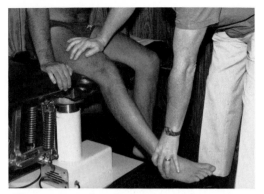

**Figure 3.69.** Quadriceps muscle testing.

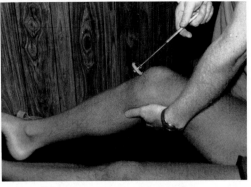

**Figure 3.70.** Patellar reflex.

The test for the straight leg raising sign may be negative in lesions of the L3-L4 disc. Pinwheel examination may reveal hyperesthesia or hypoesthesia of the L4 dermatome.

## L4-L5 DISC PROTRUSION (L5 NERVE ROOT COMPRESSION) FINDINGS

Weakness of tibialis anterior muscle, extensor digitorum and hallucis longus muscles (Fig. 3.71).

Weakness of the extensor hallucis muscle (Fig. 3.72).

Weakness of the peroneus longus and brevis muscles. Weakness in these muscles also occurs when an L5-S1 disc protrusion compresses the S1 nerve root (Fig. 3.73).

Dysesthesia of the L5 dermatome is determined by simultaneous testing of the sensation of the extremities (Fig. 3.74).

Foot and great toe dorsiflexion (ankle eversion) _inversion_ strengths depend upon the nerve supply of the peroneal nerve to the anterior tibialis and extensor muscles. The SLR will be positive in proportion to nerve compression by the disc.

## L5-S1 DISC PROTRUSION (S1 NERVE ROOT COMPRESSION) FINDINGS

Several muscles are tested for L5-S1 compression of the first and second sacral nerve roots.

Weakness of the biceps femoris, semimembranosus, or semitendinosus muscles (Fig. 3.75).

Weakness of the gluteus maximus is found by comparison of contralateral sides. The opposite pelvis should be stabilized while the thigh on the side to be tested is compressed (Fig. 3.76). The gluteus maximus muscle is innervated by the inferior gluteal nerve whose origin is in the roots of L5-S1-S2.

The gluteal skyline sign was present in 60% of patients with disc lesions of the lower lumbar spine. This sign is second only to the straight leg raising sign in frequency and was the only finding except for pain in 13% of the patients with disc protrusion (54). The patient is asked to contract his buttocks. Flaccidity is found on the side of the disc protusion (Fig. 3.77).

Diminished or absent ankle jerks

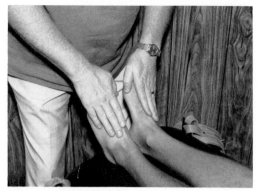

**Figure 3.71.** Dorsiflexion (ankle eversion) of the foot.

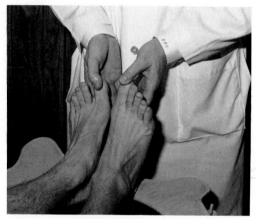

**Figure 3.72.** Dorsiflexion of the great toe.

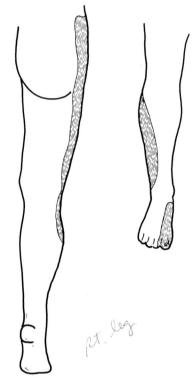

**Figure 3.74.** Dysesthesia and pain distribution of the L5 dermatome.

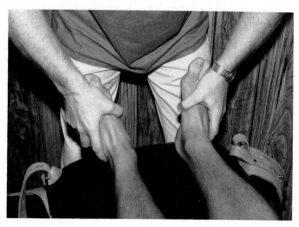

**Figure 3.73.** Eversion of foot.

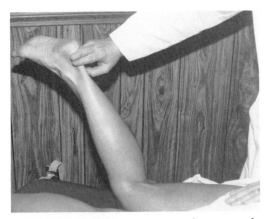

**Figure 3.75.** Hamstring muscle strength testing.

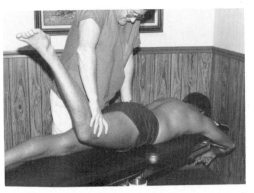

**Figure 3.76.** Gluteus maximus muscle testing.

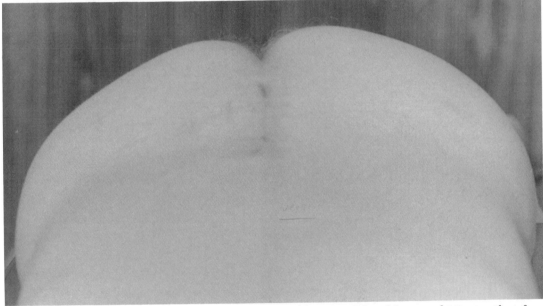

**Figure 3.77.** Gluteal skyline sign in a 36-year-old man with a history of 3½ months of right low back and first sacral nerve root sciatica. The ankle jerk reflex is absent, and there is marked loss of the tone of the gluteus maximus muscle, as noted by the flattened contour of the right gluteus maximus muscle. The CT scan and myelogram were positive for a prolapse of the L5-S1 disc on the right. Surgery was necessary to remove the fragment.

(Achilles reflexes) may be noted (Fig. 3.78).

Weakness of the calf muscles (Fig. 3.79).

Weakness of the flexor muscle of the great toe (Fig. 3.80).

Dysesthesia of the S1 dermatome by comparing the sensation of each extremity simultaneously (Fig. 3.81).

The SLR will be positive, the severity depending upon the pressure of the disc bulge or protrusion on the compressed nerve root.

It must be stated that these tests are strong indicators for disc level involvement, but there is some overlap of innervation to those muscles suppled by all three nerve roots— L4, L5, and S1.

## CASE STUDIES OF ORGANIC CAUSES OF LOW BACK AND LEG PAIN

### Ankylosing Spondylitis

**Case 1** is of a 32-year-old white married man who had low back and left hip pain and pain on movement of the cervical spine.

The pain first occurred in 1972 for no apparent reason. In 1976, he visited a chiropractor who told him he had a type of "galvanized poisoning." In 1979, he visited a neurosurgeon and underwent myelography. The results of

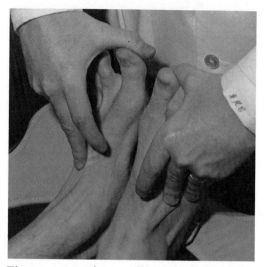

**Figure 3.80.** Plantar flexion of the great toe.

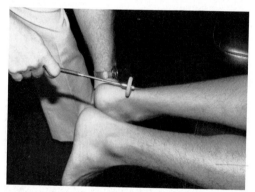

**Figure 3.78.** Ankle jerk.

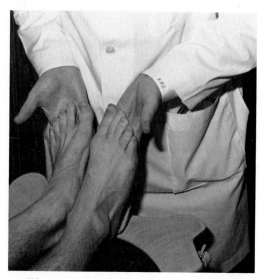

**Figure 3.79.** Plantar flexion of foot.

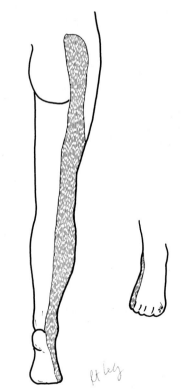

**Figure 3.81.** Dysesthesia and pain distribution of S1 dermatome.

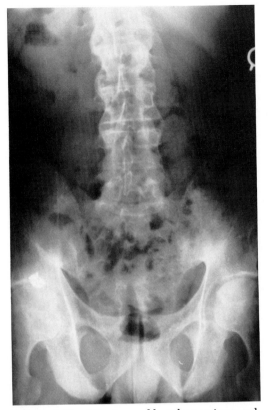

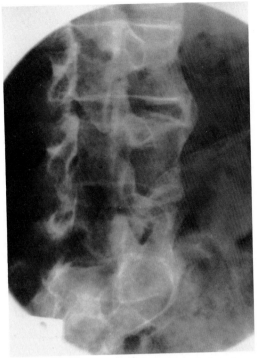

**Figure 3.83.** Oblique view of lumbar spine.

**Figure 3.82.** AP view of lumbar spine and pelvis.

the myelogram were negative. An exploratory surgery was performed following the negative myelogram; according to hospital records, the patient had lumbosacral strain and acute disc protrusion, but no relief from pain was achieved by surgery. In 1982, the pain in his back was exacerbated when he pushed a car. He was referred to us in June 1982.

Recent chiropractic care has been painful, not yielding relief.

This patient has a flattened lumbar curve and hyperkyphosis of the thoracic spine. Range of motion is 30° on flexion, 0° on extension, 10° on lateral flexion, and 10° on rotation. Motor and sensory examination are negative. Doppler examination of lower extremities is adequate.

X-rays reveal:

1. The sacroiliac joint spaces are obliterated (Fig. 3.82), and the patient has Grade III[4] ankylosis.

---

[4] Three stages of sacroiliac changes appear in ankylosing spondylitis (56):

*Stage 1 (sacroiliac stage).* The iliac border margins show increased density. There is narrowing of the joint space.

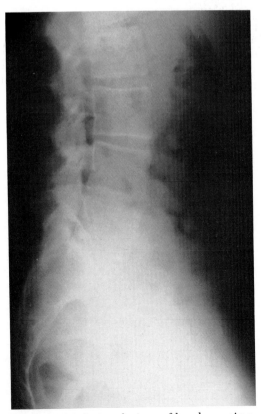

**Figure 3.84.** Lateral view of lumbar spine.

2. There is squaring of the vertebral bodies and loss of anterior concavity of the bodies (Fig. 3.84).

3. There is also a loss of bone density.

4. No calcification can be seen around the anterior longitudinal ligament or discs.

5. Oblique (Fig. 3.83) and anteroposterior (AP) (Fig. 3.82) views show ankylosis of the syndesmophytes.

6. The oblique view (Fig. 3.83) reveals articular facet loss of subchondral cortex and loss of joint space.

7. The paraspinal ligaments show ossification.

The findings suggested ankylosing spondylitis, and an HLA-B27 blood test was ordered and was positive.

The patient was referred back to his family chiropractor. If the diagnosis had been made earlier, this patient might have been saved years of frustration and surgery may have been averted. Ankylosing spondylitis is a disease that must be considered in the diagnosis of any man 20 to 40 years old with unexplained low back pain, especially if the pain and stiffness are worse at rest than at exercise.

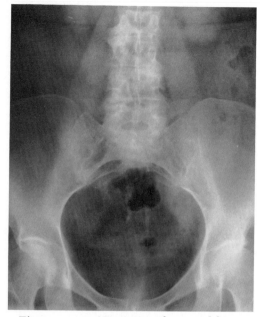

**Figure 3.85.** AP views of normal hip.

## Spondyloarthrosis

**Case 2** is of a 69-year-old white woman who had had low back and right hip pain for 2 years. The pain has been intermittent but recently has begun to bother her at night.

On examination, Patrick's sign is positive on the right, and the adductor muscles are weak and are painful at their origin.

X-ray (Fig. 3.85) reveals a worsening spondyloarthrosis at L2-L3, L3-L4, and L4-L5, with the hip joints interpreted as being normal. A follow-up x-ray (Fig. 3.86) done a year later shows that the right hip joint has degenerated.

Perhaps there was some joint space thinning indicated on the original x-ray (Fig. 3.85), but certainly 1 year later it is shown more positively on Figure 3.86. The clinician must be constantly watchful for new pathology with persistent pain.

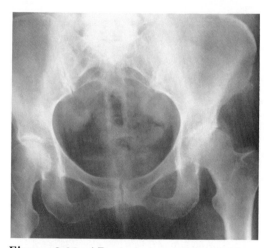

**Figure 3.86.** AP view 1 year later. Note degeneration of the right hip.

## Metastatic Carcinoma

**Case 3** is of a 47-year-old woman who had had thoracolumbar spine pain for 3 months. A mastectomy for breast cancer had been performed a year earlier.

X-rays reveal:

1. Destructive osteolytic metastases of the left L2 vertebral body and pedicle (Figs. 3.87

---

*Stage 2.* The sacroiliac joint space widens and is irregular due to cartilage destruction.

*Stage 3.* The sacroiliac joint is fused solid and bridged by bone.

and 3.88). The oblique view (Fig. 3.89) further demonstrates the lesion. Note that there is no periosteal reaction with some loss of vertebral body height.

2. Osteolytic change of the C6 spinous process and the right C6-C7 transverse processes and first rib (Figs. 3.91 and 3.93).

3. Effects of radiation therapy 3 months after application (Fig. 3.90, 3.92, 3.94, and 3.95).

This patient has carcinoma that has metastasized to bone from breast yet she complained only of lower back pain. Thus, the need for careful examination is evident. Breast carcinoma is the most probable cause of osteolytic

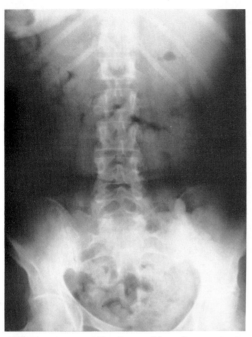

**Figure 3.87.** AP view of lumbar spine.

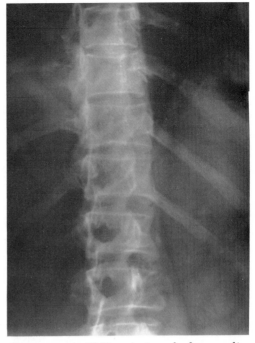

**Figure 3.89.** Oblique view before radiation.

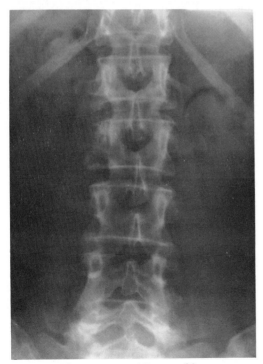

**Figure 3.88.** AP spot film.

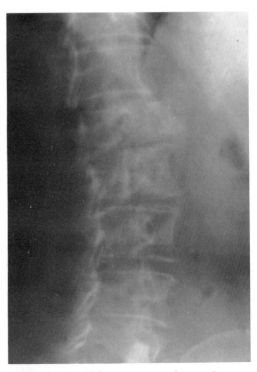

**Figure 3.90.** Oblique view after radiation.

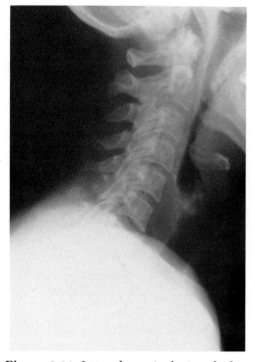

**Figure 3.91.** Lateral cervical view before radiation.

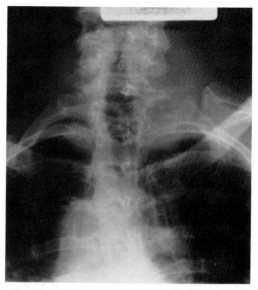

**Figure 3.93.** AP cervical view.

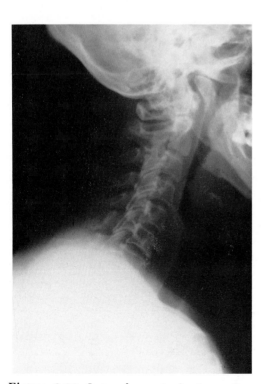

**Figure 3.92.** Lateral cervical view after radiation.

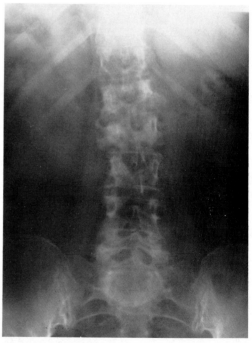

**Figure 3.94.** AP lumbar view after radiation.

metastasis in the female and is usually spread via the bloodstream.

## Fracture, Osteoporosis, and Degenerative Disease

**Case 4** is of a 69-year-old white woman who had had right low back and flank pain extend-

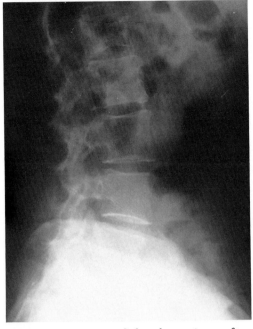

**Figure 3.95.** Lateral lumbar view after radiation.

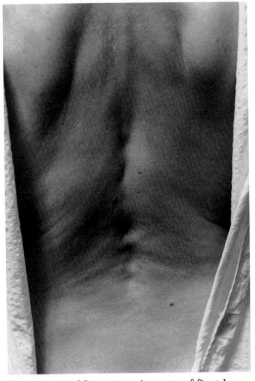

**Figure 3.96.** Note prominence of first lumbar spinous process.

ing to the pelvis following a fall on December 14, 1982. At that time she was hospitalized and told that she had a compression fracture of the spine.

Palpation reveals marked pain over the right pelvis and sacrum. The patient has been taking medication for pain.

X-ray (Fig. 3.96) reveals a prominence of the first lumbar spinous process in the lumbar lordotic curve.

Figure 3.97 is a lateral view of the spine taken on December 14, 1982. There is an approximately 30% compression deformity of the vertebral body of L1 and a nuclear invagination of the L2 disc into the inferior plate of L2. A repeat lateral view of the spine (Fig. 3.98) taken by us on February 21, 1983, shows further compression of the vertebral body to about 70%. An anteroposterior view of the lumbar spine and pelvis (Fig. 3.99) reveals generalized osteoporosis, a compression fracture of L1, and early degenerative change of the left hip joint. The opaque dye within the left hemipelvis represents barium sulfate within diverticula from a prior barium enema study.

This patient has a 70% compression fracture of the L1 vertebral body, generalized osteoporosis, and early degenerative hip disease (left).

Treatment consisted of flexion and extension manipulation of the L1-L2 articulation, followed by positive galvanism at L1-L2 and the course of the iliolumbar and iliohypogastric nerves on the pelvis and flank. A Dutch-

man roll was placed under the L1 vertebral body during flexion distraction. The osteoporosis was treated with 1,000 mg of nonphosphorous calcium daily and amino acid supplements at meals. A back support was recommended.

After the first treatment, the patient was able to sleep through the night without pain. The flank pain was greatly diminished but isolated to the right iliolumbar area. Seventy-five percent of the patient's pain was relieved after 3 weeks of treatment given 3 times weekly. She has been instructed to avoid carrying or lifting more than 15 lb, especially in the flexed waist posture.

### Unicameral Bone Cyst

**Case 5** is of a 17-year-old woman with left buttock and thigh pain. She had been receiving chiropractic manipulation for 4 weeks with no relief.

On examination, Patrick's sign is positive on the left, and there is tenderness of the left buttock, adductor muscles, and hip joint.

X-ray (Figs. 3.100 to 3.102) reveal a radiolucent area measuring 2.5 × 3.5 cm in the left femoral neck. No periosteal reaction and no

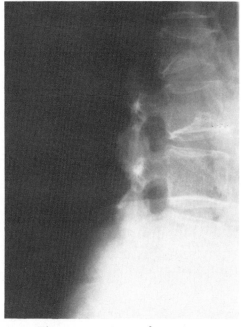

**Figure 3.97.** Lateral view.

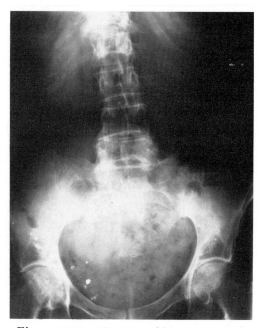

**Figure 3.99.** AP view of lumbar spine.

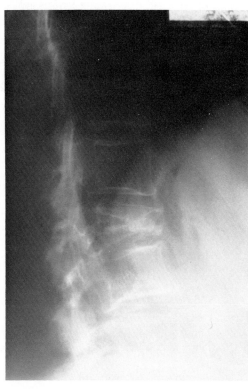

**Figure 3.98.** Lateral spot film taken 2 months after Figure 3.97.

cortical destruction are noted. The lesion is well demarcated from the normal bone. No calcific changes in the lesion are noted.

This patient had a unicameral bone cyst that was removed surgically (see Fig. 3.103). It must be remembered, however, that return of the lesion is possible.

This case is a good example of a pathological cause of pain that mimicks pain caused by a disc or facet.

## Multiple Myeloma

**Case 6** is of a 51-year-old white woman who had thoracic, lumbar, and pelvic pain, right sciatic pain into the lower extremity, and pain at night.

Serum protein electrophoresis shows a monoclonal gammopathy with elevated globulin. The A/G ratio is reversed, and Bence Jones protein is elevated in urine.

X-rays reveal:

1. Generalized osteoporosis with cortical thinning.
2. A large lesion in the right intertrochanter region has been surgically filled with bone chips (Fig. 3.105). Note the multiple, ill-defined radiolucent and opaque round lesions in the right greater trochanter. There is a suspicious-looking area near the right ilium superior to the acetabulum.

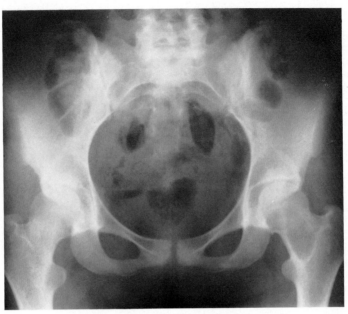

**Figure 3.100.** AP view of pelvis.

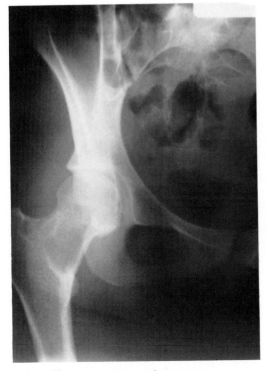

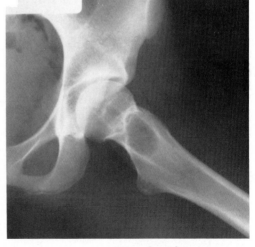

**Figure 3.102.** "Frog-leg" hip view.

**Figure 3.101.** AP hip view.

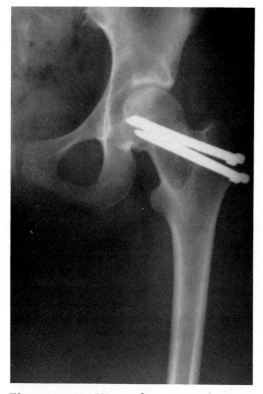

**Figure 3.103.** View after surgical repair for unicameral bone cyst.

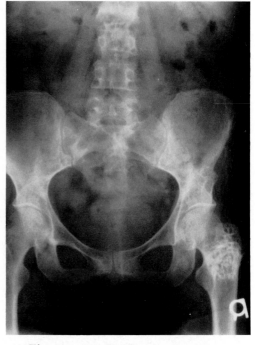

**Figure 3.105.** AP view of pelvis.

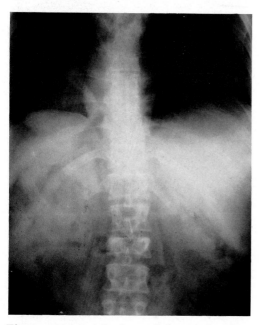

**Figure 3.104.** AP view of thoracolumbar spine.

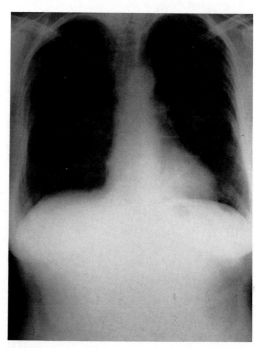

**Figure 3.106.** Posteroanterior chest view.

3. Loss of height of the 2nd lumbar vertebra with increased density of the vertebral body plates and loss of bone density (Fig. 3.104).

4. Loss of vertebral body height at the T4, T5, T7, and T9 levels (Fig. 3.107).

5. The right posterior 5th rib has a pathological fracture, and there is an extrapleural mass on the axillary lung border (Fig. 3.106).

6. The multiple teardrop configuration (punched out radiolucencies) classic to multiple myeloma is evident on Figure 3.108.

This patient has multiple myeloma which was confirmed by biopsy that revealed elevated plasma cells. Multiple myeloma is the most common primary malignant neoplasm in humans and affects bone marrow. Its onset is insidious, with vague back pain as the primary symptom. Multiple myeloma should be considered in the diagnosis of any patient over 45 years old with these symptoms.

## Abdominal Aneurysm

Case 7 is of a 58-year-old man with low back pain.

X-rays reveal an abdominal aneurysm. Note the calcific expansion of the atherosclerotic abdominal aorta, measuring 4.5 cm in diameter (normal is 1.75 cm to 3.0 cm) (Figs. 3.109 and 3.110).

Treament consisted of surgical repair.

## Kidney Disease

Case 8 is of a 46-year-old man with low back pain.

Results of laboratory studies reveal hematuria and albuminuria.

X-rays reveal:

1. Numerous opaque densities within the renal outline appear in the calyceal region (Fig. 3.111). Figure 3.112 confirms this location.

2. The intravenous pyelogram (Fig. 3.113) reveals dilation of the right ureter, dilatation of the renal pelvis, and blunting of the calyces. Both kidneys show multiple calcific densities.

This patient has renal calculi with hydro-

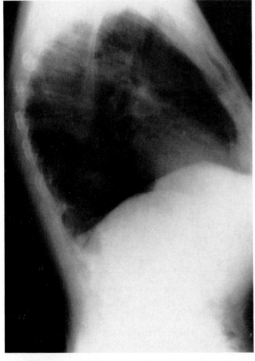

**Figure 3.107.** Lateral chest view.

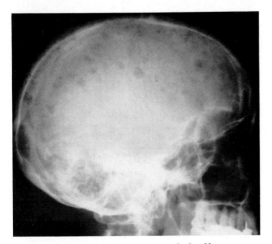

**Figure 3.108.** X-ray of skull.

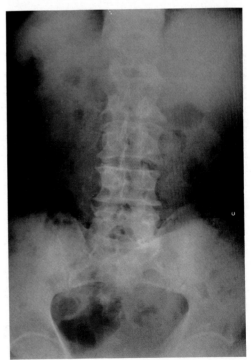

**Figure 3.109.** Left aortic expansion on AP view.

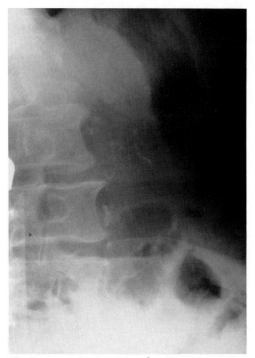

**Figure 3.110.** Arteriosclerotic expansion on oblique projection.

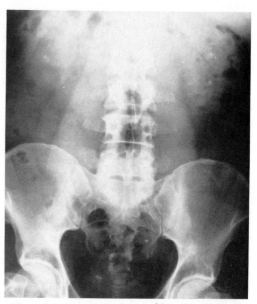

**Figure 3.111.** AP view of lumbar spine.

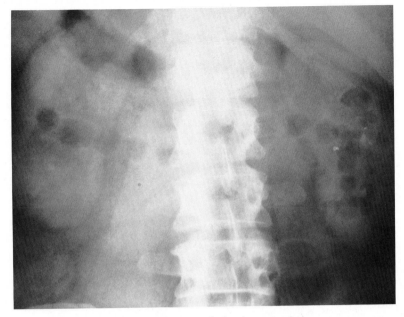

**Figure 3.112.** Renal shadow study.

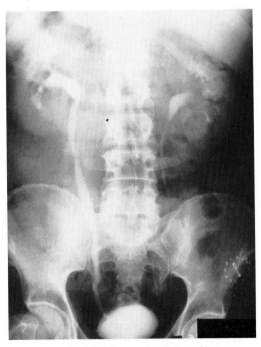

**Figure 3.113.** Intravenous pyelogram.

nephrosis of the right kidney collecting system and suspected obstruction of right ureter at the urinary bladder, which was confirmed on cystoscopy. Further tests ruled out hyperparathyroidism. This case seems a fitting end to this chapter. The most common organic condition blamed by patients for back pain is kidney disease, a condition seen not nearly as often as Doan's Pills would suggest.

## References

1. Bywater EGL: The pathological anatomy of idiopathic low back pain. In: *American Academy of Orthopaedic Surgeons Symposium on Idiopathic Low Back Pain.* St Louis, CV Mosby, 1982, 152, 153.
2. Buckwalter JA: The five structures of human intervertebral disc. In: *American Academy of Orthopaedic Surgeons Symposium on Idiopathic Low Back Pain.* St Louis, CV Mosby, 1982, pp 113–117.
2a. Hirsch C: Studies on the pathology of low back pain. *J Bone Joint Surg* 41(B):237–243, 1959.
2b. Lindblom K: Technique and results in myelography and disc rupture. *Acta Radiol* 34:321–330, 1950.
3. Rothman RH, Simeone FA: *The Spine.* Philadelphia, WB Saunders, vol II, 1975, p 451.
4. Armstrong J: *Lumbar Disc Lesion.* Baltimore, Williams & Wilkens, 1965.
5. Turek S: *Orthopaedics—Principles and Their Application.* Philadelphia, JB Lippincott, 1956, p 748.
6. White AA, Panjabi MM: *Clinical Biomechanics of the Spine.* Philadeliphia, JB Lippincott, 1978, pp 285–291.
7. Charnley J: Acute lumbago and sciatica. *Br Med J* 1:344, 1955.
8. Naylor A: Intervertebral disc prolapse and degeneration: the biochemical and biophysical approach. *Spine* 1:108, 1976.
8a. Kazarian L.: Personal communication to authors. In White AA, Panjabi MM: *Clinical Biomechanics of the Spine.* Philadelphia, JB Lippincott, 1978, pp 285.
9. Hirsch C: An attempt to diagnose the level of disc lesion clinically by disc puncture. *Acta Orthop Scand* 18:132, 1948.
10. Sprangfort EV: The lumbar disc herniation. A computer-aided analysis of 2,504 operations.

*Acta Orthop Scand [Suppl]* 142: 1972.

11. Epstein BS: *The Spine, A Radiological Text and Atlas*, ed 3. Philadelphia, Lea & Febiger, 1969, pp 35, 38, 554.

11a. Nachemson A, Morris JM: In vivo measurements of intradiscal pressure, a method for the determination of pressure in the lower lumbar discs. *J Bone Joint Surg* 46(A):1077, 1964.

12. Keele CA, Neil E: *Samson Wright's Applied Physiology*, ed 10. London, Oxford University Press, 1961, p 51.

13. Nachemson A: The lumbar spine, an orthopaedic challenge. *Spine* 1(1):59–69, 1976.

14. Fahrni WH: Conservative treatment of lumbar disc degeneration: our primary responsibility. *Orthop Clin North Am* 6(1):93–103, 1975.

15. Gresham JL, Miller R: Evaluation of the lumbar spine by diskography. *Orthop Clin* 67:29, 1969.

16. Arns W, Huter A: Conservative therapy of lumbar intervertebral disc lesions. *Dtsch Med Wochenschr* 101:587–589, 1976.

17. Semmes RE: *Rupture of the Lumbar Intervertebral Disc*. Springfield, IL, Charles C Thomas, 1964, pp 17–18.

18. Herlin L: *Sciatic and Pelvic Pain due to Lumbosacral Nerve Root Compression*. Springfield, IL, Charles C Thomas, 1966, p 19.

19. Herlin L: *Sciatic and Pelvic Pain due to Lumbosacral Nerve Root Compression*. Springfield, IL, Charles C Thomas, 1966, pp 14.

20. Herlin L: *Sciatic and Pelvic Pain due to Lumbosacral Nerve Root Compression*. Springfield, IL, Charles C Thomas, 1966, p 16.

21. Herlin L: *Sciatic and Pelvic Pain due to Lumbosacral Nerve Root Compression*. Springfield, IL, Charles C Thomas, 1966, p 31.

22. Herlin L: *Sciatic and Pelvic Pain due to Lumbosacral Nerve Root Compression*. Springfield, IL, Charles C Thomas, 1966, p 120.

23. Herlin L: *Sciatic and Pelvic Pain due to Lumbosacral Nerve Root Compression*. Springfield, IL, Charles C Thomas, 1966, p 128.

24. Herlin L: *Sciatic and Pelvic Pain due to Lumbosacral Nerve Root Compression*. Springfield, IL, Charles C Thomas, 1966, pp 168–169.

25. Emmett J, Love J: Vesical dysfunction caused by a protruded lumbar disc. *J Urol* 105:86–91, 1971.

26. Ross JC, Jackson RM: Vesical dysfunction due to prolapsed disc. *Br Med J* 3:752–754, 1971

27. Amelar R, Dubin L: Impotence in the low back syndrome. *JAMA* 216:520, 1971.

28. Gray H: *Anatomy of the Human Body*, ed 28. Philadelphia, Lea & Febiger, 1967, pp 1007–1009.

29. Rothman RH, Simeone, FA: *The Spine*. Philadelphia, WB Saunders, 1975, p 452.

30. Stoddard A: *Manual of Osteopathic Practice*. New York, Harper & Row, 1970, pp 140.

31. Falconer MA, McGeorge M, Begg CA: Observations on the cause and mechanism of symptom production in sciatica and low back pain. *J Neurol Neurosurg Psychiatry* 11:13–26, 1948.

31a. Charnley J: Orthopaedic signs in the diagnosis of disc protrusion. *Lancet* 1:186–192, 1951.

32. Finneson BE: *Low Back Pain*, ed 2. Philadelphia, JB Lippincott, 1980, p 428.

33. Raney RL: The effects of flexion, extension, Valsalva maneuver, and abdominal compression on the larger volume myelographic column. Paper presented at the International Symposium for study of the Lumbar Spine, June 1978.

34. Lasègue C: Considerations sur la Sciatique. *Arch Med (Paris)* 2:;558–580, 1864.

35. Breig A, Troup JDG: Biomechanical considerations in the straight leg raising test. *Spine* 4(3):242–250, 1979.

36. Suguira K: A study on tension signs in lumbar disc hernia. *Int Orthop* 3:225–228, 1979.

37. Goddard MD, Reed JD: Movements induced by straight leg raising in the lumbo sacral roots, nerve and plexus and in the intrapelvic section of the sciatic nerve. *J Neurol Neurosurg Psychiatry* 28:16–18, 1965.

38. O'Connell JEA: Sciatica and the mechanism of the production of the clinical syndrome in protrusion of the lumbar intervertebral disc. *Br J Surg* 30:315–327, 1963.

39. Hudgins WR: The crossed straight leg raising test: a diagnostic sign of herniated disc. *J Occup Med* 21(6):407–408, 1979.

40. Edgar MA, Park WM: Induced pain patterns on passive straight leg raising in lower lumbar disc protrusions. *J Bone Joint Surg* 56B:4, 1974.

41. Herron LD, Pheasant HC: Prone knee-flexion provocative testing for lumbar spine protrusion. *Spine* 5(1):65–67, 1980.

42. Macnab, I.: Disc degeneration without root irritation. In Macnab I: *Backache*. Baltimore, Williams & Wilkins, 1977, pp 174 and 176.

43. Waddell G, McCulloch JA, Kummel E, Venner RM: Nonorganic physical signs in low back pain, *Spine* 5(2):117–125, 1980.

44. Finneson BE: *Low Back Pain*. Philadelphia, JB Lippincott, 1973, pp 6, 25, and 163.

45. Nashold BS, Hrubec Z: *Lumbar Disc Disease, A Twenty-Year Clinical Follow-up Study*. St Louis, CV Mosby, 1971, p 63.

46. Hanrats: In Nashold BS, Hrubec Z: *Lumbar Disc Disease, A Twenty-Year Clinical Follow-up Study*. St Louis, CV Mosby, 1971, p 65.

47. Finneson BE: *Low Back Pain*, ed 2. Philadelphia, JB Lippincott, 1980, p 302.

48. Inman VT, Saunders JB: The clinico-anatomical aspects of the lumbosacral region. *Radiology* 38:669–678, 1942.

49. Perl ER: Mode of action of nociceptors, cervical pain. *Wennergren Cent Int Symp Ser* 17:157–164, 1971.

50. Hakalius A, Hindmarsh J: The significance of neurological signs and myelographic findings in the diagnosis of lumbar root compression. *Acta Orthop Scand* 43:239–346, 1972.

51. Sprangfort E: Lasèques sign in patients with lumbar disc herniation. *Acta Orthop Scand* 42:459, 1971.

52. Million R, Hall W, Nilsen KH, Baker RD, Jayson MIV: Assessment of the progress of the back pain patient. *Spine* 7(3):204, 1982.

53. Hoehler FK, Tobis JS: Low back pain and its treatment by spinal manipulation: measures of flexibility and asymmetry. *Rheumatol Rehabil* 21:21, 1982.

54. Katznelson A, Nerubay J, Lev-El A: Gluteal skyline. *Spine* 7(1):74–75, 1982.

55. McCullough JA: Chemonucleolysis. *J Bone Joint Surg* 159B:45–52, 1977.

56. Edeiken J: *Roentgen Diagnosis of Diseases of Bone*, ed 3. Baltimore, Williams & Wilkins, vol 1, 1981, pp 507–508.

CHAPTER **4**

# Short Leg Determination and Treatment

Determination of the short leg in the acute stage of low back pain is error-filled due to the antalgic posture of the patient. We wait until antalgia and pain are relieved before we x-ray for short leg. We use Chamberlain's view; i.e., the patient is standing upright, barefooted, and with the feet directly under the femoral heads. The x-ray is taken at 40 inches with the center ray through the femoral heads.

Giles and Taylor (1) report that the motion segment, meaning the vertebra itself, is conveniently subdivided into anterior and posterior elements. Some authors advance the theory that the anterior elements are the principal source of chronic low back pain, whereas others theorize that the posterior elements and adjacent soft tissues are the principal source. Most authors agree, however, that degeneration of the intervertebral discs and the associated arthrosis of the apophyseal joints cause low back pain. The objectives of this article are to clarify the controversy which has existed over the past 50 years regarding a possible relationship between leg length inequality and chronic low back pain.

We studied 1,309 patients who presented with chronic low back pain and a control group of 50 volunteers who had no history of low back pain, using erect posture radiography of the pelvis and lumbar spine. Of 1,309 patients, 244 had leg length differences greater than 9 mm. Of these 244, 217 had chronic low back pain and 27 had acute low back pain. Of the chronic sufferers, 89 were willing to participate in a survey of the effectiveness of treatment, and 50 of these patients underwent a 4-month follow-up examination.

The responses to two treatment methods were compared in this study of 50 patients with chronic low back pain who had leg length inequality of 9 mm or more. These two treatment methods were:

1. Patients received lumbosacral manipulation and a shoe-raise appropriate to the limb length discrepancy.
2. Patients received shoe-raise therapy only, but if low back pain persisted for 1 month, they received lumbosacral manipulation.

Alterations in the pain, the straight leg raise, and range of motion between the initial and the final visit were used to assess improvement. No untreated control group was used.

In the group of 15 patients who were given only a shoe-lift, 5 required manipulation to relieve their low back pain after a 1-month trial period, which may indicate that manipulation plus shoe-raise resulted in quicker remission of symptoms. The prevalence of a leg length inequality of 10 mm or more appeared to be more common in patients suffering from low back pain than in the normal population.

In the reduction of postural scoliosis in patients up to the age of 53 years the immediate response to shoe-raise was the same as the response at 4 months. The response was slower in patients over 53 than in patients under 53, and the scoliosis was never entirely eliminated.

In conclusion, some patients who had experienced chronic low back pain for 20 years or more stated that they experienced no low back pain as long as they wore their shoe-raise. The number of attacks of low back pain and the number of working days lost appeared to be reduced. The greater prevalence of short leg in patients with low back pain compared with normal controls is presented as evidence of the importance of leg length inequality in the etiology of low back pain.

## DETERMINATION OF SHORT LEG

First, study the film taken with the patient in the upright position. Draw a line across the superior femoral heads as shown in Figure 4.1 and then measure the millimeter shortness of the lower femoral head (1 inch = 25.4 mm).

## DETERMINATION OF THE PROPER LIFT

*The amount of build-up seldom equals the exact difference in femoral head shortness. If the difference is prescribed, the chance of error is significant. Therefore, use build-ups of the heel and sole to determine the exact build-up needed to level the heads.* The thickness of these build-ups increases in millimeters (see Fig. 4.20). Once the proper lift is determined place that amount on the heel and 5 mm less on the sole. For a lift of up to 6 mm, put no lift on the sole. If there is an 11-mm shortness, put 11 mm on the heel and 6 mm on the sole. A cobbler will be needed to add a lift to the sole, but for the heel, lifts of up to 6 mm can be purchased and put in at your office.

## RADIATION EXPOSURE

Two and, sometimes, three views are usually necessary to determine the proper build-up (Fig. 4.21). For protection, gonad shields are used on children and women of childbearing age (see Figs. 4.12 to 4.17).

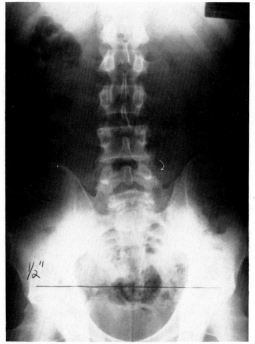

**Figure 4.1.** This x-ray taken at 40-inches through the pelvis with the feet under the femoral heads (Chamberlain's view), shows that the left femoral head is ½-inch inferior to the right with left rotation of the L3, L4, and L5 vertebral bodies.

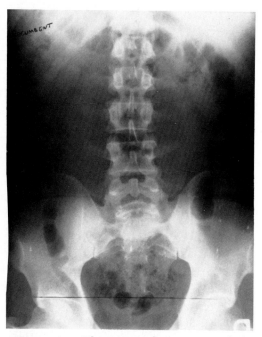

**Figure 4.2.** This recumbent view of the same patient as in Figure 4.1 shows the difficulty of using the recumbent x-ray for evaluating short leg, as here the short leg disappears.

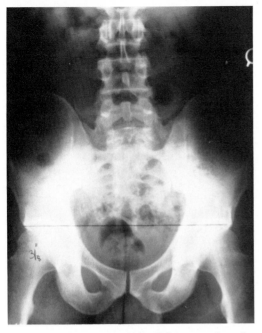

**Figure 4.3.** A ⅜-inch build-up under the patient's left heel and sole was made at the time of this x-ray. The patient can see and understand the correction of the short leg and the lumbar curve and, therefore, will wear the build-up more readily.

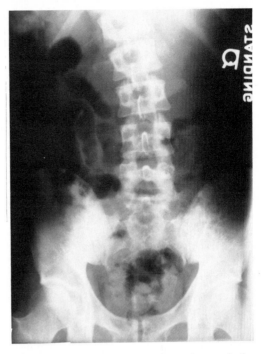

**Figure 4.5.** Posteroanterior view of the pelvis and lumbar spine of a patient with a right L4-L5 lateral disc protrusion on the first visit.

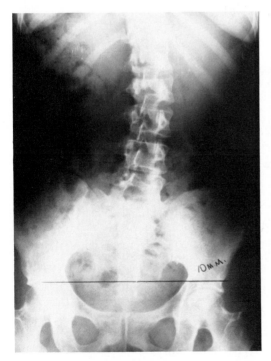

**Figure 4.4.** X-ray of a patient with a 10-mm right short leg with the resultant dextroscoliosis of the lumbar spine.

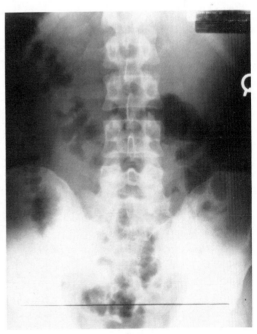

**Figure 4.6.** X-ray shows no short leg present after reduction of the L4-L5 disc. Note the straightening of the spine.

Of course, settings at the lowest mAs and at the highest kVp are used. Since these x-rays are used to determine structural changes only, the same detail as is needed on diagnostic films is not mandatory. Of course, the best technic is needed so as to glean as much bone architecture interpretation and structural fault as possible.

*Now, the disadvantages of radiation exposure are weighed against the disadvantages of using an improper build-up.* We compare the shoe lift to a tiny piece of dirt in the eye; i.e., it feels like a boulder. If the build-up corrects, it is fine, but if it overcorrects or undercorrects, it not only is less than desirable but also can result in a greater instability than existed without it.

## LEG LENGTHENING PROCEDURE

The entire spine is affected by a leg lengthening procedure, and like a rod, it is impossible to move one end without affecting the other.

Figure 4.2 is the recumbent view of the same patient as in Figure 4.1, with the short leg not shown. Figure 4.3 shows correction of the left short leg with use of a ⅜-inch heel and sole lift. Figure 4.4 shows the right rotation occurring in the lumbar spine of a patient with a 10-mm right short leg.

Figure 4.6 shows no short leg present in the same patient as in Figure 4.5 after reduction of the disc at L4-L5; the spine is now straight with reduction of the left L4 lateral flexion subluxation and disc. The patient had right L5 dermatome sciatica down the entire leg. This case shows that a disc lesion can cause the same scoliosis as does short leg. Thus careful differential diagnosis is mandatory.

Figures 4.7 and 4.8, respectively, show the changes before and after correction of a 10-mm short leg. Note the degenerative L5 disc in Figure 4.9. The patient has L5 dermatome sciatica due to an L4-L5 disc protrusion. The L5 disc degenerates first, with L4 degenerating next because the stress moves up one level. The presence of short leg may well serve to intensify the biomechanical stresses already present; thus correction can prevent stress on an already-strained low back.

Figure 4.10 shows an 8-mm shortness of the left femoral head with a left lean of the lumbar spine in a 17-year-old basketball player. Prior to this film, he had been treated unsuccessfully for 6 weeks for left leg and low back pain in the L5 derma-

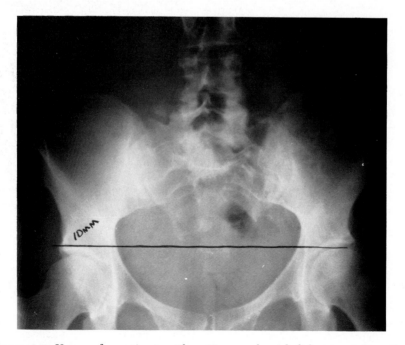

**Figure 4.7.** X-ray of a patient with a 10-mm short left lower extremity.

tome by another chiropractor who did not radiograph the boy.

Note that now the pelvis is level (Fig. 4.11) and the lumbar spine is vertically corrected. Also note that it took only 6 mm to correct an 8-mm shortness. You cannot depend on the leg length difference to be the build-up difference needed

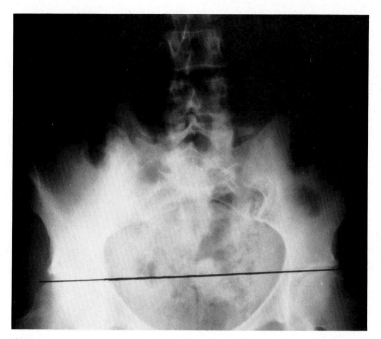

**Figure 4.8.** This x-ray is of the same patient as in Figure 4.7 but with the patient wearing a 12-mm build-up. Note the change at the L4-L5 level.

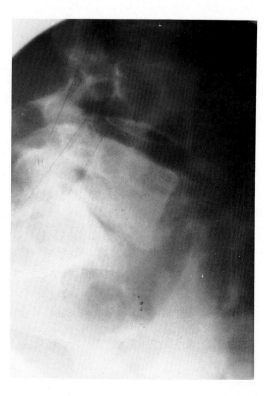

**Figure 4.9.** Lateral spot film of the same patient as in Figures 4.7 and 4.8.

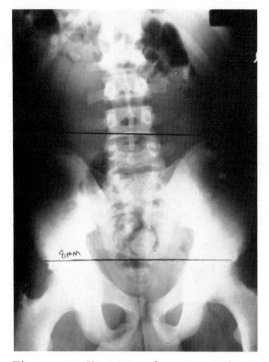

**Figure 4.10.** X-ray reveals an 8-mm shortness of the left femoral head with a left lean of the lumbar spine.

Figures 4.18, 4.19, 4.20, and 4.21 are of a patient with a 13-mm left short leg and an inferior left hemipelvis. L4 is in right flexion subluxation on L5 with a nonrotatory lean cephalad to L4 (Fig. 4.18). Note the straightening of the lumbar curve and the correction of the left short extremity shown in Figure 4.19. Figure 4.20 shows the lift used in the correction of the short leg. Figure 4.21 shows the patient during x-ray with the lift in place.

Of 576 cases reported by the International Academy on Chiropractic Low Back Pain Study, Inc. (2), in 1982, 11% had a short leg length of more than 6 mm after maximum correction of the patient's mechanical faults had been performed and maximum improvement attained. The technique outlined in this chapter can provide the final correction desired by both the doctor and the patient.

Figure 4.22 reveals the antalgic right inferior hemipelvis with right sciatic scoliosis. Figure 4.23 shows the leveling of the pelvis following reduction of a medial

to correct the shortness. *You must build up the foot at x-ray as described earlier.*

Figure 4.12 shows a 22-mm shortness in a 15-year-old who had a pinning of a slipped femoral epiphysis 1 year prior. Now the right femoral epiphysis is fused, while the left continues to grow. Figure 4.13 shows the effect of a 13-mm build-up. Note that a 19-mm build-up (Fig. 4.14) corrects the deficiency. Note how an error in correction with lifts could have been made without the proper studies. Also, observe the improvement in the patient's dextroscoliosis. The pain in the right low back has also disappeared.

Figures 4.15, 4.16, and 4.17 are studies of a 12 year old with a 10-mm short left femoral head, hemipelvis, and a levoscoliosis of the lumbar spine (Fig. 4.15). Note that the lift placed under the left shoe reduced both the short leg and the scoliosis from 13° to 7° (Fig. 4.16). Compare Figure 4.17, the recumbent x-ray, with Figure 4.15, the upright.

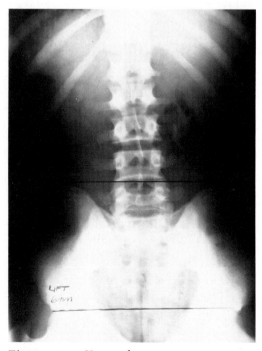

**Figure 4.11.** X-ray shows a 6-mm correction of the same patient as in Figure 4.10.

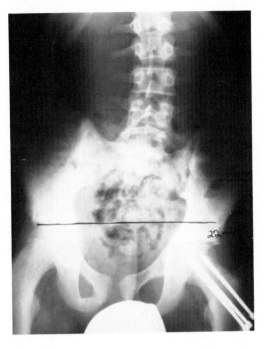

**Figure 4.12.** X-ray shows a 22-mm short-ness in a 15 year old who had pinning of a slipped femoral epiphysis 1 year prior. Now the right femoral epiphysis is fused, while the left continues to grow. Note the gonad shielding used with young people.

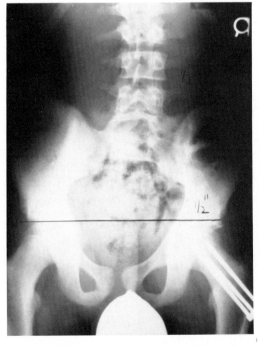

**Figure 4.13.** X-rays show that a ½-inch or 13-mm build-up is not enough.

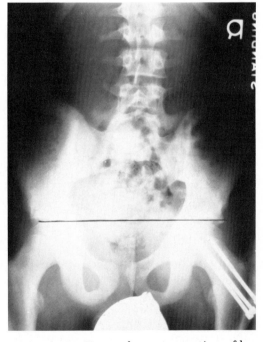

**Figure 4.14.** X-ray shows correction of leg length by use of a 19-mm build-up.

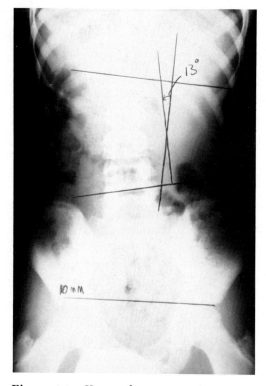

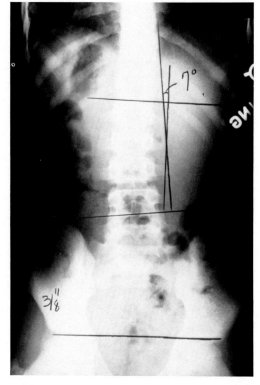

**Figure 4.15.** X-ray of a 12-year-old patient with a 10-mm left short leg.

**Figure 4.16.** A ⅜-inch lift under the left shoe reduced short leg and the scoliosis.

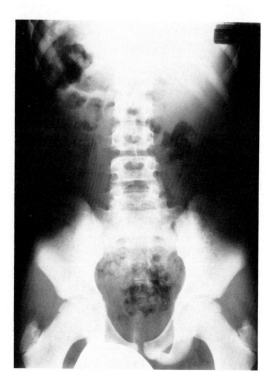

**Figure 4.17.** This recumbent view of the same patient as in Figure 4.15 shows no short leg and no scoliosis. Note how error-filled recumbent films are for structural changes.

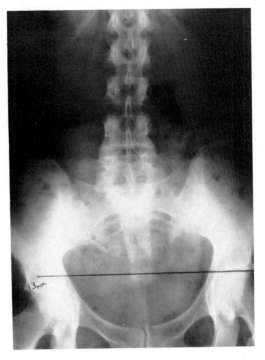

**Figure 4.18.** A 13-mm shortness in the left extremity is shown.

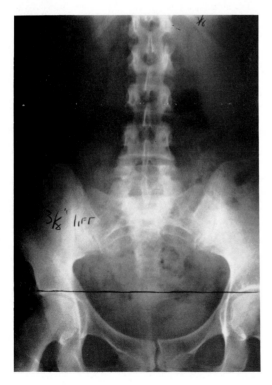

**Figure 4.19.** X-ray shows correction of short leg, achieved by use of a ⅜-inch lift.

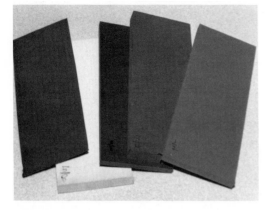

**Figure 4.20.** These build-ups are used to evaluate extremities so as to level the pelvis. Their heights range from ⅛ inch to ¾ inch.

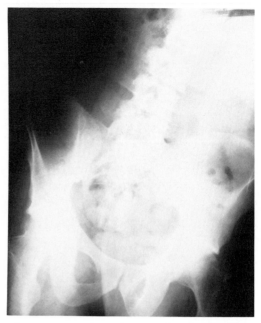

**Figure 4.22.** Antalgic right hemipelvis with right sciatic scoliosis.

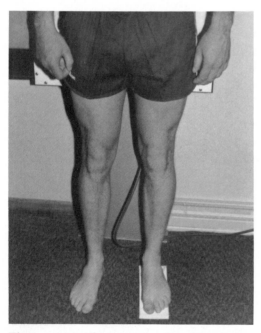

**Figure 4.21.** Photograph of patient being radiographed with the short leg build-up in place.

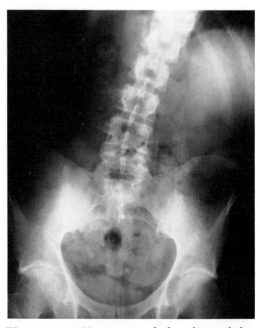

**Figure 4.23.** X-ray reveals leveling of the pelvis following reduction of a medial L5-S1 disc protrusion. No true short leg was present.

L5-S1 disc protrusion. No true short leg was present, only the muscular and discal causes of antalgia. Thus, the *clinician should evaluate the patient for short leg only after correction of biomechanical faults has been accomplished.*

Pope et al. (3) report that fetal and neonatal lower extremities are usually equal in length, but asymmetries become measurable during the second year of life, and the right leg is longer than the left in 80% of all instances. Ingelmark and Lundstrom (as discussed in Ref. 3) report that these asymmetries vanish before adolescence because the left leg usually grows faster than the right, and in adults the left leg is longer. Interestingly, Marsk (as discussed in Ref. 3) found that the left foot supports a significantly higher load than the right foot in right-handed subjects.

## References

1. Giles LGF, Taylor JR: Low back pain associated with leg length inequality. *Spine* 6(5):510–521, 1981.
2. Cox JM, Shreiner S: Chiropractic manipulation in low back pain and sciatica: statistical data on the diagnosis, treatment and response of 576 consecutive cases. *J Manip Physiolog Ther* 7(1):1–11, 1984.
3. Pope M, Wilder D, Booth J: The biomechanics of low back pain. In: *American Academy of Orthopaedic Surgeons Symposium on Idiopathic Low Back Pain.* St Louis, CV Mosby, 1982, p 272.

# CHAPTER 5

# Radiographic Biomechanics of the Lumbar Spine and Pelvis

## RELEVANCE OF THE LATERAL BENDING STUDY

The biomechanics of the lumbar spine and pelvis are best shown radiographically by use of the dynamic lateral bending study. Without it, one of the most important tools of diagnosis of lumbar mechanics is lost. Weitz (1) revealed the accuracy of lateral bending studies by comparing their findings to those of myelography and surgery. He found that of 46 patients, 12 had normal bending studies, and of these, 6 had midline disc protrusion and 2 had stenosis. Of the 34 patients with abnormal bending studies, 28 had disc protrusion confirmed at both myelography and surgery. Two of the 34 had abnormal bending studies confirmed at surgery despite negative myelography. Both patients had lateral disc protrusions with normal bending away from the protrusion and impaired bending toward the protrusion. There was no instance of a patient with an ipsilateral list and a negative myelogram.

Van Damme et al. (2) compared the relative efficacy of clinical examination, electromyography, plain film radiography, myelography, and lumbar phlebography in the diagnosis of low back pain and sciatica. They found that the *bending studies had diagnostic reliability equal to that of myelography* and lumbar phlebography.

In 1942, Duncan and Haen (3) stated that the postural attitude assumed by a patient with a disc protrusion was such as to avoid further compression of the disc: "This posture entails a list of the spine away from the side of the lesion, and since the mass is extruding posteriorly, an attitude of forward flexion is assumed." They took films of the patient in lateral flexion to each side and in flexion and extension and found that "In the majority of our cases these films have demonstrated a lack of spinal mobility localized to the involved joint." They also found that in patients with laterally placed herniation, the myelograms were consistently normal. (We believe that lateral discs can be so far lateral as not to contact the dye-filled subarachnoid space,

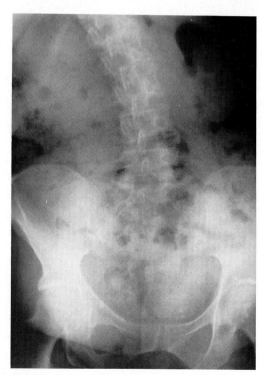

**Figure 5.1.** Posteroanterior left lateral flexion view.

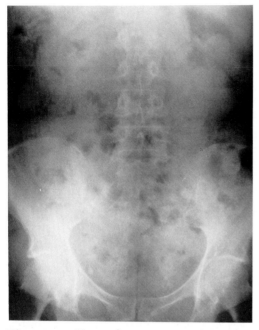

**Figure 5.2.** Neutral posteroanterior view.

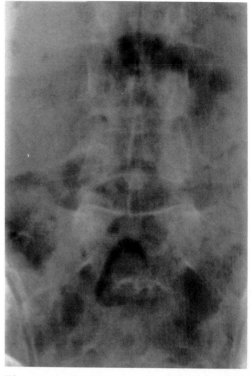

**Figure 5.4.** Posteroanterior tilt view of the L5-S1 interspace.

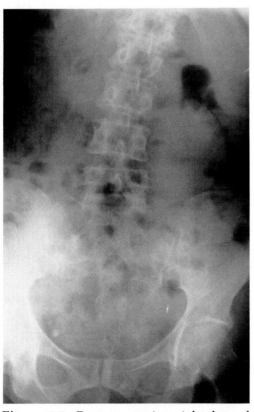

**Figure 5.3.** Posteroanterior right lateral flexion view.

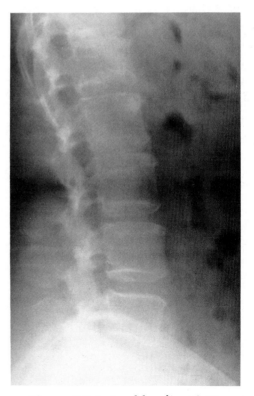

**Figure 5.5.** Lateral lumbar view.

thus giving a false negative myelogram—one reason for the 30% to 40% inaccuracy of myelography.) They also took postoperative bending films which showed that once the sequestrum had been removed from the involved joint there was immediate restoration of joint mobility.

In 1948, Falconer et al. (4) in a study of 25 patients with ipsilateral list and 17 with contralateral list, with the summit medial or lateral to the nerve root in both subgroups, discussed the importance of list in lumbar disc disease. They found that scoliosis was due to spasm designed to splint the disc prolapse so as to exert the least possible "strain" on the surrounding structures, but they were unable to correlate the direction of the curvature with the side of the symptoms. One year later, Hadley (5) noted that in certain patients with nerve root pressure the foramen is not allowed to become smaller on lateral flexion toward the affected side, although normal wedging may take place at this level when the patient bends to the opposite direction.

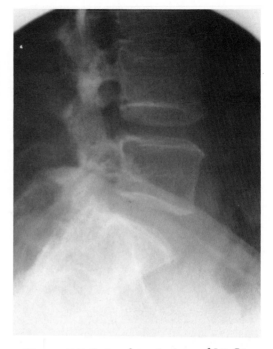

**Figure 5.6.** Lateral spot view of L5-S1.

Schalimtzek (6) and Hasner et al. (7) performed motion studies for diagnosing herniated discs. Hasner et al. discovered that if lateral bending is inhibited, either the normal angulation between vertebral bodies may be less pronounced or a state of parallelism may be noted. They (6, 7) also found that the vertebral bodies may even be divergent to each other on the side where the lateral bending takes place.

Breig (8) states that the patient's posture in an acute back disorder represents a compromise between the need to minimize tension in the dura and the root and the need to reduce the bulge of the prolapsed disc. He believes that it is not uncommon to see a patient with a flattened lumbar region flex the spine forward to minimize the herniation and ipsilaterally to relieve tension on the root, such as occurs in a patient with an axillary herniation.

Finneson (9) has demonstrated both ipsilateral and contralateral listing caused by the relationship of the protrusion to the nerve root.

Nachemson (10) believes that "the information obtained from ordinary x-rays

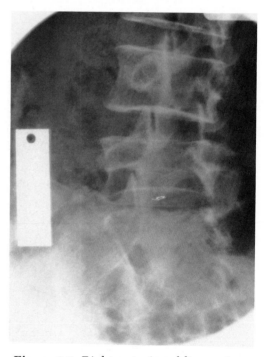

**Figure 5.7.** Right anterior oblique view.

is, however, mostly irrelevant." Weitz, therefore, states, "It is with this impetus that we urge lateral bending (dynamic) x-ray studies rather than static films in pa-

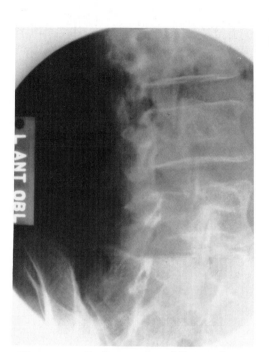

**Figure 5.8.** Left anterior oblique view.

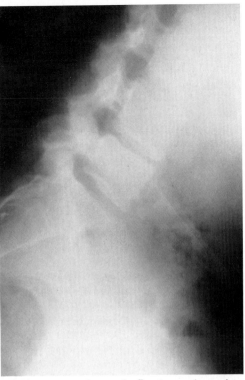

**Figure 5.10.** Lateral flexion view (optional).

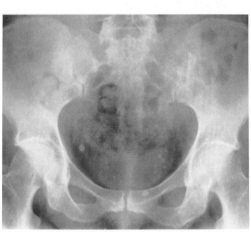

**Figure 5.9.** Anteroposterior view of pelvis (optional).

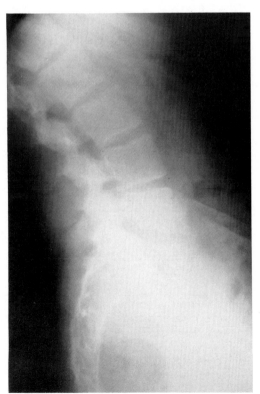

**Figure 5.11.** Lateral extension view (optional).

tients clinically suspected of having lumbar disc herniations" (1).

## RADIOGRAPHIC STUDIES

Figures 5.1 to 5.11 are routine examination views of the low back and pelvis.

Lateral bending studies are performed to determine aberrant lateral flexion of a functional spinal unit in relation to its adjacent segments. These studies are most beneficial in determining subluxation, as in hypomobility of the static subluxation accompanying intervertebral disc protrusion. For study of the L4-L5 level, routine anteroposterior views in lateral flexion are adequate, but for study of the L5-S1 level, the tilt view must be used because the sacral angle and lumbar lordosis make viewing of the lateral flexion of L5 on the sacrum impossible.

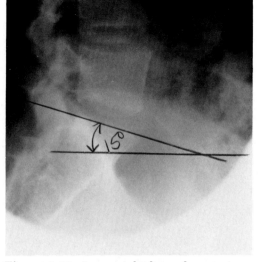

**Figure 5.12.** An upright lateral spot view. The sacral angle measured 15°.

For the tilt view, take the lateral lumbar view as shown in Figure 5.12. Next draw the sacral promontory line and measure the angle made by this line with the horizontal. Then move the x-ray tube to match this angle (Fig. 5.13), with the center ray 1½ inches inferior to the intercrestal line centered to the midline. In addition to the neutral posteroanterior view (PA), the lateral bending studies are performed by having the patient slide his hand down his thigh while keeping his feet flat on the floor directly beneath the hip joints and keeping his knees straight (Fig. 5.14). These studies may be performed with the patient either sitting or standing, depending on the doctor's preference, and provide the following information:

1. Fixation hypomobile subluxation due to either disc protrusion or facet incongruity.
2. Relief of disc or facet lesions following manipulation, as normal physiological mobility returns.

Figure 5.15 is an illustration of lateral bending antalgic postures and their effect on the medial and the lateral discs.

Figures 5.16 to 5.18 are the roentgen studies that correlate with the schematic representations in Figure 5.15 of disc protrusion causing nerve root compression. They are lateral bending studies of the

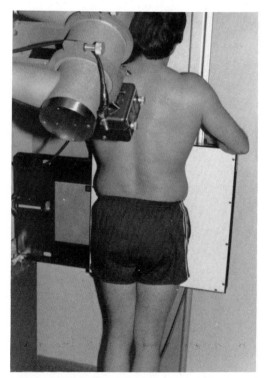

**Figure 5.13.** Tube tilted to match sacral angle and centered to L5-S1 level.

L5-S1 level in a patient with pain down the right 1st sacral dermatome and provide clinical evidence of a right lateral 5th lumbar disc protrusion. Figure 5.16 is

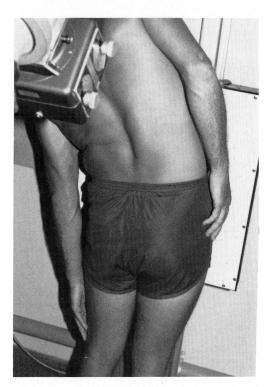

**Figure 5.14.** Lateral flexion is performed by having the patient slide his hand down his thigh while bending laterally.

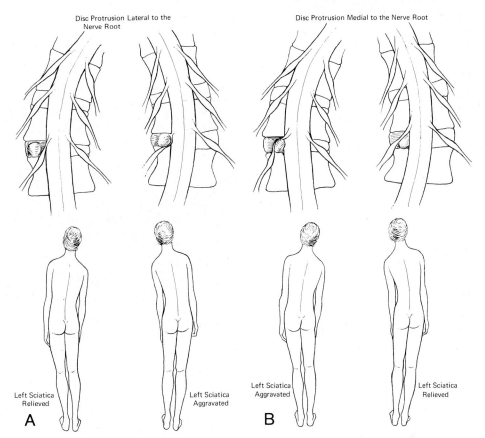

**Figure 5.15.** Relief or aggravation of pain with lateral flexion may indicate whether the disc protrusion is lateral or medial to the nerve root. (Reproduced with permission from B. E. Finneson: *Low Back Pain*. Philadelphia, J. B. Lippincott, 1973, p. 302.)

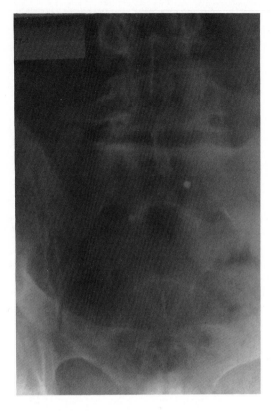

**Figure 5.16.** Left lateral flexion subluxation of L5 on the sacrum is shown. Tropism can be seen at the L5-S1 level, with the right facets faced sagitally and left facets faced coronally.

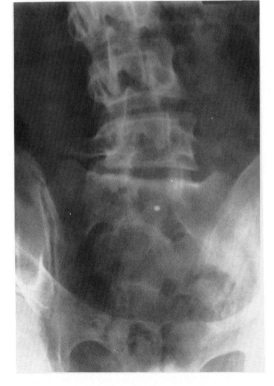

**Figure 5.17.** Left lateral flexion view of the same patient as in Figure 5.16. Good lateral mobility of each functional spinal unit is shown.

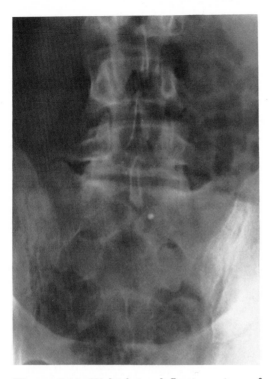

**Figure 5.18.** Right lateral flexion view of the same patient as in Figure 5.16. Note static subluxation of L5 on the sacrum and lateral movement of L3 on L4 and L4 on L5.

the PA neutral view. Note the left lateral flexion subluxation of L5 on the sacrum and the tropism at L5-S1, with the right facets being sagittal and the left facets being obliquely coronal in their planes of articulation. Dye from prior myelography can be seen in the dural root sleeve.

Figure 5.17 is the left lateral bending study. Note spinous process deviation to the left. Figure 5.18 is the right lateral bending study and shows failure of right lateral movement of L5 on the sacrum. L5 is a hypomobile fixation subluxation, as evidenced by failure of lateral flexion or spinous process motion beyond the midline, which occurs in lateral disc protrusion.

Howe (personal communication) has said that the disc lesion is an area of hypomobility on the cineradiography study. Movement occurs above or below the disc lesion subluxation, but the disc is a hypomobile segment.

Figures 5.19 and 5.20 demonstrate the mechanics of the antalgic leans shown in Figures 5.16, 5.17, and 5.18.

Figures 5.21, 5.22, and 5.23 are studies of a patient with right medial disc protrusion at L5-S1. Figure 5.21 is the neutral PA view of the L5-S1 interspace in this patient with pain down the right 1st sacral dermatome. Note the right lateral flexion of L5 on the sacrum and the tropism present, with the L5-S1 left facets being sagittal and the right facets being coronal. Figure 5.22 shows right lateral bending of the lumbar spine. Note a Lovett-positive scoliosis. Figure 5.23 shows left lateral bending of the lumbar spine with failure of lateral flexion of L5 on the sacrum and with hypomobility of the segments above to laterally flex left. This subluxation pattern is quite compatible with the motion studies observed during physical examination.

Figure 5.24 is a schematic representation of antalgia in the patient in Figures 5.21, 5.22, and 5.23.

White and Panjabi (11) state that lateral bending produces 2° to 3° of motion at L5-S1, and Tanz (12) has found that lateral bending produces 7° to 8° of motion at L4-L5 and L3-L4. Therefore, the greater mobility at the L4-L5 level than at the L5-S1 level would help to account for the greater lateral subluxation occurring in disc protrusions.

Figures 5.25, 5.26, and 5.27 are studies of L4-L5 left medial disc protrusion. Figure 5.25 is the neutral PA view of L4-L5 and shows L4 in left lateral flexion subluxation on L5. The patient has left L5 dermatome pain indicative of a left L4-L5 medial disc lesion. Figure 5.26 is the left lateral bending study of the lumbar spine, with good lateral bending shown above L4-L5. Figure 5.27 is the right lateral bending study and shows failure of lateral flexion of L4 on L5. This is a fixation hypomobile discogenic subluxation. Note the motion of the lumbar levels above L4-L5 to the right.

Figures 5.28, 5.29, and 5.30, respectively, are schematic representations of antalgia in the patient in Figures 5.25, 5.26, and 5.27.

Figure 5.31 is a standing anteroposterior lumbopelvic view of a patient who has

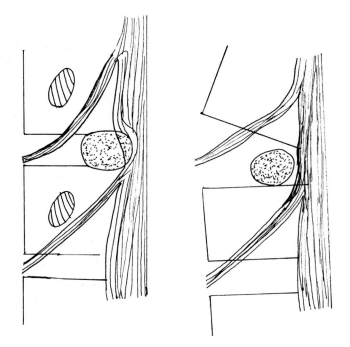

**Figure 5.19 (*left*).** A disc protrusion lateral to the nerve root.
**Figure 5.20 (*right*).** Right lean to relieve pressure caused by disc protrusion lateral to nerve root.

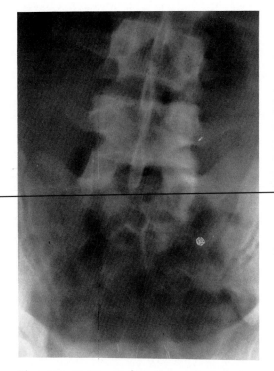

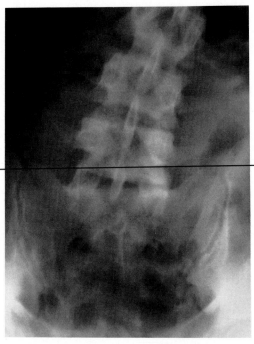

**Figure 5.21.** Neutral posteroanterior view of L5-S1. Note right lateral flexion of L5 on the sacrum. Tropism can be seen at L5-S1.

**Figure 5.22.** Right lateral flexion view showing Lovett-positive curve with spinous deviation into the concavity of the curve.

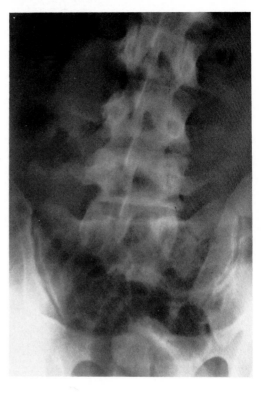

**Figure 5.23.** Left lateral flexion view showing Lovett failure curve with failure of the lumbar bodies to flex left and the spinous processes rotating left.

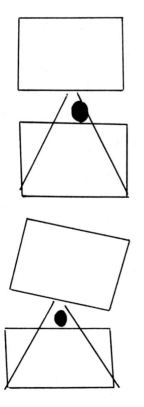

**Figure 5.24.** Schematic of L5 right medial disc protrusion in relation to the right S1 nerve root. The patient leans right to move the nerve root away from the disc; i.e., the patient leans into the side of the pain (right side) to relieve the pressure from an L5 disc protrusion medial to the S1 nerve root.

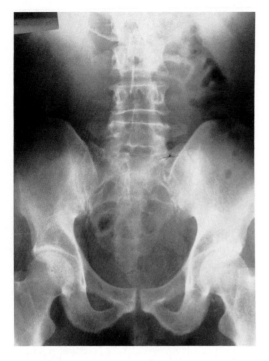

**Figure 5.25.** Posteroanterior view of the lumbar spine shows left lateral subluxation of L4 on L5.

**Figure 5.26.** Left lateral flexion view showing normal lateral flexion mechanics. All segments have spinous process rotation into the concave side (Lovett-positive motion).

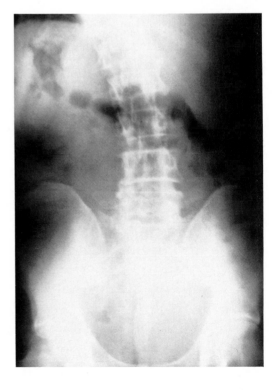

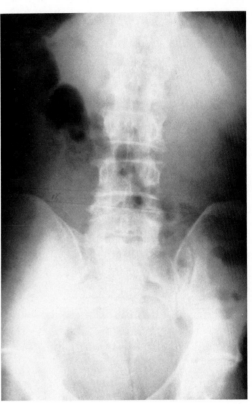

**Figure 5.27.** Right lateral flexion view. L4 fails to laterally flex right on L5. The spinous processes do not rotate right (Lovett motion failure).

had two myelograms for persistent low back and right leg 1st sacral dermatome pain. This x-ray, if read alone, might be interpreted as being relatively erect with no spinal unit subluxation patterns. There is tropism at L5-S1, with the right facet being sagittal and the left facet being coronal.

Figure 5.32 reveals normal lateral bending to the left. The spinous processes deviate to the concavity on the left and the bodies deviate to the convexity on the right.

Figure 5.33, however, is most informative; without it, misinterpretation of this spine would have occurred. In this right

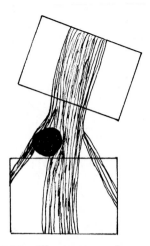

**Figure 5.30.** Illustration demonstrating how right lateral bending pulls the L5 nerve root into the left L4 medial disc protrusion and aggravates pain.

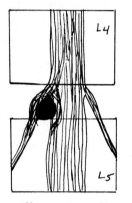

**Figure 5.28.** Illustration demonstrating how standing erect pulls the L5 nerve root into the L4 medial disc protrusion.

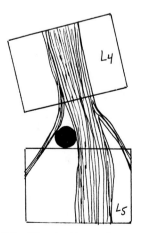

**Figure 5.29.** Illustration demonstrating how left lateral bending pulls the L5 nerve root away from the L4 medial disc protrusion and relieves pain.

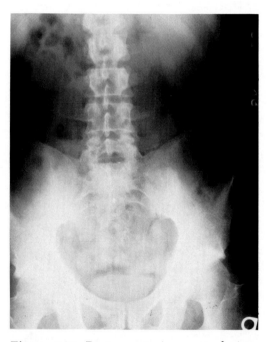

**Figure 5.31.** Posteroanterior neutral view of the lumbar spine which appears quite free of lateral curvature.

lateral flexion study, a Lovett reverse curve is shown. The spinous processes deviate to the convexity on the left and the bodies deviate to the concavity on the right. There is some right lateral flexion

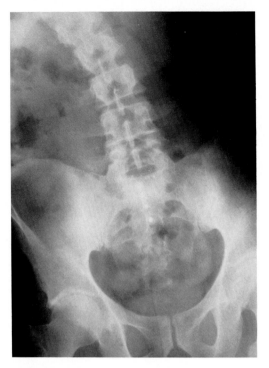

**Figure 5.32.** Left lateral flexion view of the same patient as in Figure 5.31. Normal Lovett-positive motion is shown with spinous processes rotated to the concave side.

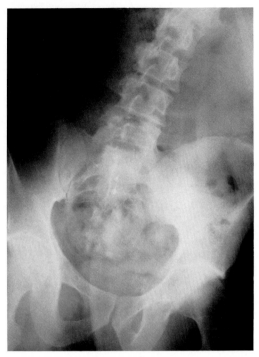

**Figure 5.33.** Right lateral flexion of the same patient as in Figure 5.32. Abnormal lateral movement with spinous process deviation to the convex side (Lovett negative) is shown. The right hemipelvis drops markedly.

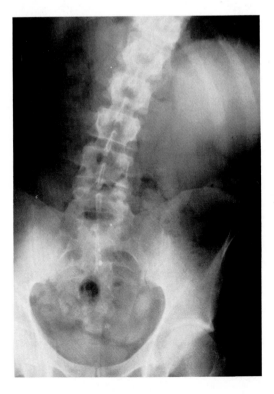

**Figure 5.34.** Repeat view of the same patient as in Figure 5.33 following 2 weeks of Cox flexion distraction manipulation. The right hemipelvis is level now. The spinous processes rotate to the midline instead of the convexity.

of L4 on L5, of L3 on L4, and of L2 on L3, but there is also marked inferiority of the right hemipelvis on right lateral bending.

Figure 5.34 is a repeat right lateral bending study of the same patient as in Figure 5.33 following 2 weeks of flexion distraction manipulation. Now the spinous processes deviate to the midline, and the pelvis no longer is inferior on lateral bending.

## References

1. Weitz EM: The lateral bending spine. *Spine* 6(4): 388–397, 1981.
2. Van Damme W, Hessels G, Verhelst M, Van Laer L, Van Es I: Relative efficacy of clinical examination, electromyography, plain film radiography, myelography and lumbar phlebography in the diagnosis of low back pain and sciatica. *Neuroradiology* 18:109–118, 1979.
3. Duncan W, Haen TI: A new approach to the diagnosis of herniation of the intervertebral disc. *Surg Gynecol Obstet* 75:257–267, 1942.
4. Falconer MA, McGeorge M, Begg AC: Surgery of lumbar intervertebral disc protrusion: study of principles and results based upon 100 consecutive cases submitted to operation. *Br J Surg* 1:225–249, 1948.
5. Hadley LA: Construction of the intervertebral foramen—a cause of nerve root pressure. *JAMA* 140:473–475, 1949.
6. Schalimtzek M: Functional roentgen exam of degenerated and normal intervertebral discs of the lumbar spine. *Acta Radiol [Suppl] (Stockh)* 116:300–306, 1954.
7. Hasner E, Schalimtzek M, Snorrason E: Roentgenographic examination of function of lumbar spine. *Acta Radiol [Diagn] (Stockh)* 37:141–149, 1952.
8. Breig A: *Adverse Mechanical Tension in the Central Nervous System.* New York, John Wiley and Sons, 1978.
9. Finneson BE: *Low Back Pain.* Philadelphia, JB Lippincott, 1973.
10. Nachemson AL: The lumbar spine, an orthopaedic challenge. *Spine* 1(1):59–69, 1976.
11. White AA, Panjabi MM: *Clinical Biomechanics of the Spine.* Philadelphia, JB Lippincott, 1978.
12. Tanz SS: Motion of the lumbar spine, a roentgenographic study. *AJR* 69:399–412, 1953.

# CHAPTER 6

*Genius may be described as the spirit of discovery. . . . It is the eye of intellect, and the wing of thought. . . . It is always in advance of its time. . . . [the] pioneer for the generation it precedes.*

*—Simms*

# Transitional Vertebrae

Except for facet tropism, a change in the number of mobile vertebrae in the lumbar spine is the most significant congenital vertebral anomaly that can cause low back pain. Lumbarization of the 1st sacral vertebra (giving the individual, in effect, six lumbar vertebrae) increases the lever arm of the lumbar spine and causes greater stress on the lumbosacral joint. In contrast, sacralization of the 5th lumbar vertebra (reducing the number of mobile vertebrae in the lumbar region to four) is unlikely to cause symptoms when the entire vertebra is solidly incorporated into the sacrum. Occasionally, only one transverse process articulates with the sacrum, altering spinal mechanics and resulting in severe instability and stress (1).

Unilateral sacralization of a lumbar vertebra or lumbarization of a sacral vertebra produces a condition known as Bertolotti's syndrome (Fig. 6.1), which has been diagnosed with increasing frequency in the past 10 years. Unilateral contact places unusual stress on the spine, and the resulting torque movements often cause herniation of the disc one level above the sacralization or lumbarization. Herniation, in turn, produces symptoms of nerve root entrapment. In the patient with Bertolotti's sydrome, surgery to decompress the herniated disc should always include spinal fusion to weld the affected vertebrae together so that further torque stresses are eliminated.

## TREATMENT

In the research paper on 576 patients with back pain, it was reported that it was more difficult to relieve pain caused by transitional segments than that caused by any other condition (3). Wigh (2) found that none of the 42 patients who had disc surgery had any sign of disc protrusion under the transitional segment. The disc at the transitional segment is hypoplastic, and the stress is placed on the segment above; i.e., if L5 is transitional, the L4-L5 disc is under stress and will bulge after annular failure. Treatment, therefore, may not provide the desired outcome.

We treat patients with transitional vertebrae by first eliminating rotatory movements of the lumbar spine and pelvis, especially if severe pain is present. This is accomplished by having the patient wear a 10-inch lumbar support until pain is relieved by 50%. The patient is advised to wear the support whenever he performs any activity in which twisting is involved, even when he feels no pain.

Further, the patient is sent to the Low Back Wellness School, where he learns how to lift weight without hurting his back and how to avoid rotatory movements that exacerbate his back pain. All of the nine Cox exercises are also recommended.

## Manipulation

Figure 6.2 shows hand contact on the spinous process one level above the transitional segment and not more than 1 finger pressure on the caudal section of the table. This opens the discal space, and the articular facets can be put through their normal ranges of motion. Figure 6.3 shows a Dutchman roll under the abdomen to increase the fulcrum force. It also gives relief to the patient when in pain.

**Lumbosacral Transitional Vertebrae (sacralization of L5)**

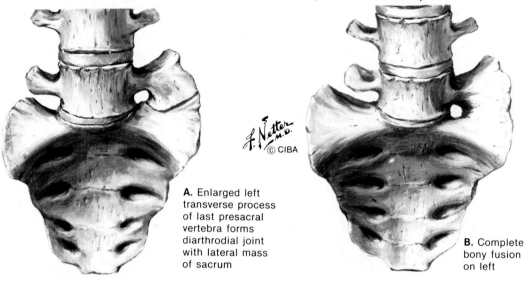

**A.** Enlarged left transverse process of last presacral vertebra forms diarthrodial joint with lateral mass of sacrum

**B.** Complete bony fusion on left

**Figure 6.1.** Illustration of lumbosacral transitional vertebrae (sacralization of L5) by Frank H. Netter, M.D. (Reproduced with permission from H. A. Keim and W. H. Kirkaldy-Willis: Clinical Symposia. *Ciba Found Symp* (32)6:89, 1980 (1). © 1980, CIBA Pharmaceutical Company, Division of CIBA-GEIGY Corporation. All rights reserved.)

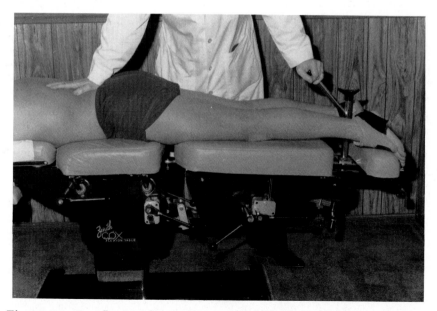

**Figure 6.2.** Cox flexion distraction applied to the transitional segment.

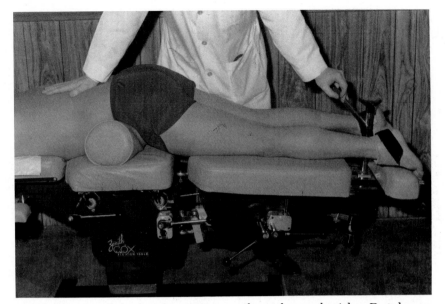

**Figure 6.3.** Flexion of the lumbar spine can be enhanced with a Dutchman role.

The same therapy applied to the patient with a transitional segment is applied as to the patient with disc protrusion following manipulation.

## CASE STUDIES

**Case 1** is of a 17-year-old white woman who for the past 2 years has experienced low back pain following gymnastics, especially after bending and hyperextension exercise. The pain has worsened in last few months.

Range of motion is beyond normal. The straight leg raising test is negative. Kemp's sign and Déjérine's triad are negative. No motor or sensory changes are noted.

X-rays reveal:

1. Spatulization L5 transverse processes forming pseudoarthrosis with the sacrum (Fig. 6.4).
2. Dextrorotation of lumbar vertebral bodies (Fig. 6.4).
3. An 8-mm short left femoral head (corrected by a 6-mm lift) (Fig. 6.4).
4. Rudimentary disc at the transitional L5-S1 level (Figs. 6.5 and 6.6).

This patient has transitional L5 vertebra with pseudosacralization and left short leg (8 mm) with dextrorotation of the lumbar vertebral bodies.

She was advised to avoid hyperextension in gymnastics and to wear a left 6-mm heel build-up, which provided good relief from pain.

**Case 2** is of a 39-year-old white man who has had right low back pain for 1 week after bending forward to wash his hair. Since his teenage years he has had progressively worsening episodes of low back pain. In 1979, while bent over a drawer, he felt immediate low back pain which was the most severe of his life. It was diagnosed as a partial slipped disc. Drugs in addition to bed rest have been his only treatment. Finally, over the objections of his family, he consulted a chiropractic physician.

Déjérine's triad is positive for low back pain. The straight leg raise is positive on the right at 50°, causing low back pain. Kemp's sign is bilaterally positive. Range of motion on flexion is 65°, on extension is 22°, on right lateral flexion is 12°, on left lateral flexion is 8°, on right rotation is 20°, and on left rotation is 20°.

X-rays reveal:

1. Sacralization of L5, which is bilaterally false, forming pseudoarthrosis with the sacrum (Fig. 6.7).
2. Lovett-positive motion, with the spinous processes deviating to the concavity on the left and the bodies deviating to the convexity on the right (Fig. 6.8).
3. Lovett reverse motion, with the spinous process deviating to the convexity on the left and the bodies deviating to the concavity on the right (Fig. 6.9), which represents severe psoas or multifidus spasm.
4. A large L5 left superior facet that closely approximates the L4 pedicle (Fig. 6.10).
5. Tropism at the L4-L5 facets, with the left facets being coronal and right facets being semisagittal.

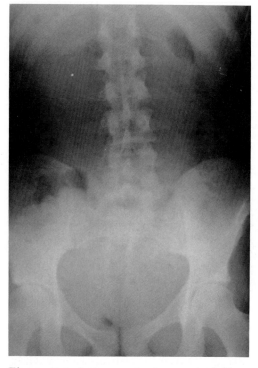

**Figure 6.4.** Anteroposterior neutral film.

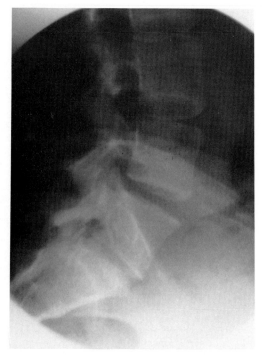

**Figure 6.6.** Lateral spot film.

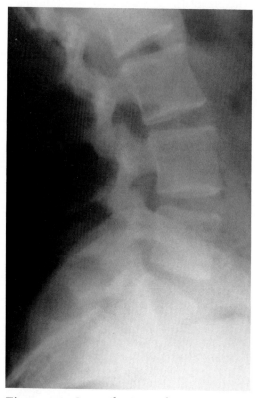

**Figure 6.5.** Lateral view of same patient as in Figure 6.4.

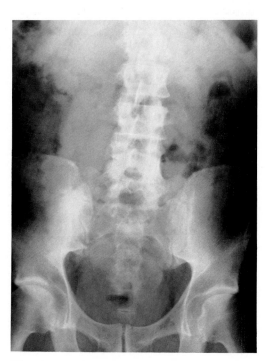

**Figure 6.7.** Anteroposterior neutral view.

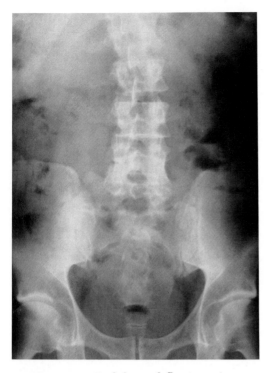

Figure 6.8. Left lateral flexion view.

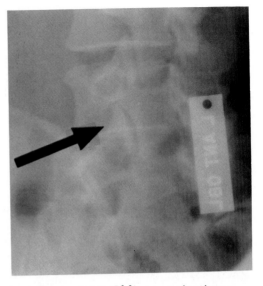

Figur☉ 6.10. Oblique projection.

This patient has Bertolotti's syndrome, i.e., a transitional L5 segment (sacralization) with annular discal irritation at the L4-L5 disc; Lovett reverse scoliosis on lateral flexion to the right side; a hyperplastic left superior L5 facet forming possible pseudoarthrosis with the L4 pedicle; and tropism at L4-L5.

The biomechanics of this spine are interesting in that there is a lateral bending aberrancy with an accompanying L5 transitional bilateral pseudosacralization. This condition places great stress on the L4-L5 articulation and, coupled with the tropism at L4-L5, results in an unstable articulation at this level. Remember that the disc of a transitional segment does not prolapse and that it is common for the disc directly above this segment to be damaged. The combination of a transitional segment and a disc lesion above is called Bertolotti's syndrome.

One session of distraction manipulation resulted in complete relief from pain. The patient went through Low Back Wellness School to learn to avoid movements in daily living that aggravate his condition.

**Case 3** is of an 83-year-old white woman who has low back and left leg pain. She had sought neurosurgical consultation and was told that she had a congenital defect and that surgery could be done if she wanted it. She was advised to wait until the pain became bad enough to warrant surgery.

On examination, a left rotation of the lumbar vertebral bodies is noted. Range of motion is 60° on flexion, 10° on extension, 20° on right lateral bending, 10° on left lateral bending, 20° on right rotation, and 10° on left

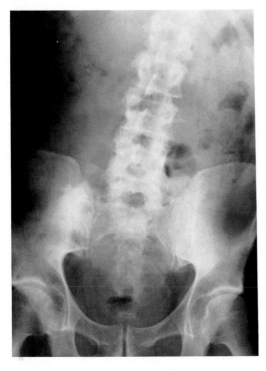

Figure 6.9. Right lateral flexion view.

rotation. Straight leg raise is normal. Kemp's sign is bilaterally positive. Deep ankle jerks are active and 3+ equal. Muscle strength is equal in the lower extremities. Pain on palpation is present at the left L5-S1 level and radiates into the left buttock.

X-rays reveal:

1. Levoscoliosis of the lumbar spine (Fig. 6.11).

2. A transitional S1 segment on the left with true fusion of the left S1 transverse process with the sacrum (Fig. 6.12).

3. A 25% spondylolisthesis of L5 on the sacrum (Fig. 6.13).

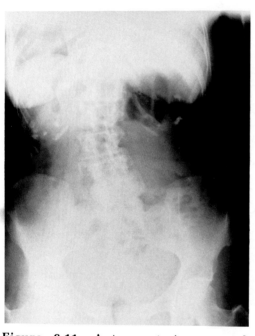

**Figure 6.11.** Anteroposterior neutral view.

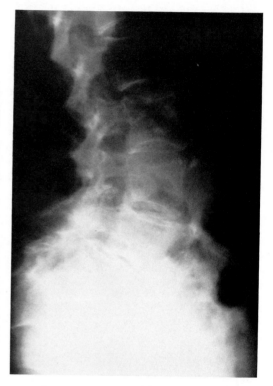

**Figure 6.13.** Lateral lumbar film.

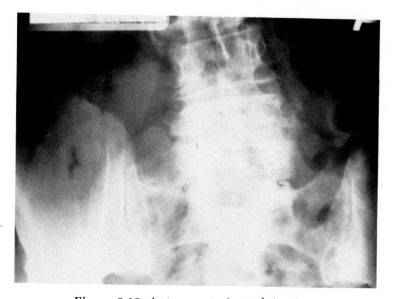

**Figure 6.12.** Anteroposterior pelvic view.

This patient has levoscoliosis of the lumbar spine, a 25% spondylolisthesis at L5, and left lumbarization of the S1 transverse process. This combination of lumbarization and spondylolisthesis is very uncommon.

After 3 weeks of care, the patient did not feel relief from pain and stopped treatment.

## References

1. Keim HA, Kirkaldy-Willis WH: Clinical symposia. *Ciba Found Symp* 32(6):89, 1980.
2. Wigh RE: Transitional lumbosacral discs. *Spine*, March/April 1981.
3. Cox J, Shreiner S: Chiropractic manipulation in low back pain and sciatica: statistical data on the diagnosis, treatment and response of 576 consecutive cases. *J Manip Physiolog Ther* 7(1):1–11, 1984.

# CHAPTER 7

# Stenosis

Many in the chiropractic profession remember the work of Earl Rich, D.C., radiologist for the Lincoln Chiropractic College, on pedicogenic spondylosis. This man, who died prior to the full impact of his efforts in this field being felt, contributed greatly to our understanding of a very important aspect of low back pain. This article highlights the implications of Rich's work on pedicogenic stenosis in the further study of the etiology of low back pain.

Lumbar spondylosis is the lipping or marginal vertebral osteophytic formation secondary to degenerative disc disease. It is not observed in the absence of disc degeneration and collapse (1–3); i.e., it is not noted in the presence of a normal disc. Vernon-Roberts and Pirie (4) believe that there is a direct relationship between the degree of disc degeneration, the marginal osteophyte formation on the vertebral bodies, and the apophyseal joint changes which suggest that disc degeneration is the primary event leading to degenerative spondylosis. Dics degeneration is the genesis of osteoarthrosis of the apophyseal joints, as well as of the spondylosis seen commonly in the lumbar spine. Figure 7.1 shows the spondylotic change seen so typically in the lumbar spine, which follows collapse of the disc and protrusion of the annulus. According to Collins (5), spondylosis primarily refers to separation of the annulus fibers from their firmly embedded attachments to the margins of the vertebral bodies. Periosteal elevation stimulates osteoblastic activity, resulting in the anterolateral osteophytic change and the possible bridging that follow. Osteophytosis, therefore, is the spondylotic effect of intervertebral nuclear protrusion through the annulus, elevating the periosteum and resulting in subperiosteal osteogenesis.

The term arthrosis describes the sclerosis and loss of joint space that accompanies a synovial lined joint, namely, the articular facets. Thus, we refer to discogenic spondylosis as an early change in disc degeneration and to discogenic spondyloarthrosis as a later manifestation. Interestingly, according to Schmorl and Junghanns (6) the marginal osteophytes may appear within 4 to 8 weeks following injury. Remember, therefore, that the term osteoarthrosis of the spine is used to refer only to the degenerative changes occurring in the synovial lined joints, namely, the articular facets, not to changes occurring in the anterolateral vertebral plates following disc degeneration.

## PEDICOGENIC STENOSIS

Figures 7.2 and 7.3 are photographs of two lumbar vertebrae. Figure 7.2 shows the typical round vertebral canal with fairly well developed pedicles, whereas Figure 7.3 shows a trefoil canal with underdeveloped pedicles.

Various clinicians have measured the

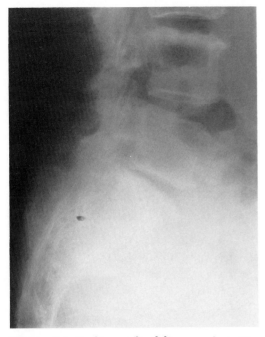

**Figure 7.1.** Radiograph of discogenic spondyloarthrosis at the L5-S1 level. The facet syndrome is present at both the L4 and the L5 level.

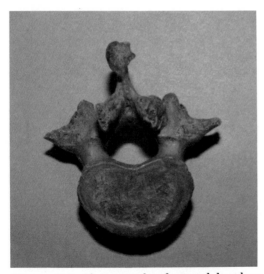

**Figure 7.2.** Photograph of actual lumbar vertebra showing a rounded vertebral canal with well-developed pedicles.

interpedicular and sagittal diameters of the canal. Epstein et al. (7) found the sagittal diameter normally to be 15 to 23 mm, with a measurement of less than 13

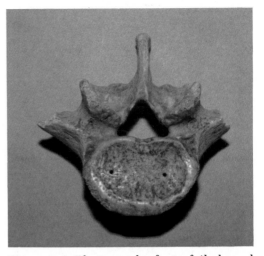

**Figure 7.3.** Photograph of a trefoil-shaped vertebral canal with underdeveloped pedicles.

mm to be clinically significant of narrowing. He further noted that accompanying the shortened pedicles are thickened neural arches and prominent facets which further narrow the diameter. Paine and Haung (1) report that the sagittal diameter of canals in patients with stenosis is 8 mm. The pioneer and perhaps the best authority on stenosis of the canal is Verbiest (8) who states that a sagittal diameter of less than 12 mm is definitely too short. His conclusion is based on the measurements of the vertebrae of American (9), Dutch (10), Norwegian and Lapp (11), and White and Zulu skeletons (12). According to Verbiest (8), absolute stenosis is indicated when the sagittal diameter is 10 mm or less, and which may produce signs of radicular compression in the absence of any additional compressive agent, such as disc protrusion, ligamentum flavum hypertrophy, and lamina hypertrophy. Midsagittal diameters between 10 and 12 mm are classified as relative stenosis and serve as warnings of possible future disturbances caused by the development of spondylosis and its accompanying arthritic changes in the facets. According to Verbiest, the narrow canal in the presence of mild disc protrusion or minimal ventral osteophytosis produces symptoms which could be well tolerated in a lumbar canal of normal size.

In our clinical investigation, we used

the technic of Eisenstein (12), which is illustrated in Figure 7.4. Figure 7.5 and 7.6 demonstrate the use of this technic on actual x-rays. Figure 7.5 reveals the sagittal diameter of a well-formed canal. According to Epstein et al. (7), the sagittal diameter of a good-sized canal is equal to one half of the diameter of the vertebral body. Application of the Eisenstein technic in Figure 7.6 reveals stenosis of the L5 level, since the sagittal diameter of the canal measures less than 12 mm; this underdevelopment can be seen by scanning the radiograph even if one does not meas-

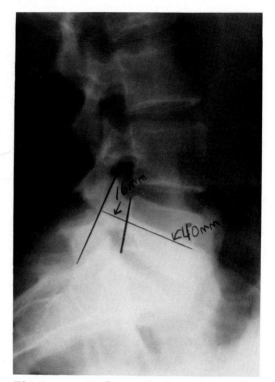

**Figure 7.5.** Radiograph demonstrating a well-developed sagittal diameter of the vertebral canal.

ure the diameter. It is well to remember that the L5-S1 intervertebral foramina are the smallest in the lumbar spine and that the size of the L5 nerve root exiting through them is the largest of the lumbar cauda equina. Rabinovitch (13) observed that the L3 through S5 nerve roots are less mobile than those above these levels, making these nerve roots more susceptible to compression by disc protrusion and osteophyte formation than those in the levels above. According to Hadley (14), the lumbar nerve roots occupy from 17% to 25% of the upper aspect of the foramina. Epstein et al. (7) found that intervertebral foramina in normal cadavers have a sagittal diameter roughly equal to that of both the foramen and neural canal but that they are consistently 2 to 3 mm less in the lower three lumbar segments where the nerve roots are larger.

## Symptoms of a Stenotic Canal

Until recently, the term intermittent claudication was believed to be associated

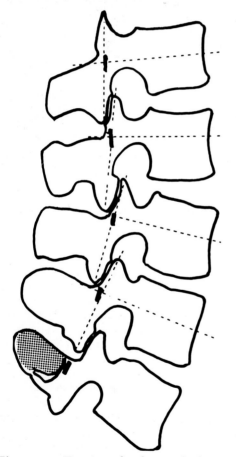

**Figure 7.4.** Tracing of radiograph showing the method of locating the posterior border of the spinal canal. The posterior border of the canal at the 5th lumbar vertebra is consistently more posterior than is expected. (Reproduced with permission from S. Eisenstein: *Clinical Orthopaedics and Related Research* 115:43, 1976, (12).)

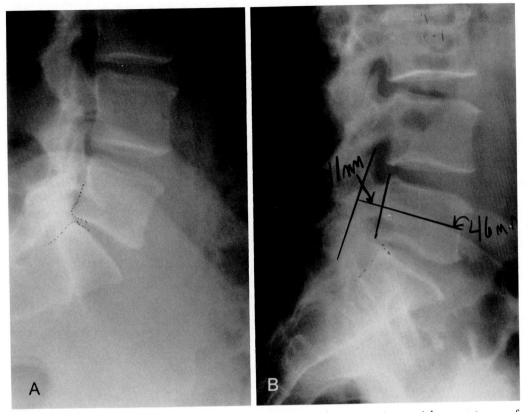

**Figure 7.6.** Radiographs of a stenotic vertebral canal in a patient with symptoms of intermittent neurogenic claudication. *A*, retrolisthesis of L5 on the sacrum; *B*, stenosis measurements.

with reduced blood flow to the lower extremities, resulting in hypoxia of the muscles with attendant cramping and pain in the lower extremities. The French applied this term to the atheroscleromatous plaqueing of the arteries in old carriage horses when these horses were unable to walk due to limp. This concept was applied to humans with similar plaqueing until vascular surgeons found that there was no interference with the blood supply of the lower extremities and further explanation for this phenomenon had to be made. Today, the term neurogenic intermittent claudication is used and applies to those conditions found in people who have such lower extremity pain and who have no ischemia to the leg muscles but have compression of the cauda equina in the lumbar spine.

In the conclusion to their article, Dyck et al. (15) state that the diagnosis of neu-

rogenic intermittent claudication can be made on the clinical findings alone and that demonstration of a deformity by myelography is not diagnostic proof of the syndrome.

The pain of intermittent claudication may be unilateral or bilateral and may be more severe in one leg than in the other. It is caused by or aggravated by walking or standing for a long period of time. The pain is relieved by flexion of the lumbar spine and is aggravated by extension of the spine. It is interesting to note that in 1911 Goldthwaite (15a) was credited with paralysis of a patient when he placed that patient in a hyperextension plaster cast for the treatment of low back pain.

Figure 7.7 is a diagnostic differential chart of the lower extremity pain as caused by arterial insufficiency and neurogenic claudication. According to Weinstein et al. (16), the most classic clinical

| Finding | Arterial Insufficient Claudication | Neurogenic Claudication |
|---|---|---|
| Arterial pulses of femoral, popliteal, post, tibial, and dorsalis pedis | One or more diminished | Normal |
| Pain in legs induced by | Exercise such as walking but not by posture change | Walking, standing kneeling, hyperextension |
| Relieved by | Rest | Bend forward, squat, flexion |
| Accompanied by low back, buttock, thigh pain | Rare | Common |
| Type pain | Cramping is severe if exercise is continued | Dysesthesia such as numbness, tingling, and burning |
| Comes at rest | No | Yes |
| Sensory loss | Rare | Mild |
| Leg raise | Normal | Normal |
| Arterial murmur | Yes | No |
| Plain x-ray findings | Arteriosclerosis of abdominal aorta or iliac and femoral vessels | Discogenic spondyloarthrosis |

**Figure 7.7.** Differential diagnostic factors of intermittent claudication.

symptom of a narrowed lumbar canal is aggravation of the pain in the lower extremities following exaggerated lordosis of the lumbar spine. This classical clinical symptom is one of numbness and tingling or a feeling that the legs are asleep. It may be brought on by standing, bending backward, or reaching overhead. Ehni (17) has shown that during myelography the extension of the lumbar spine produces total block of the column, whereas flexion permits the dye to pass through the lumbar spine.

An interesting diagnostic point is presented by Dyck et al. (15) who say that the ankle reflex, when accompanying intermittent claudication, may be absent after exercise and present when at rest. Furthermore, Weinstein et al. (18) noted that there were two patients in the claudication groups who when ambulatory had urinary retention but following rest were able to void normally.

Although an exact neurological explanation for the changes in lumbar stenosis is difficult, certain facts have been established. Sunderland (19) believes that ischemia of a nerve root must accompany any compression that is great enough to alter its nerve function. Such compression produces nerve sheath constriction, axonal narrowing, and partial obstruction of the vasa nervorum. Nerve roots are more vulnerable to stretch than are peripheral nerves (20). The pain of neurogenic claudication is that of paresthesias and numbness in the legs due to the mechanical compression of the nerve roots. While documenting this phenomenon, Ehni (17) found simultaneous impairment of the perceptions of touch, pressure, and pain stimuli applied to the area supplied by the affected nerves. He believes that this may explain the imprecise and puzzling complaint of the patient who reports that his painful legs "go dead" or "go out" when he walks or stands.

Sebolt and Elies (21) report that 28 patients in the neurology department of the University of Tubingen who underwent disc surgery were found to have a 25% increase of blood supply to the lower extremities within 2 to 3 weeks following surgical root decompression. An explanation for the relief of leg pain and for the increased blood flow in the lower extremity is that the irritation of the cauda equina by disc protrusion or a narrowed canal also creates a relative ischemia of the involved nerve roots. This results in hypoxia which is further aggravated by exercise and the increased oxygen consumption in the activated nerves (22). Evans (23) found that his patients could walk farther before claudication symptoms appeared when they breathed 100% pure oxygen rather than room air or 12% oxygen. Experimental studies have demonstrated that oxygen uptake in nerves increases proportionately with an increase in frequency of fiber stimulation (24).

Therefore, in summary, true intermittent claudication due to arterial blockage, as in atheroscleromatous plaqueing of the femoral arteries, results in lower extremity pain at exercise, which is relieved by rest. Hyperextension of the lumbar spine does not aggravate the pain associated with true intermittent claudication. In neurogenic intermittent claudication, the pain not only is brought about by walking but also is brought about by hyperextension of the lumbar spine and by standing and is not relieved by rest. Always remember that the patient with neurogenic intermittent claudication tends to stand in a bent-forward posture, so as to relieve the pressure on the cauda-equina. This is not true of the patient with true intermittent claudication.

## Impressions and Conclusions

The existence of the stenotic lumbar canal is another factor to be considered in the effectiveness of manipulation of the lumbar spine. Certainly, the congenital presence of this abnormality cannot be reversed without surgical relief. Yet, the best of manipulation may well render a measure of relief for the patients without providing 100% relief from symptoms. The changes occurring with the stenotic changes, namely, ligamentum flavum hypertrophy and disc degeneration, may not be reversible. Ehni, Weinstein (16), and others have had a 70% success rate with surgery in decompression laminotomy of patients with a stenotic lumbar spine. Thus, clinical investigation and statistic keeping eventually will provide an answer to the effectiveness of manipulation versus that of surgery in the treatment of patients with this condition.

With the technics of measurement outlined in this article, it certainly is possible to determine the existence of lumbar canal stenosis and the prevalence of spondylotic canal radiculopathy by clinical investigation. Clinically, follow-up will show the effectiveness of manipulation. In a report in the *Journal of the Canadian Chiropractic Association* (25), 744 patients with neck and back pain were treated with spinal manipulation. These patients were referred from the Orthopedic Clinic at the University Hospital in Saskatoon. The reports covered only those suffering with low back and leg pain and the effects of manipulation. It was found that 70% of the patients did well and that spinal manipulation now receives top priority in the conservative management of back

problems at the University center. One of the main points that I wish to stress to you is that the postsurgical patient did very well under chiropractic care and that center patients were routinely referred back 3 months after surgery for manipulative care. Spinal surgery was regarded not as the end but rather as the beginning of manipulative involvement. Thus, there is the strong possibility that in the treatment of the patient with a stenotic lumbar canal, the combination of surgical decompression and manipulation may render the greatest benefit.

A sophisticated study (26) of various methods of measuring the inner diameter of the lumbar vertebral canal was presented in the June, 1978, issue of the *Jour-*

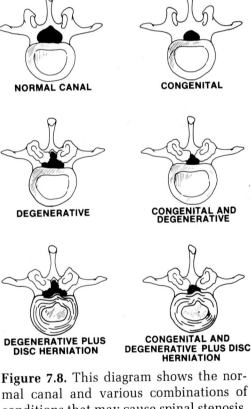

**Figure 7.8.** This diagram shows the normal canal and various combinations of conditions that may cause spinal stenosis. Congenital stenosis with disc herniation alone, not pictured here, is another possibility. (Reproduced with permission from A. A. White and M. M. Panjabi: *Clinical Biomechanics of the Spine.* Philadelphia, J. B. Lippincott, 1978, p. 293.)

*nal of Manipulative and Physiological Therapeutics* by Michael T. Buehler, D.C., former Chief of Radiology, National College of Chiropractic. You are urged to read it for an excellent study of lumbar canal mensuration.

Figure 7.8 shows various stenotic formations. X-ray may reveal the osteoarthritic involvement of facets that enter and reduce the lateral recess of the vertebral canal. Myelographic studies to define it are performed by injecting 30 ml of dye into the subarachnoid space and taking films with the patient upright. An anteroposterior diameter of less than 14 mm is suggestive of stenosis (27). The lumbar spinal canal usually becomes progressively wider from L1 to L5 (28) and is shallowest at L5.

Figure 7.9 illustrates the formula of Jones and Thomson (29) for measuring the ratio of the canal to the vertebral body, which is an accurate radiographic indicator of lumbar stenosis. This technic eliminated misinterpretation of the plain radiographs due to patient size, magnification, and rotation and provided good clinical correlation in 12 of 13 patients. Ratios of 1:2 to 1:4 (small normal) were considered normal, and ratios of 1:4 to 1:6

were considered stenotic. Of course, this technic does not provide as accurate a measurement as does CT scan, but it is a good indicator that more detailed tests such as CT or myelography are needed.

According to Epstein et al. (30), an anteroposterior spinal canal diameter of less than 13 mm (from the posterior margin of the intervertebral foramen to the posterior surface of the vertebral body) indicates stenosis. Hypertrophic osteoarthritic spurs may be tolerated in a normal canal but create severe compression of nerve roots in stenosis. Considerably more spurring can be tolerated at L5-S1 than at L4-L5 because of a "snug" bony confine at L4-L5 and a "great" amount of space at L5-S1 between neural elements and bone.

Figures 7.10 and 7.11 reveal why patients with stenosis stand in a flexed posture; i.e., to maximize the sagittal diameter of the spinal canal.

## Categories of Spinal Stenosis

Spinal stenosis is generally categorized into two types: congenital-developmental and acquired (28). Ordinarily, the interpedicular distance widens from the upper lumbar spine to the lower lumbar spine.

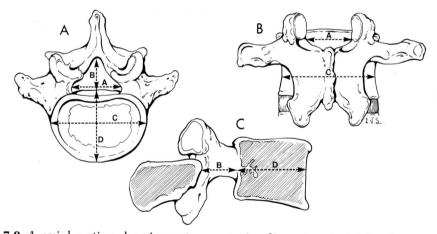

**Figure. 7.9.** *A,* axial section showing anteroposterior diameter of a 5th lumbar vertebra; *B,* superior view; *C,* median sagittal view. A, interpedicular distance; B, anteroposterior diameter of spinal canal; C, transverse diameter of vertebral body; D, anteroposterior diameter of vertebral body. The products AB and CD are compared. (Reproduced with permission from D. L. McRae: Radiology of the Lumbar Spinal Canal. In P. R. Weinstein et al.: *Lumbar Spondylosis: Diagnosis, Management and Surgical Treatment.* Year Book Medical Publishers, © Chicago, 1977.)

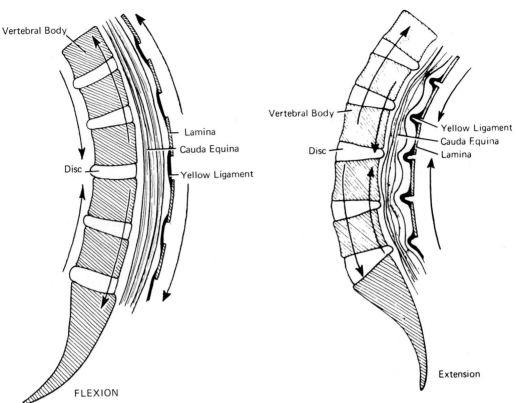

Vertebral Body

Lamina
Cauda Equina
Disc
Yellow Ligament

FLEXION

Vertebral Body

Yellow Ligament
Cauda Equina
Disc
Lamina

Extension

**Figure 7.10.** Increased spinal canal volume and decreased nerve root (cauda equina) bulk with flexion. (Reproduced with permission from B. E. Finneson: *Low Back Pain*, edition 2. Philadelphia, J. B. Lippincott, 1980, p. 432.)

**Figure 7.11.** Decreased spinal canal volume and increased nerve root bulk with extension. (Reproduced with permission from B. E. Finneson: *Low Back Pain*, edition 2. Philadelphia, J. B. Lippincott, 1980, p. 432.)

The most common cause of spinal stenosis is from degenerative disease. As the articular processes hypertrophy and bulge inwardly, the lower lumbar spine takes on a trefoil appearance. This appearance is often associated with lateral recess disease. In fact, in degenerative disease causing lumbar spinal stenosis, it is difficult to differentiate facet joint disease, lateral recess disease, and central canal stenosis, as they often occur simultaneously.

Spinal stenosis can be caused by thickening of the ligamentum flavum, which may account for some of the cases of clinical spinal stenosis with normal bony measurements. Soft-tissue windows should be used to best visualize the ligamentum flavum on CT examinations.

In facet joint disease, lumbar facet arthropathy can cause low back and sciatic pain almost indistinguishable from that due to a herniated nucleus pulposus. It is not unusual to have a combination of facet disease and disc disease at a single level. Osteophyte formation in the lumbar facet joints was defined by Carrera et al. (32) as excrescent new bone lacking a medullary space and arising from the margin of the joint. Hypertrophy is defined as an enlarged articular process with normal proportions of the medullary cavity and cortex.

The lateral recess has also been called the nerve root canal or tunnel. Anatomically, it is an area bordered laterally by the pedicle, posteriorly by the superior articular facet, and anteriorly by the posterior lateral surface of the vertebral body and the intervertebral disc. The nerve lies adjacent to the thecal sac in this recess and tends to exit the central canal immediately beneath the pedicle. The narrowest part of the lateral recess is at the superior border of each pedicle, due to the anterior slanting of the superior articular facet. Therefore, hypertrophy of the superior articular facet is more likely to cause nerve root compression at the superior border of the pedicle, and it is at this point that the height of the lateral recess should be measured. Although measurements for lateral recess stenosis are available, they should be used as guidelines only. A lateral recess of 2 mm or less is said to be diagnostic of lateral recess stenosis, a height of 3 mm or less is said to be highly indicative of lateral recess stenosis, and a lateral recess of 5 mm or more in height should rule out the possibility of a lateral recess stenosis. The clinical symptoms vary in these patients, and it can be difficult to diagnose lateral recess stenosis on clinical grounds alone. In the patient with lateral recess stenosis, typically, leg pain and paresthesia are brought on by standing and walking, and the pain is usually completely relieved by squatting or sitting, whereas in the patient with a herniated lumbar disc the symptoms are generally made worse by sitting. The intermittent compression of an entrapped nerve root from lateral recess stenosis during standing or walking is said to be most likely the result of a slight forward shift of the superior articular facet when the lumbar spine lordosis is accentuated. Thus, with more hypertrophy of the superior articular facet, lateral recess stenosis becomes more pronounced.

Narrowing of a neuroforamen at any level can cause nerve root symptoms. This can occur because of actual bony narrowing or from encroachment on the neuroforamen by an extruded disc fragment or a herniated nucleus pulposus. Postoperative fibrosis can also encroach on the neuroforamen and cause symptoms identical with those of bony stenosis. The posterior wall or roof is formed by the pars interarticularis.

Spondylolisthesis can be a cause of bilateral neuroforaminal stenosis. The pars interarticularis forms the posterior roof of the neuroforamen, and a break through the pars with subsequent slippage forward of the superior portion can occasionally pinch the exiting spinal nerve root.

Exertional leg pain may be secondary to a variety of problems. A systematic approach allows early, accurate diagnosis of patients with such pain. Noninvasive technics allow the differentiation between claudication due to vascular disease and that due to spinal stenosis (33).

Warren (as discussed in Ref. 33) set forth three criteria that define what he called true claudication. First, the pain must begin as a muscle cramp in the calf or thigh after the patient has walked a predictable distance. Second, it must be relieved by rest in the standing position after a predictable period of time. Finally, the pain must occur again after the patient walks a similar distance, and the pain must be relieved again by rest in the standing position after the same period of time as before. Exertional leg pain that does not satisfy all of these criteria must be suspected of being neuromuscular in origin. Pain of neuromuscular or skeleton etiology is generally much less consistent than arterial claudication. In contrast to true vascular claudication, the pain may begin in the lower back with radiation into the thigh, calf, and foot. The pain may begin after walking an unpredictable distance or may even occur with the patient in a standing or a sitting position. The history of pain that occurs with standing or sitting should alert the astute clinician to a diagnosis other than vascular claudication. The patient often states that he has good and bad days. He may give a history of being able to walk a prolonged distance on one day and only a few steps on a subsequent day. This pattern of inconsistency argues strongly against a vascular etiology. The pain of musculoskeletal etiology is also relieved if the patient assumes a supine or specific sitting position. Again, this is very uncharacteristic of vascular pain.

## VASCULAR CLAUDICATION

The patient with advanced peripheral vascular insufficiency shows evidence of hair loss and skin atrophy. Transcutaneous flow detection based on the principle of the Doppler effect uses blood pressure determination as a standard part of the physical examination for vascular disease. This is routinely measured in both upper extremities. A differential blood pressure between the upper extremities suggests vascular disease in the large branches of the aorta. Doppler testing has made it possible to determine the blood pressure at the ankle level in both the dorsalis pedis and the posterior tibialis artery. Pressure at the ankle should be equal to or slightly greater than arm pressure with the patient in the supine position. A systolic pressure in the ankle less than the systolic pressure in the arm suggests peripheral arterial disease. Comparison of the systolic pressures obtained at the ankle with those in the arm provides the ankle-to-arm index. This index is used to define the presence of hemodynamically significant vascular disease. An index of 0.6 or less has been determined to be diagnostic of vascular insufficiency significant enough to cause intermittent claudication. The index may be as low as 0.26 in the presence of rest, pain, and gangrene. Once it has been established that there is an abnormal index, the next step in this noninvasive evaluation is to measure the postexercise ankle pressure. The normal physiologic response to moderate exercise is a slight increase in the ankle pressure. In the presence of occlusive disease to the lower extremities, the major inflow vessels are unable to accommodate the increased demand to the lower extremities. The increased demand results in a lower peripheral resistance, opening of the collateral vascular beds, and a subsequent drop in perfusion pressure in the ankle. As a result of a limited inflow secondary to hemodynamically significant disease, the ankle pressure in patients with claudication falls after a period of exercise. This allows a documentation of the physiological events causing claudication. Exertional leg pain that occurs with walking but does not occur on the exercise bicycle is most characteristic of spinal stenosis. Verbiest (8) in 1954 described a leg pain that was similar to that in the patient with true claudication and was associated with developmental narrowing of the lumbar spinal canal and

called it spinal stenosis. Patients with leg pain due to spinal stenosis often experience the onset of symptoms while walking. These patients obtain relief by sitting down or bending at the waist. It is for this reason that these patients do not experience leg pain while pedaling the exercise bicycle.

The lateral recess syndrome (LRS) represents stenosis of the lateral subarticular gutter that will often lead to nerve root compression. The most common etiology is hypertrophy of the superior articular facets, which is associated with lumbar instability and arthrosis of the posterior joint complex. The diagnosis may be made clinically with a routine lumbosacral x-ray series but is not definitive without the use of CT scanning. Recent studies show that spinal manipulation can provide relief and should be considered before surgical referral for decompression is made (35).

## STOOP TEST

Dyck (36) states that in claudication patients, stooping increases the sagittal diameter of the vertebral canal and relieves back and leg pain.

It was found that there is a trend toward a narrower-than-normal canal in patients with a prolapsed disc (37). Thus, it has been concluded that in patients with a prolapsed lumbar intervertebral disc such narrowing enhances the effect of any disc protrusion, leading to severe symptoms of back and leg pain. Plain film lateral radiographs were made to measure the anteroposterior diameter of the spinal canal from the midline of the back of the vertebral body to the base of the opposing spinous process. Ratios of body to canal were made, with 1:2.5 being normal and 1:4.5 being narrow.

CT scanning has shown that the smallest normal anteroposterior diameters of the lumbar spinal canal occur between the posterior wall of the vertebral body and the anterosuperior margin of the spinous process and that the largest diameters occur at a level at which the inferior margin of the spinous process is opposite the posterosuperior margin of the next lower vertebral body. The smallest anteroposterior diameter that was normal was 11.5 mm (38).

Porter (as discussed in Ref. 39) found that 10% of the healthy population had lumbar spinal canals less than 1.4 cm wide. Of 154 patients with sciatica, 56% had spinal canals less than 1.4 cm wide. The implication is that individuals with narrow canals are more prone to back pain, since the main cause of severe back pain is intervertebral disc damage.

## VALUE OF PLAIN RADIOGRAPHIC EVALUATION FOR STENOSIS

This study indicates that plain films are of great usefulness in the diagnosis of lumbar spinal stenosis, contrary to the opinions of some authorities who believe that plain films are of little value. In a large number of cases, clinical presentation with careful analysis of plain films is sufficient to reach an almost certain diagnosis. *In spinal stenosis, the superior articular process is more sagitally oriented* (40).

## CONSERVATIVE VERSUS SURGICAL CARE OF STENOSIS

Surgical treatment of lumbar stenosis should be considered only after an adequate trial of conservative therapy has failed. This includes exercises, supports, medications, and manipulation. Conservative therapy should be continued indefinitely as long as pain is tolerated (41). According to Wiltsie et al. (43), neurologic changes alone are rarely indications for surgery.

## CASE STUDIES

**Case 1** is of a 50-year-old white man who has had low back pain for 12 days. His history reveals that he had had low back and leg pain 10 years ago.

Straight leg raise is negative except for the hamstrings, which are extremely short. Déjérine's triad is negative. Kemp's sign is negative. Range of motion is 80° on flexion and 20° on extension. All other movements are normal.

X-rays reveal:

1. The intercrestal line cuts the L4 body (Fig. 7.12). This means that maximum mobility is at the L4-L5 disc level, based on the work of MacGibbon and Farfan (42). Interestingly, the L4-L5 and L3-L4 discs show more degenerative changes than does the L5-S1 disc. Note the sagittal facet facings at L4-L5 and L5-S1.

2. Schmorl's nodes can be seen at the T12-

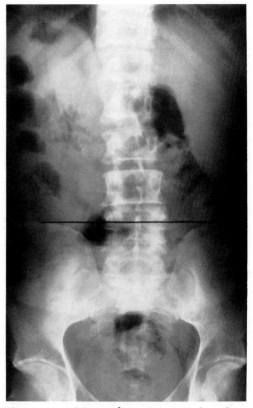

**Figure 7.12.** Neutral anteroposterior view. The intercrestal line cuts the L4 vertebral body.

L1 level, and discogenic spondyloarthrosis can be seen at the L3-L4 and L4-L5 levels (Fig. 7.13). The lumbar angle is 37° and the sacral angle is 38°. The lumbar angle is formed by drawing two lines perpendicular to the superior plate of L1 and the inferior plate of L5 to their intersection, with the resultant angle being the lumbar angle.

3. Stenosis is evident as measurement shows (Fig. 7.14). The ratio of body to canal at L4 and L5 is 5:1, with the L5 sagittal diameter being 8 mm (80% of 10 mm) and the L4 sagittal diameter being 10 mm (80% of 12 mm).

4. Osteophytic changes of the anterolateral body plates can be seen at L3-L4 and L4-L5, as can reduction in the facet joint space at L5-S1 and telescoping of the superior S1 facet into the intervertebral foramen at L5-S1 (Fig. 7.15).

This patient has discogenic spondyloarthrosis at L2-L3, L3-L4, L4-L5, and L5-S1 and stenosis of the vertebral canal at the L4-L5 levels and of the sagittal facet facings at the L5-S1 and L4-L5 levels. Thus, he has a combination of mechanical faults—stenosis, sagittal facets, and degenerative discs.

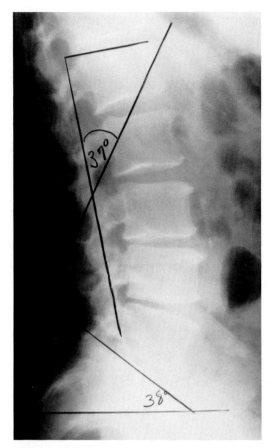

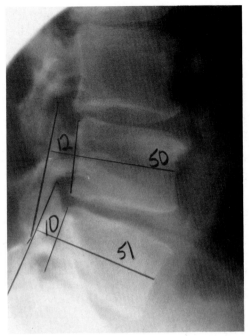

**Figure 7.14.** Lateral spot view. Note the stenosis at the L5 vertebral canal.

**Figure 7.13.** Lateral projection. Schmorl's nodes can be seen at the T12-L1 level.

Cox flexion distraction was applied to each level of the lumbar and lower thoracic spine. Positive galvanism and tetanizing current was applied to the L4-L5 and L5-S1 discs and the paravertebral muscles, respectively. Exercises were prescribed, especially hamstring stretching exercises. The patient was sent to Low Back School to learn ergonomics of the lumbar spine. He obtained excellent relief from pain and was able to learn to prevent irritation of his low back.

**Case 2** is of a 55-year-old white man who had low back and bilateral leg pain that was worse on the left than on the right. He also described numbness made worse on walking, leg pain aggravated by sitting and pain in the testicles. He had been to chiropractors and was referred to us by his last doctor.

Straight leg raise is bilaterally positive at 45°, creating low back pain. Range of motion is normal. Kemp's sign is negative. Muscle strengths are normal in the lower extremities. Right ankle jerk is absent. Atrophy of the right

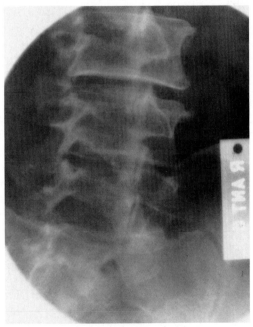

**Figure 7.15.** Oblique view. Note the loss of the L5-S1 facet joint space and telescoping of the 1st sacral facet superiorly into the intervertebral foramen at L5-S1.

thigh and calf are present, with the circumference being 30 mm less in the right thigh than in the left thigh and 17 mm less in the right calf than in the left calf. Milgram's sign is positive bilaterally. Nachlas', Yeoman's, and Ely's maneuvers and prone lumbar flexion all increase low back pain. Doppler testing reveals a reading of 110 mm at the left posterior tibialis (upper arm, 130 systolic) and a reading of 50 mm at the right posterior tibialis. Varicose veins of the left leg are noted. Laboratory tests (CBC, sedimentation rate, and SMAC) are normal. Triglycerides are 291 mg/dl (normal is 30 to 175). The prostate is normal. There are external hemorrhoids. X-rays reveal:

1. Over 50% reduction in L5-S1 disc space height can be seen, with retrolisthesis of L5 and lipping and spurring of the anterolateral body plates at L3-L4, L4-L5, and L5-S1 (Fig. 7.16).
2. Stenosis as determined by Eisenstein's measurement is evident, with the sagittal canal being 11 mm, and the body being 46 mm, the body to canal ratio being 4:1 (Fig. 7.16).

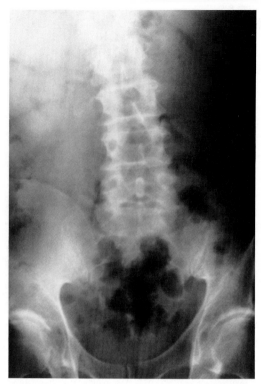

**Figure 7.17.** Posteroanterior left lateral bending view. Normal lateral bending is shown.

3. Lateral bending is normal (Fig. 7.17, 7.18, and 7.19).

This patient has:

1. L5 stenosis with retrolisthesis subluxation of L5 on S1.
2. Discogenic spondyloarthrosis at L3-L4, L4-L5, and L5-S1.
3. An old, healed L5 disc rupture, as evidenced by an absent right ankle reflex, and past untreated leg pain.
4. Intermittent claudication pain in both legs, with a marked insufficiency in the right leg where blood pressure could not be found at the posterior tibialis artery. The stenosis may cause neurogenic claudication in both legs.
5. Left L5-S1 medial disc protrusion causing S1 dermatome sciatica.

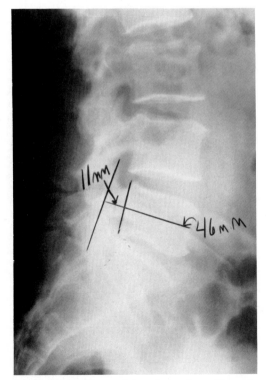

**Figure 7.16.** Lateral lumbar view. Retrolisthesis subluxation of L5 on the sacrum, with stenosis of the vertebral canal at L5 determined by Eisenstein's measurement.

Following the above diagnosis, it was decided to apply treatment 4 times daily at the outset, for 3 weeks. If 50% relief was obtained, both subjectively as evidenced by patient re-

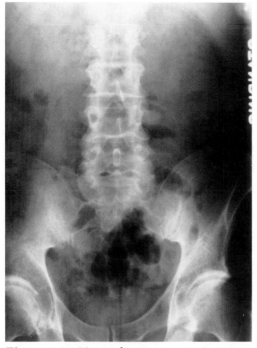

**Figure 7.18.** Neutral posteroanterior view.

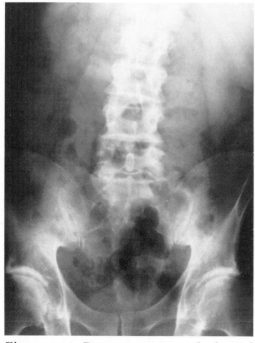

**Figure 7.19.** Posteroanterior right lateral bending view. Normal lateral bending is shown.

sponse and objectively as evidenced, by tests for Kemp's sign, Déjérine's triad, range of motion, and the straight leg raise, 2 more months of treatment would be given. If there was no relief, a vascular surgeon and, possibly, a neurosurgeon would be consulted.

Cox distraction manipulation was given, followed by therapy 4 times daily for 3 weeks. The result was a right lower extremity blood pressure of 90 mm, which was approximately 50% the blood pressure of the left leg. The leg pain ceased and the back pain localized in the gluteus maximus muscle.

Treatment consisted of 3 or 4 distractions daily with positive galvanic current to the L5-S1 disc and B54. Tetanizing current was applied to the adductor and gluteus medius muscles. Acupressure points B24 through B31 were goaded. A belt was worn on the low back 24 hours daily. Sitting was prohibited and exercises for the low back were given.

The patient was sent home to be treated by his family chiropractor.

Prior to returning to work 3 months after the onset of treatment, the patient went through our Low Back Pain School where he was taught the movements dangerous to the low back, how to lift and bend, how to pick up objects from the floor or from shelves, and how to protect the back in activities of daily living.

At the end of 3 months, the patient had obtained 75% relief from pain. The major symptom was left hip and buttock stiffness on standing or walking.

**Case 3** is of a 32-year-old woman who had low back pain for 6 years following delivery of triplets. She also experienced painful menstruation and an increase of back pain at menstruation. Treatments by two chiropractors had previously rendered some relief. She was a mesomorph, was 70 inches tall, and weighed 142 lb.

Range of motion is 90° on flexion, 20° on extension, 10° on right lateral flexion, 10° on left lateral flexion, 20° on right rotation, and 20° on left rotation. Straight leg raise is positive on the right at 80°. Kemp's sign is bilaterally positive. Déjérine's triad is positive for low back pain. No motor or sensory changes are noted.

X-rays reveal:

1. Left inferior hemipelvis with 20-mm short left femoral head (Fig. 7.20).
2. Levoscoliosis of the lumbar spine (Fig. 7.20).

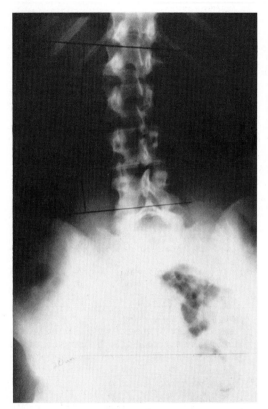

**Figure 7.20.** Neutral posteroanterior (Chamberlain's) view of the lumbar spine and pelvis reveals a 20-mm inferior left hemipelvis and femoral head with levoscoliosis of the lumbar spine.

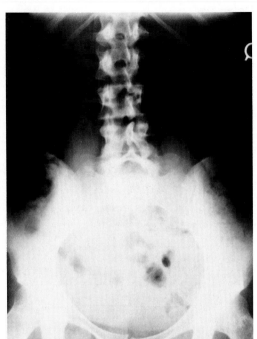

**Figure 7.21.** A 15-mm left heel and sole lift levels the pelvis and partially corrects the levoscoliosis.

3. A 15-mm heel and sole lift to the left shoe (Fig. 7.21).

4. Spondylolisthesis at L5 and a 25% slippage with a pars interarticularis separation (Fig. 7.22).

This patient has true spondylolisthesis at L5 and a 20-mm short left lower extremity with concomitant levoscoliosis of the lumbar spine.

Treatment consisted of Cox flexion distraction for spondylolisthesis (see Chapter 12). Acupressure points B24 to B54 were goaded. A 15-mm heel and sole lift was added to the left shoe, and the patient was advised not to wear high heel shoes. Cox exercises 1 to 4 were advised. The patient was given Discat supplement. She was advised to use hot and cold alternating packs in acute stage and was sent to our Low Back Pain School to learn to lift, bend, and carry out activities of normal daily life.

This patient obtained complete relief from pain after 7 office visits over 22 days.

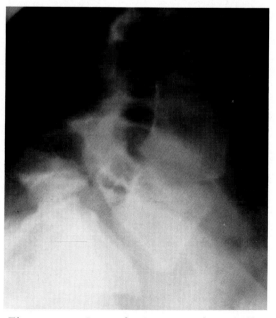

**Figure 7.22.** Lateral view reveals a 25% spondylolisthesis of L5 on the sacrum. A 20-mm short leg could add to this instability.

# References

1. Paine K, Haung P: Lumbar disc syndrome. *J Neurosurg* 37:75, 1972.
2. Sarpyener MA: Congenital stricture of that canal. *J Bone Joint Surg* 27:70, 1945.
3. Verbiest H: A radicular syndrome from developmental narrowing of the lumbar vertebral canal. *J Bone Joint Surg* 36B:230, 1954.
4. Vernon-Roberts B, Pirie C: Degenerative changes in the invertebral discs of the lumbar spine and their sequelae. *Rheumatol Rehabil* 16:13, 1977.
5. Collins DH: Degenerative diseases. In Nassim R, Burrows JH (eds): *Modern Trends in Diseases of the Vertebral Column.* London, Butterworth & Co, 1959.
6. Schmorl, C, Junghanns H: *The Human Spine in Health and Disease.* New York, Grune & Stratton, 1959.
7. Epstein BS, Epstein JA, Lavine L: The effect of anatomic variations in the lumbar vertebrae and spinal canal on cauda equina nerve root syndromes. *Am J Roentgenol Radium Ther Nucl Med* 91:105, 1964.
8. Verbiest H: Fallacies of the present definition, nomenclature, and classification of the stenoses of the lumbar vertebral canal. *Spine* 1(4):217–225, 1976.
9. Elsberg CA, Dyke CG: The diagnosis and localization of tumors of the spinal cord by means of measurements made on x-ray films of the vertebrae, and the correlation of the clinical and x-ray findings. *Bull Neurol Inst NY* 3:359–394, 1934.
10. Huizinga J, Heiden JA vd, Vinken PJG: The human vertebral canal: a biometric study. *Proc R Netherlands Acad Sci C* 55:22–33, 1952.
11. Sand PG: The human lumbo-sacral vertebral column: an osteometric study. Oslo Universitets forlaget Trynkningssentral. 1970.
12. Eisenstein S: Measurements of the lumbar spinal canal in 2 racial groups. *Clin Orthop* 115:42–45, 1976.
13. Rabinovitch R: *Diseases of the Intervertebral Disc and Its Surrounding Tissues.* Springfield, IL, Charles C Thomas, 1961.
14. Hadley LA: *Anatomico-Roentgenographic Studies of the Spine.* Springfield, IL, Charles C Thomas, 1964.
15. Dyck P, Pheasant HC, Doyle JB, Rieder JJ: Intermittent cauda equina compression syndrome. *Spine* 2(1):75, 1977.
15a. Goldthwait JE: The lumbosacral articulation: an explanation of many cases of "lumbago," "sciatica" and paraplegia. *Bost Med Surg J* 164:365–372, 1911.
16. Weinstein P, Ehni G, Wilson C: *Lumbar Spondylosis.* Chicago, Year Book Medical Publishers 1977, p 119.
17. Ehni G: Spondylitic cauda equina radiculopathy. *Tex J Med* 61:746, 1965.
18. Weinstein P, Ehni G, Wilson C: *Lumbar Spondylosis.* Chicago, Year Book Medical Publishers, 1977, p 131.
19. Sunderland S: *Nerves and Nerve Injuries.* Baltimore, Williams & Wilkins, 1968.
20. Sunderland S, Bradley KC: Stress-strain phenomena in human spinal nerve roots. *Brain* 94:120, 1971.
21. Sebolt H, Elies W: The method of surgical root decompression on patients with unilateral lumbar disc prolapse and muscle blood flow of the lower extremities. *VASA,* Band 5, Heft 3, 1976.
22. Wilson CB: Significance of the small lumbar spinal canal: cauda equina syndromes due to spondylosis. Part III. Intermittent claudication. *J Neurosurg* 31:499, 1969.
23. Evans JG: Neurologic intermittent claudication. *Br Med J* 2:985, 1964.
24. Blau JN, Rushworth G: Observation on the blood vessels of the spinal cord and their responses to motor activity. *Brain* 81:354, 1958.
25. Potter G: A story of 744 cases of neck and back pain treated with spinal manipulation. *J Can Chiropractic Assoc* 154, December 1977.
26. Buehler MT: Spinal stenosis. *J Manip Physiolog Ther* 2:103–112, 1978.
27. White AA, Panjabi MM: *Basic Biomechanics of the Spine.* Philadelphia, JB Lippincott, 1978, p 292.
28. Helms CA: CT of the lumbar spine stenosis and arthrosis. *Comput Radiol* 6:359–369, 1982.
29. Jones RAC, Thomson JLG: The narrow lumbar canal, a clinical and radiological review. *J Bone Joint Surg* 50B:595, 1968.
30. Epstein JA, Epstein BS, Levine L: Nerve root compression associated with narrowing of the lumbar spinal canal. *J Neurol Neurosurg Psychiatry* 25:165, 1962.
31. Deleted in proof.
32. Carrera GF, Haughton VM, Syvertsen MD, Williams AL: Computed tomography of the lumbar facet joints. *Radiology* 134:145–148, 1980.
33. Greenfield GQ, Anderson CA: Evaluation of exertional leg pain—claudication or neuromuscular pain. *Orthopedics* 5(11):34, 1982.
34. Deleted in proof.
35. Ben-Eliyahu DJ, Rutili MM, Przbysz JA: Lateral recess syndrome: diagnosis and chiropractic management. *J Manip Physiolog Ther* 6(1):25, 1983.
36. Dyck P: The stoop test in lumbar entrapment radiculopathy. *Spine* 4:89, 1979.
37. Ramani P: Variations in the size of the bony lumbar canal in patients with prolapse of lumbar intervertebral discs. *Clin Radiol* 27:301–307, 1976.
38. Ullrich CG, Binet ER, Sanecki MG, Kieffer SA: Quantitative assessment of the lumbar spinal canal by computed tomography. *Radiology* 134:137–143, 1980.
39. Eagle R: A pain in the back. *New Scientist* pp 170–173, October 18, 1979.
40. Chynn KY, Altman WI, Finby N: The roentgenographic manifestations and clinical features of lumbar spinal stenosis with special emphasis on the superior articular facet. *Neuroradiology* 16:378–380, 1978.
41. Echeverria T, Lockwood R: Lumbar spinal stenosis. *NY J Med,* 872–873, May 1979.
42. MacGibbon B, Farfan H: A radiologic survey of various configurations of the lumbar spine. *Spine* 4(3):258–266, 1979.
43. Wiltse LL, Kirkaldy-Willis WH, McIvor GW: The treatment of spinal stenosis. *Clin Orthop* 115:483, 1976.

*If you treat a person as he is, he will stay as
he is; but if you treat him as if he were what
he ought to be and could be, he will become
what he ought to be and could be.*

**—Source unknown**

# Care of the Intervertebral Disc

Splendid research in the biomechanics of the low back is presently being performed, and varying technics in the surgical treatment of low back conditions are being investigated and tried. Therefore, it is incumbent on chiropractic to develop manipulative care of the low back to its utmost perfection.

"The last part of surgery, namely operations, is a reflection on the healing arts. No surgeon should approach an operation without reluctance." John Hunter made this statement in 1749 (1), and it seems just as applicable today to the chiropractic physician utilizing manipulation to the low back. Manipulation can be a great tool when used properly or an iatrogenic nightmare if abused.

According to Dommisse and Grabe (1), a spinal surgeon rather than an orthopedic or a neurosurgeon is the appropriate leader of the surgical team in an operation on the spine. This reflects the idea that a surgeon whose training is primarily in spinal surgery is the appropriate physician to enter the spine. It might also be said that some chiropractic physicians should specialize in the care of the low back and make this their primary study and practice. To this end, the manipulative care of other specialists throughout the world is briefly examined.

## MANIPULATION AND DISTRACTION TECHNICS FOR LOW BACK PAIN

According to Hirschberg (2), herniation of a nucleus pulposus causing nerve compression can heal spontaneously, provided that low intradiscal pressure can be maintained for 3 months. He described two regimens: one of complete continuous bed rest, and an ambulatory regimen which includes the use of a canvas corset or plastic body jacket and specific exercise. The use of the ambulatory regimen alone or in combination with the bed rest regimen has produced complete disappearance of symptoms in more than 90% of patients.

Furthermore, he states that conservative management in the treatment of patients suffering from symptoms of a herniated nucleus pulposus should be tried before resorting to a surgical procedure and that this concept is commonly accepted. The danger of surgical complications, the certainty that laminectomy causes damage to the stability of the spine, and the occasional failure of surgical procedures to relieve symptoms indicate the advisability of an initial trial of conservative treatment.

According to Hirschberg, under favorable circumstances the protruded portion of the nucleus pulposus shrinks by dehydration, and the symptoms of nerve root compression are relieved. Over a period of months the posterior wall of the annulus fibrosus heals, which may result in complete clinical recovery. If excessive pressure on the disc occurs before healing of the annulus fibrosus has progressed sufficiently, however, the tear will recur, additional disc material will be expelled, and symptoms will return or become aggravated. Conservative management, therefore, keeps the intradiscal pressure low enough for a period long enough to permit adequate healing of the annulus fibrosus. In our experience, it is approximately 3 months before a patient can carry out the activities of daily living without the danger of recurrence.

Neugebauer (3) who has treated more than 30,000 patients in 14 years has proved that a disc prolapse can be converted into a disc relapse. He has achieved a 99% incidence of healing and believes that decompression treatment provides the only lasting recovery for the patient with a disc prolapse. Neugebauer has found that, as evidenced by x-ray measurement, he can increase the height of the L5 disc and has increased the intervertebral disc distance from 3 mm dorsally and 9 mm ventrally to 6 mm dorsally and 15 mm ventrally over a course of treatment of 6 months. He is the first person to document that a disc can be reestablished by decompression treatment.

Neugebauer achieves three therapeutic effects by his decompression treatment:

1. The disc is reestablished.
2. The intervertebral foramen is enlarged, giving enough space for the nerve root to escape the prolapse.
3. Restretching of the anterior and posterior longitudinal ligaments brings the vertebra back into its normal position.

Tien-You (4) writing in the *Chinese Medical Journal* states that manipulative reduction is the key to the treatment of patients with a protruded nucleus but asks the question: Can a protruded nucleus be reduced by simple manipulation? His answer is that a specific feature of the nucleus pulposus is its strong elasticity. This elasticity has been used during manipulative reduction to change the shape of the space between the affected vertebrae and to produce a retractile force by which the prolapsed nucleus is pulled back to its original position.

Others (5–12) using similar technics have provided strong documentary evidence as to the effectiveness of manipulative treatment and/or the nonsurgical approach to the care of patients with myelographically proven disc protrusion who are awaiting surgery.

How much can the intervertebral disc space be opened on distraction? Gupta and Ramarao (13) write that traction by various methods was a very popular form of treatment for lumbar disc prolapse in the early years of this century. Subsequently, it fell into disrepute until the middle of the century when more modern and sophisticated traction technics were introduced and became popular. For example, Mathews (8) is reported to have demonstrated the efficacy of traction in the reduction of lumbar disc prolapse in 3 patients, with the help of epidurography. In his series, symptoms persisted and there was no change in the patterns on epidurograms in only 2 of 14 patients, supporting the popular belief that disc protrusion may safely be treated by traction.

According to Gupta and Ramarao (13), DeSeze and Levernieux reported a distraction of 1.5 mm/disc space after lumbar traction, and Mathews reported a vertebral distraction of 2 mm/disc after traction. Gupta and Ramarao, however, could demonstrate a vertebral distraction of only 0.5 mm/disc space.

Lind (14) documented a 20.7% increase in the intervertebral disc space during manipulative reduction of lumbar disc protrusion. Furthermore, of 20 patients awaiting surgery for lumbar disc protrusion, 14 received complete relief from pain within 1 hour of application of her autotraction technic.

In an article from China (15) on the treatment of lumbar disc protrusion by an automatic chiropractic traction instrument, it is reported that 73% of the 400 patients treated were completely cured of disc protrusion. Also, myelography showed that the defects reduced spontaneously; it was believed that the increased forward pressure of the longitudinal ligaments caused the protruded disc to return to its proper place.

Myelography has consistently shown that flexion of the lumbar spine causes disappearance of the bulge of the posterior annulus and longitudinal ligament as the anterior margins of the vertebral bodies approach each other and the posterior margins separate. The myelographic column becomes flat, and the dural sac closely approximates the back of the posterior longitudinal ligament and annulus. Even though flexion increases the force propulsing the disc posteriorly, it also tightens the posterior annulus and posterior longitudinal ligament and improves the barrier, with the net effect being reduction of the posterior protrusion. Raney (16) points out that complete prolapse is not helped by this procedure and that *abdominal compression and the Valsalva maneuver also diminish the amount of protrusion of the bulging disc.*

Discs absorb shock in two ways: (a) by squeezing fluid out of the nucleus and/or (b) by allowing the fibers of the outer shell to stretch (17). Hukins and Hickey (18) show that the disc fibers have limited elasticity and suffer irreparable damage at 1.04 times their initial length. When a person is standing upright, the discs can withstand 10 times more compression as the vertebrae can, so a heavy load crushes the bones before it ruptures the disc. Disc fibers are less capable of coping with torsion because the stress then concentrates at points of maximum curvature. It has been reported that astronauts are 5 cm taller on their return to earth than they were when they left (17); Nachemson (19) reports that they are 10 cm taller.

Protrusion or rupture of the disc is usually preceded by degenerative changes characterized structurally by radiating cracks in the annulus that develop and weaken its resistance to nuclear herniation. As Tindall (20) points out, the sinuvertebral nerve supplies the posterior longitudinal ligament, periosteum, meninges, articular connective tissue, annulus, and vascular structures of the vertebral canal. The characteristic clinical features of back and leg pain, therefore, are related to irritation and stretching of the sinuvertebral nerve by the bulging annulus and by direct pressure on the nerve root, respectively (20).

## Gauging Patient Response to Surgery and Manipulation

Of the 200,000 back surgeries done in the United States annually, 30% fail to relieve any pain, and at 5-year follow-up, only 10% of the remainder have provided satisfactory relief (22). Malec et al. (21) define success from back surgery thusly: The patient is free from the use of pain medication and is more active than he was before treatment, i.e., working, training, running a house, or capable of continued exercise 50% to 100% of the time with no increase in pain. Trief (22), however, defines success as being improvement in the straight leg raise of 20° and the ability to bring the knee 10 cm closer to the chest.

Recent interest in manipulation as an adjunct to the conservative treatment of low back and sciatic pain led us to study the effects of this procedure on a group of patients who had this typical syndrome and have received little relief from ordinary conservative care (23).

In an analysis of 205 patients with clinically diagnosed ruptured intervertebral disc who were treated conservatively, which included rotatory manipulation, Mensor (24) reports prompt and satisfactory relief of symptoms in 64% of his private patients and 45% of his patients injured in industrial accidents. These results are considerably better than those reported by Colonna and Friedenberg (25), who found that only 29% of 28 patients whose myelograms were positive for disc rupture were pain-free after conservative treatment without manipulation. It should be noted that these two series are not necessarily comparable because Mensor did not use myelograms as an aid in establishing diagnosis. It is possible that patients with the best manipulative results did not have myelographically demonstrable protrusions.

In an attempt to determine how manipulative treatment alleviates symptoms, Wilson and Ilfeld (26) studied 18 patients with a ruptured intervertebral disc, the diagnosis of which was clinically firmly established; myelography was performed both before and after rotatory manipulation. Only 2 of the 18 patients received anesthesia for the manipulation. Thirteen showed myelographic defects before manipulation; 5 did not. Myelographic changes after manipulation were seen in only one patient whose myelogram was positive and in whom the size of the defect increased slightly. Three of the patients had brief improvement, and 12 of the 18 subsequently underwent operation.

The following conclusions can be drawn from these last studies.

1. Twenty of 39 patients (51%) who were unequivocally diagnosed as having a ruptured intervertebral disc unrelieved by conservative care had good or excellent results after rotatory manipulation of the spine under anesthesia, thus confirming Mensor's results (51.2%) with this method.

2. The appearance of the myelograms of these patients before and after manipulation, whether positive or negative, were unchanged.

3. Ten of the 27 patients whose myelograms were positive had good to excellent results 3 years or more after manipulation.

4. Patients whose myelograms were negative consistently did better after manipulation than those whose myelograms showed a defect.

The examination and treatment results of 576 patients treated by chiropractic manipulation as well as other clinical treatment results are included in Chapter 15.

## Intervertebral Disc Pain Sensitivity and Production

The sinuvertebral nerve supplies the posterior longitudinal ligament, annulus fibrosus, and neurovascular contents of the epidural space (27, 28). The outer annulus and the nerve root are the most pain-sensitive and can reproduce the patient's presurgical symptoms when stimulated 3 to 4 weeks postsurgically (19).

The existence of unmyelinated nerve endings, usually associated with pain reception in the posterior annulus and even penetrating the nucleus, are increasingly evident. The posterior longitudinal ligament is well innervated (29).

When a radial tear penetrates the outer annulus, there is an attempt at healing by ingrowth of granulation tissue. Naked endings of the sinuvertebral nerve have been identified in this granulation tissue. These endings may be pain receptors, which would explain discogenic pain in the absence of herniation (30).

Tsukada (31) believes that there are nerve fibers not only in the posterior longitudinal ligament but also in the nucleus

and notochord. Malinsky (32) and Hirsch et al. (33) suggest that nerve fibers accompany granulation tissue in free nerve endings within the inner layers of the annulus and in the nucleus of some degenerated discs. In this same article, Yoshizawa et al. (33a) are reported to have found profuse free nerve terminals in the outer half of the annulus but no such terminals in the nucleus. According to Sunderland (34), the recurrent meningeal nerve supplies the dura, the intervertebral disc, and associated structures.

The sinuvertebral nerve divides into ascending, descending, and transverse branches adjacent to the posterior longitudinal ligament (35). According to Lazorthes (36), this nerve supplies the neural laminae, the intervertebral disc at adjacent levels, the posterior longitudinal ligaments, the internal vertebral plexus, the epidural tissue, and the dura mater. It should be noted, however, that although there is still disagreement concerning what tissue is supplied by this nerve, some investigators believe that there is such a wide distribution. Tsukada (31) and Shinohara (37) have found that in a normal disc the outer annulus is innervated but that in a degenerated disc, fine nerve fibers accompany granulation tissue present in degenerating nuclear material.

According to Macnab (38), the pain of osteoporosis can be ascribed to trabecular buckling or fracture. Pain is also due to the venous spaces in the vertebral body spongiosa. The intraosseous venous pressure of a normal vertebra is 20 mm and that of an osteoporotic vertebra is about 40 mm.

Farfan (39) points out that the disc contains A, B, and G nerve fibers and that the G nerve fibers are found in high-velocity communicating networks. If the disc is not sensory, why then are they present?

One series (40) reports that in at least some circumstances low back pain is provoked by direct mechanical stimuli. This effect was demonstrated in experiments made during spine surgery when the patient was under local anesthesia. According to Spurling and Grantham (41), patients often complained of back pain when the annulus fibrosus was manipulated. Falconer et al. (42) report that during spine surgery, pressing on a disc prolapse produced low back pain, whereas pressing on a nerve root produced sciatica. Longitudinal nerve root stretching did not produce pain. Hirsch (43) found that lumbar pain was sometimes elicited by pressing on an intervertebral disc. According to Wiberg (44), however, pressing on the nerve root caused acute "root pain," whereas pressing on the intervertebral disc caused back pain. Disc palpation caused pain whether or not the area was anesthesized. At surgery, Smyth and Wright (44a) tied threads into various structures of the low back. After the surgery, the effects of pulling on these threads was recorded. "*Pulling on the dura mater, the ligamentum flavum, or the interspinous ligaments provoked no pain. Pressing on the nerve root caused pain, and the nerve root involved in the herniation was much more sensitive than the uninvolved nerve root. Pressure on the annulus fibrosus caused sciatic pain and sometimes caused backache*" (44a).

A second series concerns studies of pain accompanying fluid injection into an intervertebral disc during discography. Although not all authors are in agreement, there is a significant amount of literature on the subject.

For example, Hirsch (43) found that pain typical of back pain was produced in 16 patients by injection of normal saline into the lumbar disc, especially if considerable pressure was needed for the injection. This pain disappeared after a few minutes. Lindblom (45) found that on discography in 150 patients, back pain occurred when the needle passed through the posterior surface of the disc but not when the needle entered the center of the disc. Injection of contrast medium and an anesthetic produced pain similar to low back pain. If the disc did not hold the fluid, no pain was produced. According to Hirsch (43), when normal saline was injected, pain was elicited only in the presence of raised pressure. When the pressure dropped, the pain disappeared. These reports imply that the pain was due to the pressure increase rather than to the chemical irritation.

Cloward and Buzaid (46) found that injection of contrast medium into a disc was often painful and frequently elicited back pain similar to that elicited by bending or lifting. *Collis and Gardner (47) injected contrast medium into the lumbar discs of 400 patients with surgically verified herniated discs. Of these injections, 68% produced both back and leg pain, 26% produced only back pain, and only 6% produced no pain at all.* On injection of contrast medium into 148 cervical discs in 50 volunteer subjects who were free of any cervical pathology, Holt (48) found that needle insertion produced only slight discomfort but that injection produced severe pain in every subject at every disc space injected! This pain lasted about 5 minutes, then disappeared completely. Again, this seems to point to mechanical rather than chemical pain receptors.

In a later report on lumbar discography, however, Holt found that little discomfort resulted from injection of a normal lumbar disc. Discomfort resulted only when the contrast medium came into contact with any tissue having sensory innervation, implying that the irritation was chemical rather than mechanical. Hudgins (49) also found that the pain response elicited by lumbar discography was inconstant and unreliable. Occasionally, injection reproduced back pain.

A third series concerns studies of pain referred from the low back regions. The objectives of these studies were to determine when pain was referred and from what structures. Injections of hypertonic saline solution into structures superficial to the disc were the stimuli. The original work was done by Kellgren (50), and several investigators (50a) did follow-up studies. Considerable controversy has arisen over some of the issues. Aside from the controversy, all authors seem to agree that the injections caused pain much of the time. Sometimes it was local pain, and sometimes it was referred pain. Whether the pain resulted from the mechanical pressure of the injected fluid or from chemical irritation is not clear.

Perhaps more work on injection responses and pain-sensing mechanisms would be of value, if it could be done without excessive risk. Attempts should be made to distinguish chemical stimuli from mechanical stimuli. Only Hirsch's results seem to allow this distinction to be made, if one assumes that normal saline would not produce any chemical irritation (43).

According to LaMotte (51), the word "nociceptors" is defined broadly as those endings of certain peripheral nerve fibers in humans, and by inference in animals, which when active are associated with sensations of pain. There are numerous peripheral sources of low back pain. Distortion of the annulus and facet joints could stretch the posterior longitudinal ligament and activate nociceptors in the ligament. There is evidence that the outer border of the annulus fibrosus is supplied with nerve endings and that pain can arise from intradiscal injection of a contrast material. Also, intradiscal injection of chymopapain in the treatment of lumbar disc herniations can, in certain cases, relieve pain in minutes.

The observations and illustrative cases surgically explored by Torkildsen (52) give support to the idea that cervical spondylosis giving rise to brachialgia may simultaneously be the cause of pains in the leg that resemble sciatica. This may be the case even if spondyloarthritic changes are limited to the cervical intervertebral canal. This type of sciatica—brachialgic sciatica—differs in nature from true sciatica as seen in cases of lumbar disc lesion. The differential diagnostic points are pyramidal tract signs; i.e., deep reflexes of the painful leg are increased, the plantar reflex is extensor in response, and the tone of the painful leg extends beyond the limits of one or two dermatomes, with the Achilles reflexes being bilaterally equal. These signs occur in addition to the peripheral nerve lesions of the arm.

The sources of pain in various structures associated with ruptured discs have been identified by Murphy (53). *The sequence of events as involves pain in the lumbar region is as follows: When an incomplete tear in the annulus occurs, and if the tear is in the midline posteriorly, a fragment of nucleus will protrude into this tear, stretching the annulus and posterior longitudinal ligament, causing midline back pain. If the tear in the annulus is lateral, then the pain will be over the sacroiliac joint and in the buttock and hip,* *with nerve root compression, and depending on the level, it will cause radiation of pain down the leg. For example, if a patient claims that his back pain stopped when his leg pain began, it is almost a certainty that the disc fragment has extruded through the posterior longitudinal ligament into the canal and will have to be removed.*

## Case Studies: Lateral Flexion Subluxations in Disc Cases

**Case 1** is of a 51-year-old man who developed right-sided sciatica on the lateral side of the thigh, leg, and foot after lifting a generator.

Leg raise is positive at 45° on the right side, with palpation revealing pain over the right buttock, thigh, and calf. The paravertebral musculature is tender over the L4-L5 and the L5-S1 areas, and there is a burning sensation in the right L5 nerve root distribution. X-ray (Fig. 8.1) reveals a left lumbar inclination from L4 cephalad, with coronal facet development occurring at the L4-L5 and the L5-S1 levels.

A correlative diagnosis of a right 4th lumbar disc protrusion lateral to the 5th lumbar disc

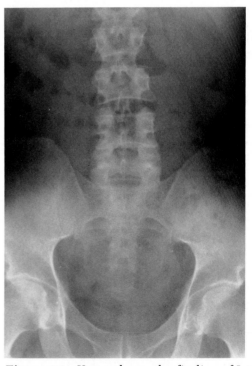

**Figure 8.1.** X-ray shows the finding of L4 right lateral disc protrusion with L4 left lateral flexion subluxation on L5.

was made. Treatment for a lateral disc protrusion yielded relief from pain after 2 months.

**Case 2** is of a 27-year-old man who had low back pain of 3 months duration, with left-sided sciatica becoming progressively worse in the buttock and radiating down the lateral thigh and leg into the lateral foot.

The Lasègue test reveals pain in the left gluteal area overlying the sacroiliac joint area. Pain is elicited over the lumbosacral area and over the 4th and 5th lumbar spinous and transverse processes and musculature. Neurological examination reveals that the deep reflexes are active and equal. The patient leans to the right side in the lumbar spine area.

X-ray (Fig. 8.2) reveals right lumbar spine inclination from L4 cephalad with the coronal facets at the L5-S1 and the L4-L5 articulations. Physical examination reveals a Grade II swelling of the prostate gland.

A correlative diagnosis of a left lateral 4th lumbar disc protrusion compressing the 5th lumbar nerve root was made. Treatment for a lateral disc protrusion resulted in complete remission of sciatica and back pain in 1 month.

**Case 3** is of a 31-year-old white woman who developed low back pain after stooping. She

has had the low back pain for 3 months and has subsequently complained of pain radiating down the posterolateral aspect of the right thigh and leg.

Her posture is antalgic to the left from L5 cephalad. Kemp's sign is positive on the right side, and anterior flexion causes pain. The right leg raise sign is positive at 40°. Nothing unusual is noted on neurological examination. Figure 8.3, a special tilt view of the lumbosacral spine, shows a left lateral flexion subluxation of L5 on the sacrum, indicating a correlative diagnosis of right lateral 5th lumbar disc protrusion compressing the 1st sacral nerve root.

Figure 8.4, an x-ray of the same patient taken in a similar lumbosacral tilt position 3 weeks later, shows that the flexion subluxation has been completely reduced. The patient is symptom-free.

**Case 4** is of a 52-year-old white woman who has had left low back pain of 2 weeks duration following a fall from the bathroom stool after a dizzy spell. She had had two gallbladder surgeries and a hysterectomy for removal of a fibroid tumor in 1968. Both parents had died of carcinoma—the mother of duodenal and the

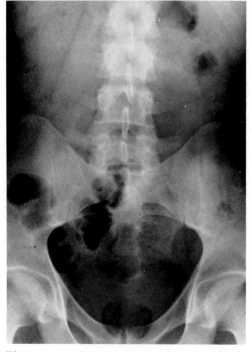

**Figure 8.2.** Posteroanterior view shows L4 right lateral flexion subluxation on L5. Clinical diagnosis: L4 left lateral disc protrusion.

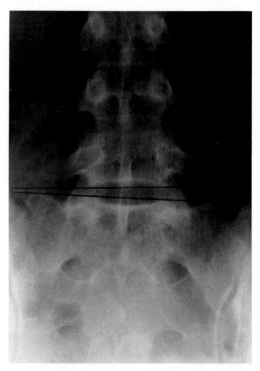

**Figure 8.3.** Posteroanterior tilt view through L5-S1 reveals left lateral flexion of L5 on the sacrum. Clinical diagnosis: L5 right lateral disc protrusion.

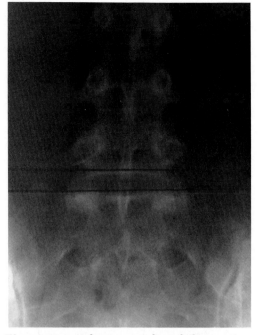

**Figure 8.4.** After 3 weeks of distraction the left lateral flexion subluxation of L5 on the sacrum (same patient as in Fig. 8.3) was relieved.

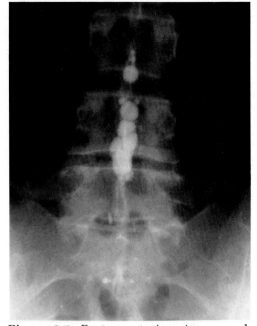

**Figure 8.5.** Posteroanterior view reveals right lateral flexion of L4 on L5 in a patient who has had both L4 and L5 discs removed surgically.

father of prostatic carcinoma. The patient had a skin carcinoma removed from the face in 1969. When she came to the center, she was being treated for nephritis by her medical doctor. She had been told that she had diverticulitis of the colon. She was referred to the Chiropractic Associates Diagnostic and Treatment Center by another chiropractor who refused to treat her because of her history of two previous lumbar disc surgeries. These surgeries were performed 9 and 2 years previously.

Examination reveals a positive leg raise sign on both sides at 45° with Kemp's sign being positive on the right side. There is tenderness over the 4th vertebral musculature, with pain radiating into the left buttock and along the lateral thigh and anterior leg and sometimes into the foot and great toe. Neurological examination reveals nothing unusual after disc surgery.

X-ray films reveal a right lateral flexion subluxation of the 4th lumbar vertebra. This can be seen on Figure 8.5.

A correlative diagnosis of a 4th lumbar left lateral disc protrusion compressing the 5th lumbar nerve root, resulting in the typical sciatic radiculitis, was made. Treatment for a 4th lumbar lateral disc protrusion resulted in a progressive relief of symptoms. The x-ray 2 weeks later (Fig. 8.6) revealed that although

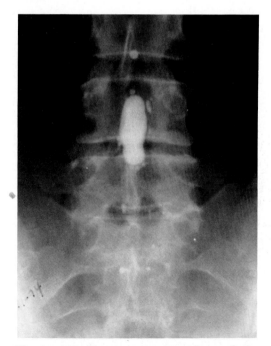

**Figure 8.6.** Posteroanterior view of the same patient as in Figure 8.5 after 2 weeks of care. Straightening of the spine and some relief of the right lateral flexion of L4 on L5 are noted.

the right lateral flexion subluxation of L4 was still in evidence, some reduction could be seen. Considering the complex surgical history of the patient and the presence of the dye from the previous myelography, relief of symptoms coupled with the partial reduction of the lateral flexion subluxation was considered an effective clinical response.

**Case 5** is of a 33-year-old white man who worked as a grain elevator operator and developed right 5th lumbar dermatome sciatica after lifting. He had been treated with classic lumbar rotation manipulation adjustment which progressively worsened his condition. After 1 month of this care, he had come to our facility.

Straight leg raise is positive at 20° for the right leg and is negative for the left leg. Range of motion is limited to 10° on flexion, 5° on extension, 5° on right lateral flexion, and 20° on left lateral flexion. Déjérine's triad is positive, as is Kemp's sign bilaterally.

Figure 8.7, a posteroanterior neutral view taken on first visit, reveals left lateral flexion

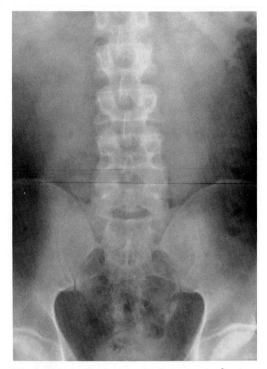

**Figure 8.8.** Posteroanterior neutral view of the same patient as in Figure 8.7 after nine distraction manipulations. There is reduction of the L4 left lateral flexion subluxation and increase in the disc space at L4-L5.

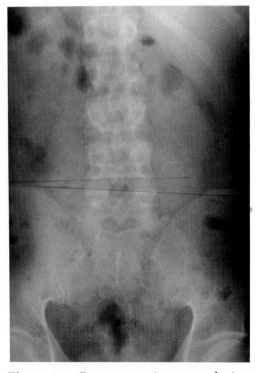

**Figure 8.7.** Posteroanterior neutral view of left lateral flexion subluxation of L4 on L5. Clinical diagnosis: L4 right lateral disc protrusion.

subluxation of L4 on L5. Figure 8.8, a repeat posteroanterior view taken after nine flexion distraction manipulations on the Cox table over 1 week, shows reduction of the L4 left lateral flexion and some increase in the disc space at L4-L5.

The patient's leg pain was completely relieved.

Note: Figure 8.9 serves as a reminder of the sciatic scoliosis that patients develop in order to relieve their low back and sciatic pain.

X-ray examination provides an excellent method for study of lateral flexion discogenic subluxation. The following are some classic examples of its use.

Figures 8.10, 8.11, and 8.12 are from the motion study of a patient with 5th lumbar right lateral disc protrusion creating right S1 dermatome sciatica. Note the hypomobility of L5 on S1 and the hypermobility of the segments above in the right and left lateral bending views. The patient will not bend into the side of lateral disc lesion. Note also the vertebral body rotation.

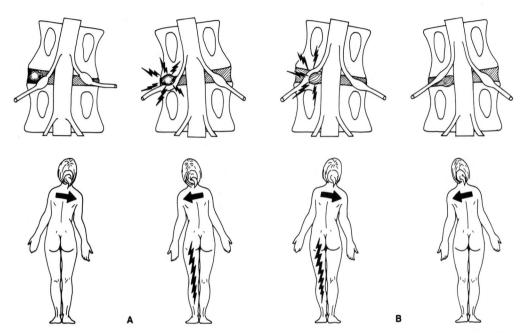

**Figure 8.9.** Patients with herniated disc disease may sometimes list to one side. This is a voluntary or unvoluntary mechanism to alleviate nerve root irritation. The list in some patients is toward the side of the sciatica; in others it is toward the opposite side. A reasonable hypothesis suggests that when herniation is lateral to the nerve root (A), the list is to the side opposite the sciatica because a list to the same side would elicit pain. Conversely, when the herniation is medial to the nerve root (B), the list is toward the side of the sciatica because tilting away would irritate the root and cause pain. If this hypothesis could be documented in clinical practice, it would be helpful at the time of surgical exploration. (Reproduced with permission from A. A. White and M. M. Panjabi: *Clinical Biomechanics of the Spine*. Philadelphia, J. B. Lippincott, 1978, p. 299.)

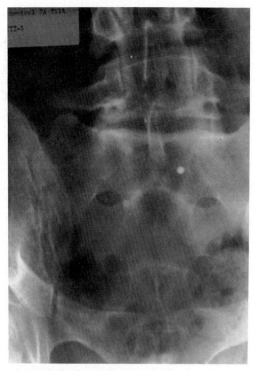

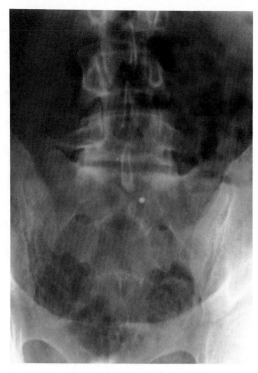

**Figure 8.10.** Neutral posteroanterior 20° tilt view of the L5-S1 disc space. Note left lateral flexion discogenic subluxation of L5 on S1. Also note tropism of the facets which predisposes a disc problem by altering rotatory motion, thus adding stress to the annulus fibrosus.

**Figure 8.12.** Right lateral bending view shows maintenance and hypomotility of the L4 left lateral flexion discogenic subluxation. The segments above L4-L5 are mobile or hypermobile.

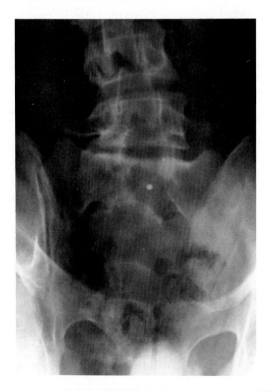

**Figure 8.11.** Left lateral bending view with 20° posteroanterior tilt. Note hypermotility above the L5-S1 level and hypomotility at L5-S1. Note the maintenance of left lateral flexion of L5 on S1.

Figures 8.13, 8.14, and 8.15 are neutral lateral and right and left lateral bending views of a patient with L4-L5 left medial disc protrusion. Following disc reduction, the subluxations shown in these figures were found to be corrected or to show improved range of motion.

**Case 6** is of a patient with sciatic pain down the left 5th lumbar dermatome.

Figure 8.16 reveals right lateral flexion subluxation of L4 on L5. The diagnosis, therefore, is a left lateral L4-L5 disc protrusion.

Figure 8.17 was taken following relief of the left leg pain after nine flexion distraction manipulations. The L4 right lateral flexion subluxation had been relieved and no right lean of the lumbar spine was noted.

**Case 7** is of a 32-year-old woman who had developed left leg sciatica following placement of a Harrington rod for scoliosis.

In Figure 8.18, a discogram of this patient, the hook of the rod can be seen to insert at the laminae of L3. The bone fragments in the pos-

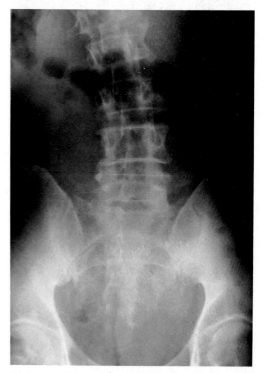

**Figure 8.14.** Left lateral bending view shows hypermotility above the disc lesion at L4-L5 and maintenance of the left lateral flexion discogenic subluxation of L4 on L5.

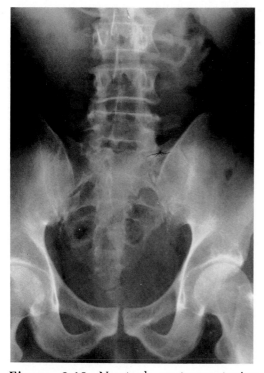

**Figure 8.13.** Neutral posteroanterior view of the L4-L5 disc space. Note the left lateral flexion discogenic subluxation of L4 on L5.

terior L4-L5 disc space may represent displaced bone from the surgery. Note that the Harrington rod has fused the thoracic and lumbar spine, placing all movement at the lower lumbar segments. Note also the small nuclear extension posteriorly and superiorly into the vertebral body plate on discography.

Figure 8.20, a CT scan at the L5-S1 disc level, shows that epidural fat surrounds the 1st sacral nerve roots in the lateral recesses. Contrast the L5-S1 nerve root and its epidural fat with the L5 nerve root at L4-L5 (Fig. 8.19).

Figure 8.19, a CT scan at the L4-L5 disc level, reveals a disc protrusion to the left midline and lateral recess. Note how large the annular protrusion appears on CT and how small the nuclear protrusion appears on the discogram. This demonstrates the need to correlate diagnostic procedures and not to be dogmatic in clinical impressions based on single test results.

Due to persistent pain, it was suggested that this patient have a myelogram done; no follow-up with our office has been made.

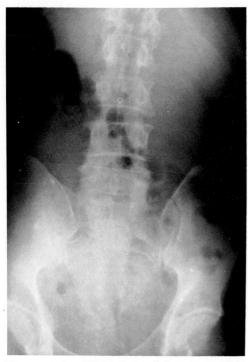

**Figure 8.15.** Right lateral bending view shows maintenance and hypomotility of the L4 left lateral flexion discogenic subluxation. The segments above L4-L5 are mobile or hypermobile.

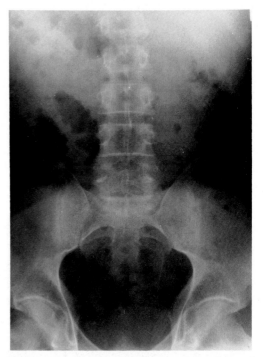

**Figure 8.17.** Relief of the right lateral flexion of L4 on L5 and the leg pain following 3 weeks of distraction manipulation. The spine no longer leans to the right.

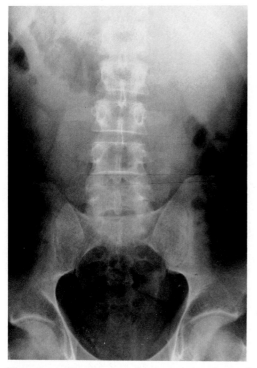

**Figure 8.16.** X-ray shows right lateral flexion subluxation of L4 on L5 in a patient with left L5 dermatome pain.

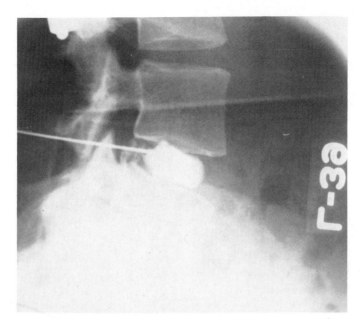

**Figure 8.18.**  Discogram performed prior to chemonucleolysis reveals a small posterior and superior nuclear bulge.

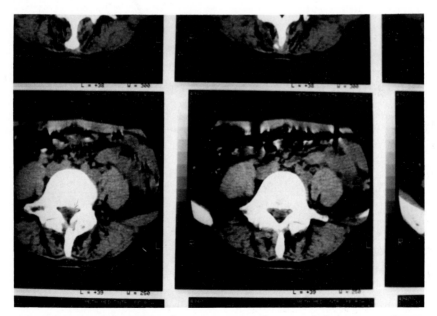

**Figure 8.19.**  CT scan of the L4-L5 disc space reveals a much larger annular protrusion into the canal than was suggested by the discogram (Fig. 8.18).

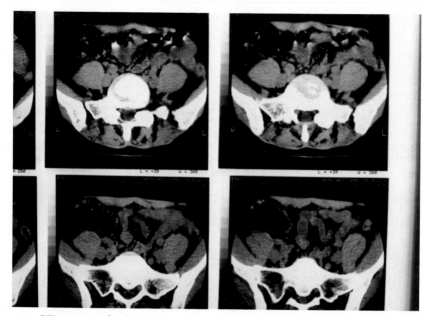

**Figure 8.20.** CT scan at the L5-S1 level reveals the S1 nerve roots in the lateral recess with good epidural fat density.

## COX CLOSED REDUCTION OF DISC PROTRUSION

### The Cox Table

In the early 1970s, this author developed the Cox table which was a blending of osteopathic and chiropractic principles into one instrument. This table has application in the treatment of lumbar disc protrusion, spondylolisthesis, facet syndrome, subluxation, and scoliotic curves of a nonsurgical nature and can be used to place the articulations of the spine through the normal ranges of motion. These normal ranges of motion are *flexion, extension, lateral bending, rotation, and circumduction* (Figures 8.21 to 8.25).

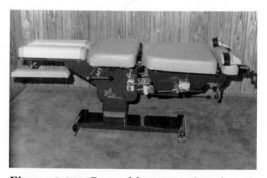

**Figure 8.21.** Cox table in its closed position.

### Closed Reduction: Its Definition and Use in the Patient with an Acute Disc Lesion

*Cox flexion distraction manipulation* is a form of chiropractic spinal manipulative therapy allowing the following benefits:

1. Increase of the intervertebral disc height to remove annual distortion in the pain-sensitive peripheral annular fibers.

2. Allow the nucleus pulposus to assume its central position within the an-

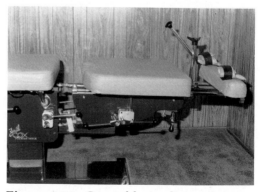

**Figure 8.22.** Cox table in distraction position.

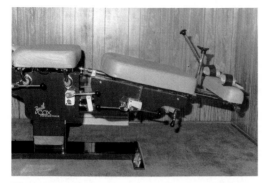

**Figure 8.23.** Cox table in flexion distraction position.

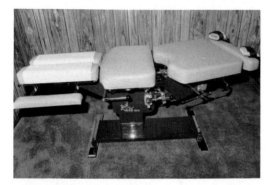

**Figure 8.24.** Cox table in lateral flexion position.

nulus and relieve irritation of the pain-sensitive annular fibers.

3. Restore vertebral joints to their physiological relationships of motion.

4. Improve posture and locomotion while relieving pain, improving body functions, and creating a state of well-being.

Note that we use the term closed reduction. This term has been used in much of the literature as well as by this author. Frankly, it has met with some misunderstanding, in that it has been mistaken for a surgical procedure, such as setting a broken bone. Closed reduction should be understood to be in opposition to a surgical open reduction or surgical removal of a disc protrusion or prolapse.

Treatment of the patient with acute disc protrusion or prolapse demands specific care. The steps preparatory to distraction are explained below.

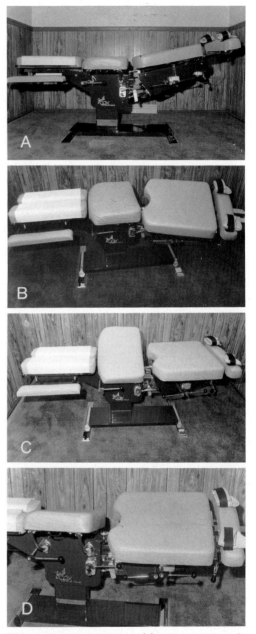

**Figure 8.25.** A, Cox table in position for application of extension to the spine. B, Cox table with caudal section in rotation position for lumbar spine rotation. C, Cox table with thoracic rotation section for motion palpation of the thoracic spine. D, Cox table with combined lumbar and thoracic rotation section for manipulation of "S" scoliotic thoracolumbar curves.

A deep goading pressure is applied as shown in Figure 8.26, in preparation for distraction. The goading pressure is applied over the paravertebral areas of the upper lumbar spine through the coccyx. These areas coincide with bladder meridian points B24 through B35 at the coccyx.

The goading is then applied into the belly of the gluteus maximus muscle (Fig. 8.27). Further information on the treatment of this muscle is given in a later chapter; suffice it here to state that the gluteus maximus is supplied by the inferior gluteal nerve having a common spinal origin with the sciatic nerve. The pain and spasm of the gluteus maximus muscle will recede as the disc lesion heals and the sciatic nerve is relieved. Therefore, a deep goading pressure is placed into the belly of this muscle for 15 to 20 seconds both before and after treatment. The relaxation and loss of pain in this muscle is an indicator of patient response.

Next, the gluteus medius and minimus muscles are goaded (Fig. 8.28) at their origin and insertion prior to distraction. These are abductor muscles of the lower extremity, are quite painful to palpation, and are usually weak to muscle testing.

Bladder meridian point B54 in the popliteal space is goaded vigorously for 15 to 20 seconds (Fig. 8.29). This point is used in acupuncture to relieve sciatic pain.

The goading of the adductores and gracilis muscles at their origins and insertions is shown in Figs. 8.30, 8.31, and 8.32. These muscles are supplied by the obturator nerve from the 2nd, 3rd, and 4th lumbar nerve roots. They are extremely tight and painful in the patient with a disc lesion. These muscles are also discussed in a later chapter on muscle treatment.

The first step in distraction manipulation of a patient with an acute disc lesion is demonstrated by A and B of Figure 8.33. The patient's ankles are not placed in the ankle cuffs but are left free. Note that the

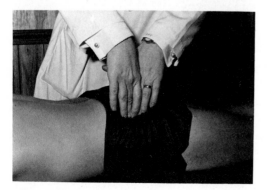

**Figure 8.26.** Paravertebral bladder meridian acupressure points being goaded.

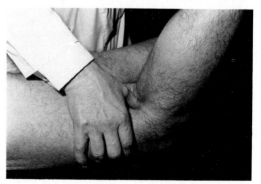

**Figure 8.28.** Abductor muscle origin and insertion pressure applied.

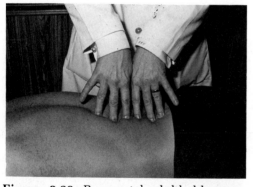

**Figure 8.27.** Gluteus maximus B49 acupressure point being goaded.

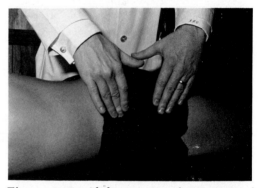

**Figure 8.29.** Bladder meridian point B54 being goaded.

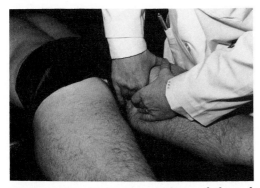

**Figure 8.30.** Pressure goading of the adductores muscle origins.

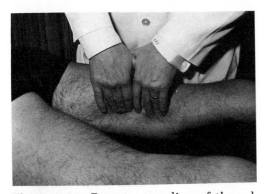

**Figure 8.31.** Pressure goading of the adductor insertions.

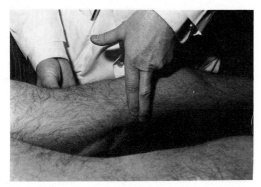

**Figure 8.32.** Goading of the gracilis insertion.

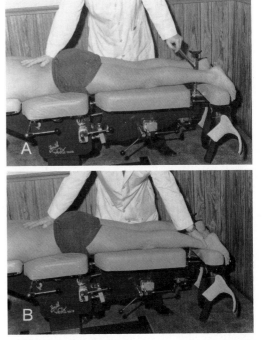

**Figure 8.33.** A and B, testing patient's tolerance to distraction.

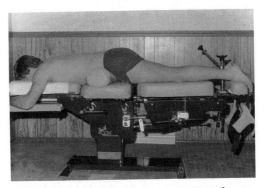

**Figure 8.34.** Patient lying over Dutchman roll in acute pain.

doctor's hand is placed upon the spinous process directly above the disc to be treated and the patient's ability to tolerate traction is tested. While holding the contact hand on the spinous process, gentle downward pressure is placed on the caudal end of the table. The patient is asked if this causes any pain. If the patient says "yes," stop traction, leave the table locked at that point in flexion, and place a Dutchman roll under the abdomen as shown in Figure 8.34, until the patient can tolerate this tractive force. It may be hours or days before he is able to withstand much tractive force.

The patient with an acute disc lesion may not be able to lie flat upon the table; therefore, placement of the Dutchman roll under the abdomen (Fig. 8.34) opens up the dorsal intervertebral disc space so as to allow them to lie prone. This may be the most comfortable position that the patient with an acute disc lesion is capable of assuming. If this is the case, apply hot and cold therapy to the disc area in the following manner. Moist heat is applied for 10 minutes, followed by application of a cold pack for 5 minutes. Moist heat is applied a total of 4 times and is applied at both the beginning and the end of the therapy, with the cold applied between the heat applications; i.e., heat is applied 4 times and the cold is applied 3 times.

Once the patient can tolerate traction without ankle cuffs, ankle cuffs are then applied (Fig. 8.35). Please note the amount of tractive force used in opening the intervertebral disc space. The hand is held in contact with the spine so that the spinous process directly above the disc to be tractioned is held static while the caudal section of the table is moved downward. Approximately one third of the doctor's weight is placed upon the spinous process, and the other two thirds is distributed directly toward the patient's head. The spinous process is very tender due to the irritation of the posterior ramus of the involved nerve root, so the pressure should be distributed over as broad an area as possible by the contact hand. *Note that no greater than 2 finger pressure should ever be applied to the caudal section of the table, so that it should never go down over 2 inches at maximum tractive force.* More traction than this can aggravate the patient's problem and is not needed in the treatment of the disc lesion. *Doctors who sometimes have adverse ef-*

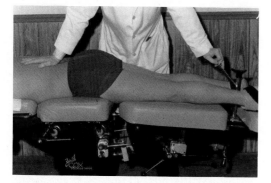

**Figure 8.35.** Cuffs are placed on the ankles and distraction is applied.

*fects from traction find that they are applying too much tractive force.*

Note that *no other treatment is utilized in the patient with an acute disc lesion until all leg pain is gone.* Depending upon the severity of the lesion, this may be hours or days.

## Treatment of the Patient with Only Low Back Pain

There are two basic causes of low back pain: the disc itself and the articular facets. The doctor who can effectively relieve these two sources of pain will get rid of the majority of back pain for the patient. *In the patient with an acute disc lesion, we utilize no movement other than traction and flexion of the table. Once the leg pain is relieved, the disc patient is treated in the same manner as any patient who comes in strictly complaining of low back pain.*

Each articulation of the spine is capable of flexion, extension, lateral bending, circumduction, and rotation to various degrees, depending upon the level of the spine. In the patient with low back pain, the articulations are gently put through their normal range of motion. As we proceed with this discussion, please note that any fixation subluxations can be determined while putting the facet through its normal range of motion. Such fixation is relieved by placing this articulation through its normal movements.

Hold the spinous process with your thenar contact or grasp the spinous process between the thumb and index finger in order to keep it in place as lateral bending is performed (Figs. 8.36 and 8.37). The facets that will move are those between the grasped spinous process and the vertebra below; i.e., if you grasp the spinous process of L5, the facets between L5 and S1 will bend laterally.

Note that the rotation movement should not be used at the lower two levels, since rotation is minimally executed at these levels (Fig. 8.38). The L4-L5 and L5-S1 levels rotate only 6°. The degree of rotation can be increased as you proceed upward into the lumbar spine and into the thoracic spine.

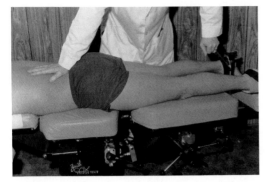

**Figure 8.36.** Lateral bending is applied for motion palpation of the facets and for regaining of range of facet motion.

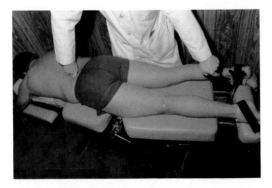

**Figure 8.37.** The spinous process is held between the index fingers and the thumb while lateral bending is applied.

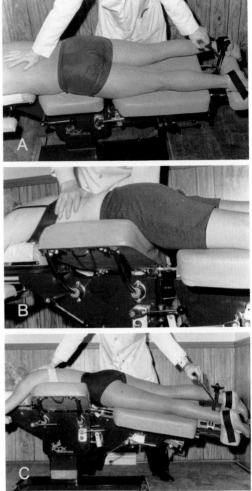

**Figure 8.38.** A, B, and C, rotation movements applied.

Note also that the table can be locked in any degree of rotation motion needed, so the doctor is not forced to control rotation movement during application of flexion.

## Postreduction and Manipulative Care

Following distraction or manipulation, the muscles are treated as they were prior to the Cox treatment.

A positive galvanic pad is placed over the disc lesion and over bladder point B54 behind the knee. Heat is applied over these pads for 10 minutes and then cold applied for 5 minutes, alternating hot and cold circulatory stimulation as described earlier.

## APPLICATION OF GALVANISM

Galvanism is a continuous, waveless, undirectional current of low voltage, commercially spoken of as a *direct current*. Galvanic current is decidedly chemical in action and, as it passes through the body, breaks up some of the molecules that it encounters into their component atoms or *ions* as they are more properly called. All ions have either a *positive* or *negative* electric charge and attract or repel each other with *like* charges repelling and *unlike* charges attracting. When two dissimilar ions unite, a neutral molecule is formed, but when the galvanic current breaks this union, the original positive and negative ions are liberated.

Table 8.1 outlines the action produced at the respective poles.

The active pole, either positive or negative, is the one that produces the effects desired. The other is the inactive or indifferent pole. The active should be the smaller in order to concentrate the current locally and thus intensify the action.

The milliamperes to be used depends on the smoothness of the current and the susceptibility of the patient, with from 5 to 20 ma being the average. The length of the treatment is determined by the milliamperes used, with from 5 to 15 minutes usually being sufficient time for application of the current.

Rules for the Application of Galvanic Current

1. Caution should be used to prevent galvanic burns.

2. Never dispute the patient. If he complains, investigate.

3. Be careful with paralyzed patients.

4. Avoid shocks.

5. See that the pads are properly placed, i.e. active and indifferent.

6. See that the intensity control is completely turned off before placing the pads.

7. Do not place or remove the pads while the instrument is running.

8. Be sure to have pads thoroughly moist but not dripping wet.

9. Turn current on and off slowly.

10. Have the patient remove enough clothing and protect the remainder from getting damp.

11. Never change poles while the current is flowing, except when testing.

12. Protect scars or wounds.

*Remember: Positive* ions are driven in under the positive pole.
*Negative* ions are driven in under the negative pole.

Polarity

The most important feature of the galvanic current is its *polarity*, with each pole having distinctive attributes and, consequently, being productive of certain specifically definite therapeutic effects. The action of one pole is opposed to that of the other pole. This matter of polarity must be well understood. The direct current (DC) decomposes liquid as it passes through it. This decomposing of a liquid by an electric current is termed *electrophoresis*. The liquid decomposed is the *electrolyte*; and the parts of the separated electrolyte are the *ions*. The current enters the electrode by the *anode (positive pole)* and leaves it by the *cathode (negative pole)*.

There are *positive ions* and *negative ions*. Those ions possessing an excess negative charge are termed *electronegative* and those possessing an excess positive charge are termed *electropositive*. It is a *universal law of electrical physics that like poles repel and unlike poles attract, therefore negative ions will travel toward the positive pole and positive ions will travel toward the negative pole*. Oxygen, being electonegative, is repelled from the negative pole and forms at the positive pole; hydrogen, being electropositive, is repelled from the positive pole and collects

**Table 8.1.**
**Actions Produced by Galvanic Content**

| Positive | Negative |
|---|---|
| Attracts acids | Attracts alkali |
| Repels alkali | Repels acid |
| Hardens tissue | Softens tissue |
| Contracts tissue | Dilates tissue |
| Stops hemorrhage | Increases hemorrhage |
| Diminishes congestion | Increases congestion |
| Sedative | Stimulating |
| Relieves pain in acute conditions due to reduction of congestion. If scar is formed, it is hard and firm. | Reduces pain in chronic conditions to softening of tissues and increase of circulation. If scar is formed, it is soft and pliable. |

at the negative. Consequently, when we treat a pain, we use the *positive* pole over the seat of pain because the positive pole is a sedative and is acid in reaction. We desire this reaction because where there is pain, there is always an alkaline reaction and by using the positive pole the alkalinity is driven toward the negative pole.

The slogan for pain is *positive pole*; however, there are exceptions. For instance, if inflammation has been prolonged sufficiently to cause distinct organic tissue changes (fibrosis, adhesions) that, in turn, cause pain on motion of the parts involved, the *negative* pole is used because of its liquefying and vasodilative properties.

Application of Electrodes

The active electrode is always the smaller of the two electrodes; the opposite electrode is known as the indifferent electrode and should be placed as nearly opposite to the active electrode as possible (Fig. 8.39). The indifferent electrode is usually a well-moistened pad.

Electrodes must be secured or must be held in contact with the patient before the instrument is turned on and current is allowed to flow. Also, contact between the patient and the electrode must not be broken while the current is flowing. Lastly, the current must not be turned off until it has been reduced to zero; otherwise the patient will receive a *shock*.

Patients with an acute disc lesion are best kept in the office throughout the day

so that treatment can be given 2 or 3 times. The patient should avoid sitting which increases the intradiscal pressure and slows healing. By lying recumbent the patient enhances healing. It is far superior to have the patient lie recumbent than to have the patient leave the office, get in a car, and drive home; the driving posture can destroy what you have accomplished through manipulation.

Following treatment of the disc, the patient is fitted with a lumbosacral support which he must wear for 24 hours a day until the leg pain eases. The patient is weaned from wearing of the support and is allowed to remove the support permanently when his back pain has ceased.

All patients with an acute disc lesion are treated for 3 months. At the outset, these patients are told to be prepared to come into the office every day for treatment. As they begin to respond, the length of time between treatments is then extended.

*As a rule, all patients are told that when they have low back and leg pain due to a disc protrusion, they must show at least a 50% relief from pain within 3 weeks or a neurosurgical consultation will be requested.* This statement relieves the patient of the worry as to what to do if treatment is not effective. Secondly, it lessens the chance that the patient will come for 3 or 4 visits and then stop coming for treatment. Lastly, it allows you to have the patient's complete confidence because he knows that, regardless of what it takes to fix this condition, you will see to it that it is done, which makes for an excellent doctor-patient relationship.

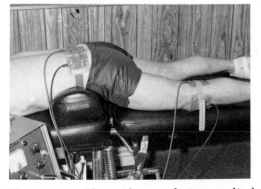

**Figure 8.39.** Physiotherapy being applied after distraction manipulation.

EXERCISES

The patient is started on the first 3 of the Cox exercises (see pages 194 and 195) at the outset of treatment, regardless of the severity of his pain. Following the relief of Déjérine's triad, i.e., relief of pain in the low back on coughing, sneezing, and straining at the stool, he is given the remainder of the exercises to do. These exercises must be chosen carefully by the doctor with regard to the patient's condition.

## THE COX EXERCISES

### TO ACCOMPANY CHIROPRACTIC MANAGEMENT OF LOW BACK PAIN

# General Instruction

Exercises for the acute severe low back pain patient.

Exercise 1.

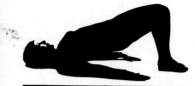

Lie on your back with your knees flexed and your feet flat on the floor as close to the buttocks as possible. Keep the knees together. Tighten the muscles of the lower abdoman and buttocks so as to flatten your low back against the floor. Slowly raise your hips up from the floor and hold for slow count of 8. Repeat this exercise 4 times. If you cannot raise your hips from the floor, merely tighten the belly, the abdominal and buttock muscles and wait until you can raise the hips.

Do Not Sit when you have low back pain. This increases the pressure within the disc and the joint of your spine. If your doctor prescribes a belt to wear, remove it to do these exercises. If your doctor agrees, it is good to alternate hot and cold on your low back before doing these exercises. This is done by applying moist heat in the form of a hot towel for 10 minutes followed by 5 minutes of ice therapy in which a moist cool towel is placed on the skin with an ice bag on top of it. Place the heat on the back 4 times and ice on the back 3 times beginning and ending with heat.

Exercise 2.

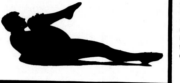

Lie on back and draw the right knee up to the chest and pull the knee down upon chest while attempting to touch the chin to the knee. Do this for a slow count of 8 and repeat 4 times. Repeat the same exercise with left knee brought to the chest. Relax between each session. Repeat with both knees brought up to the chest.

If your doctor suggests nutritional supplementation, be sure to follow it closely.

Exercise 3.

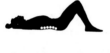

While standing or lying tighten the abdominal and buttock muscles so as to flatten your back. Repeat this several times throughout the day. Contract the muscles and relax the approximately 8 times at each session.

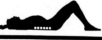

Do these exercise on a firm surface such as the floor or a mat. Do not be alarmed if discomfort is noted during exercise. If this pain is great, stop it and consult your doctor before continuing.

Exercises after the acute pain has diminished. Do the following exercises if you feel no pain in your low back upon coughing, sneezing, or straining to move the bowel.

Exercise 4.

Repeat #1 exercise above but be sure to hold the knees firmly together.

The Cox exercises are to be used in conjunction with your chiropractic care and should be discussed with the chiropractic physician before use.

Exercise 5.

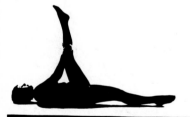

Do the exercises marked (x) in numerical order _____times a day.

Lie flat on your back and raise the right leg straight upward without bending the knee. Place your hands behind the knee while keeping the knee straight, pull the leg straight up so as to stretch the muscles behind your thigh. Repeat this 8 times on the right leg and then do it on the left. Relax your low back muscles following this exercise.

Exercise 6.

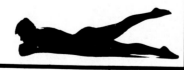

Lie on stomach and raise the right leg off of floor while keeping the knee straight. Hold the leg up in this position for a count of 4 and slowly let it down. Repeat this 4 times. Repeat the same exercise with the opposite leg. Relax following this exercise.

**Exercise 7.**

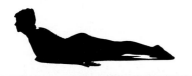

Lie flat on stomach with arms along side, palms down. Slowly raise chest from floor. Feel the muscles of the low back tighten. Hold the chest up from the floor for a slow count of 6 and slowly let it down. Rest between each session. Repeat this 6 times.

**Exercise 8.**

Sit on floor on your knees. Extend your right leg as far to the side as possible, keeping the knee straight and the arch of the foot on the floor. Slide your foot along the floor until you feel the stretch of the muscles inside your thigh. Do it slowly and hold for a count of 5. Repeat it 3 times on the right leg and then repeat with the left side. These muscles, which are tight at the beginning, will loosen and stretch with subsequent exercise sessions.

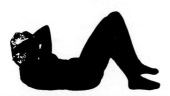

**Exercise 9.**

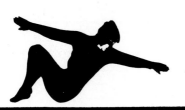

Abdominal Strengthening Exercises. Lie on Back with Knees bent and feet on floor. Bring chin to chest as shown. Now tighten the abdominal muscles so as to lift and curl the shoulders up to about 1 foot off the floor. Remember - curl up the spine from the neck downward to between the shoulder blade. Feel the abdominals tighten. Do this 10 to 30 times depending on your stamina.

**Exercise 10.**

Lie on side. Turn the toes inward on the right foot and lift leg upward. Repeat this 6 times on right and then 6 times on the left. You will feel pulling in the outer thigh and pelvis.

**Exercise 11.**

Lie on back and draw knees to chest, arms extended level with shoulders, roll hips to side in attempt to touch the knees to floor. Turn your head, in the opposite direction to which your knees are bending. Repeat this 4 times going first to the right and then to the left. This exercise brings all spinal movements together in a smooth forceful manipulation of the spinal articulations. Since the exercise involves rotation, it should only be done under physician instruction.

**Exercise 12.**

Lie on back. Bend knees and bring feet up to the buttocks. Now lift and straighten the legs so that the legs are at a right angle to the body. Raise the buttocks from the floor and place the hand beside the buttocks and support your pelvis as you raise the pelvis from the floor. Allow the legs to go over the head with feet over the head and the legs parallel to the floor. Hold this position for 10 seconds and repeat 2 - 3 times. Slowly lower your pelvis and legs to the original starting position. This exercise should only be used by those who have been working with the exercises for some time and have their low back pain under control.

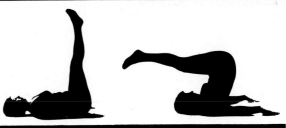

## NUTRITION

The patient is told to eat foods that will help him to avoid constipation and is instructed to take *Discat,* which contains 150 mg manganese sulfate, 150 mg calcium, 50 mg potassium, 75 mg magnesium, 4 mg iron, 10 mg zinc, and 50 mg perna canaliculus. Discat contains the minerals that research has found to be in the intervertebral disc. At the outset of treatment, 6 to 8 tablets/day are prescribed; at the end of 3 months a maintenance dosage of 2 tablets/day is prescribed.

## HOME CARE

According to Hirschberg (2), recent studies in which the intradiscal pressures have been measured in vivo have shown that intradiscal pressure is lowest when the patient lies supine with the hips flexed. Pressure increases when the subject lies on the side, sits, stands, bends forward, or lifts an object. Pressure is also increased when the subject strains, coughs, or laughs.

On the other hand, strong compression on the abdomen by means of a tight corset decreases the load on the lumbar discs and lowers the intradiscal pressure at the L3 level up to 50% when the subject stands or sits. These studies of intradiscal pressure explain the empirical fact that bed rest and a tight corset relieve the pain of lumbar disc lesion.

The patient is told to continue applications of heat and cold to his back every 4 hours at home, to avoid sitting, and, as much as possible, either to lie recumbent in the supine position or to stand. The effects of sitting, which are deleterious to the intervertebral disc, are explained, and the booklet, *Low Back and Leg Pain, What It Is and How It Is Treated,* which fully explains home care, is given to the patient. He is then sent to Low Back Pain School to learn the basic causes of low back pain and how to minimize its risk.

## Details on Manipulation of the Lumbar Spine

As explained earlier, the articulations of the patient who has no leg pain are put through the normal ranges of motion. This is done in a gentle manner, and each movement is performed approximately 6 times; i.e., if you are treating the L5-S1 facets, place them in flexion 6 times, in extension 6 times, in lateral bending to the right and to the left each 6 times, and in circumduction 6 times. Remember that circumduction is a combination of lateral bending and flexion and is perhaps the most effective means of placing a facet through its normal ranges of motion. It certainly is effective at releasing fixation subluxation.

## EFFECTS OF DISTRACTION OF THE INTERVERTEBRAL DISC

According to Cyriax (54), there are three effects from traction and its attendant distraction on the intervertebral disc (Fig. 8.40):

1. Increase in the interval between the vertebral bodies, thus enlarging the space into which the protrusion must recede.
2. Tautening of the joint capsule, which allows the ligaments joining the vertebral bodies to exert centripetal force all around the joint, thus tending to squeeze the pulp back into place.
3. Suction.

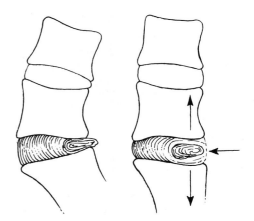

**Figure 8.40.** Positive effect of traction (lumbar flexion) upon protruding fragment of disc. (Reproduced with permission of B. E. Finneson: *Low Back Pain,* edition 2. Philadelphia, J. B. Lippincott, 1980, p. 312.)

## ACUTE SYMPTOMATIC DISC PROTRUSION

Kessler (55), in a discussion on the effects of pelvic traction, states that "*static pelvic traction must not be used in the acute stage of a disc prolapse*" The patient may feel less pain while the distractive force is applied, but as the traction is released, he often experiences a marked increase in pain. He may have some difficulty in rising from the treatment table. Such an effect is probably due to absorption of additional fluid by the nucleus while the traction is applied and the development of a high intradiscal pressure as the distractive force is relaxed. This unfortunate result is less likely to occur with intermittent traction, but few patients in the acute stage tolerate this well. We often hear of the patient with low back pain who enters the hospital and is placed in pelvic traction. How often these patients are the same or even worse following such traction! In clinical practice we often see patients who have been hospitalized, had every test done, and were discharged in the same or worse condition. Static traction actually opens the intervertebral disc space, can allow the nucleus to imbibe fluids, and can thereby increase the intradiscal pressure which will cause a worsening of pressure against the already-compressed nerve root.

According to Kessler (55), if a patient is hospitalized or can attend therapy sessions without risking worsening of the lesion from increased intradiscal pressure, treatment may include specific segmental manual distraction technics by a therapist skilled in such technics. Oscillatory technics may relieve pain by increasing large fiber and proprioceptive input and thus by relieving some of the protective muscle spasm. Possibly, decreasing the longitudinal slack in the posterior longitudinal ligament and annular lamellae overlying the bulge in the disc effects a centripetal movement of the disc material away from the pain-sensitive structures.

Thus, Kessler (55) believes that the management of the patient with an acute disc protrusion should include

1. Bed rest with short periods of ambulation.

2. Avoidance of positions or activity that may increase intradiscal pressure, especially sitting, forward bending, and the Valsalva maneuver.

3. Relaxation of reflexed muscle splinting.

4. *Specific segmental distraction technics.*

Please note that the Cox technic is a specific intermittent distraction. Distraction of the disc provides a push-pull pumping effect on the intervertebral disc space as the caudal section of the table is gently moved up and down during traction. This movement creates a milking action on the intervertebral disc space. Remember that in the acute stage of a disc lesion, the patient may not tolerate traction until some of the swelling and inflammation has dissipated.

## FURTHER DETAILS ON DISTRACTION MANIPULATION OF THE PATIENT WITH AN ACUTE DISC PROTRUSION

Many chiropractic physicians have found wanting the diagnosis and treatment of disc protrusion and its resultant sciatica. Our past knowledge was not rendering satisfactory regimes for this condition. The side posture adjustment of a disc protrusion, for any doctor who has experienced it, can be a nightmare. As a posteroanterior thrust or side posture adjustment is attempted, it is as if a hard piece of rubber with little flexibility were being encountered, and a lot of pain is being transmitted to the patient. Indeed, the patient often could not get off the table following the treatment and had great apprehension and perhaps disgust with the treatment.

Never, in the first 251 patients with disc protrusion and sciatica, have we hurt a patient; actually, it is by far the rule that the patient feels a degree of immediate relief and a feeling of confidence in the doctor and his treatment.

## Mechanics of Applying Cox Distraction Manipulation

The patient with a medial disc protrusion receives the same basic treatment as the patient with a lateral disc protrusion.

First, the patient is placed on the table
with the disc area over a split between
the front and rear sections (Fig. 8.41). The
ankle straps are placed over the ankles
after the patient has been tested for the
ability to withstand tractive force. The
patient pulls himself cephalad until his
ankles are tight in the cuffs. He may hold
the bar during traction. Following opening of the caudal section of the table as
traction is applied to the disc (Fig. 8.42),
the patient feels traction in the lumbar
area and often states that this affords relief.

Note that some patients (Figs. 8.41) hold
the armrest at the head of the table. The
armrest may be used to pull upward
against the ankle straps prior to traction;
some patients then prefer to continue to
hold the armrest at the head.

Next, flexion traction is applied (Fig.
8.43) while the spinous process directly
superior to the disc protrusion is held
with a thenar contact. This opens the disc

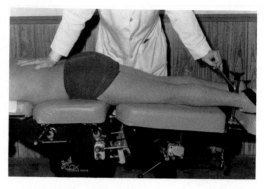

**Figure 8.43.** Flexion distraction being applied.

space, allowing reduction of the protruded disc material, stimulation of circulation, and decompression of the nerve
roots. The traction so applied is held for a
slow count of 8 to 10 or for 20 seconds,
depending upon patient tolerance. The
caudal section of the table is then moved
up and down slowly to create a milking
action on the disc space. Release of the
traction is performed slowly.

This traction is applied 3 times for approximately 20 seconds each time, for a
total of 1 minute of distraction. (A fine
differential point should be noted: The
patient with a protruding disc usually
states that he feels mild pain from traction, whereas the patient with a prolapsed
disc will not.) *Remember to not use a
strong traction.* Most doctors tend to use
too much force in applying the traction
technic. Start gently and increase the
traction as patient relaxation and confidence take place. Understand that following the traction the patient may have a
feeling of weakness or perhaps discomfort
in the low back. This is because swollen
irritated tissues are being tractioned during the reduction of the disc.

Medial and lateral disc protrusions are
treated in the same ways. After initial
plane traction at the specified disc level,
the lateral disc may be flexed, via the
caudal section of the table, away from the
side of pain so as to increase the lateral
flexion of the vertebra above the site of
disc protrusion, as is shown in Figure 8.44.
This flexion increases the distraction effect and hastens reduction of the lateral
disc.

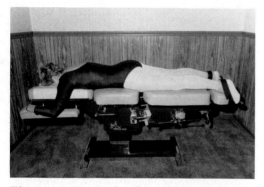

**Figure 8.41.** With the ankle cuffs attached, the patient pulls cephalad.

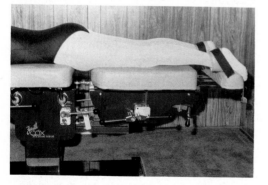

**Figure 8.42.** Caudal section of Cox table
is opened for traction.

For treatment of a left lateral L4 or L5 disc protrusion, the caudal end of the table is bent to the right so as to accentuate the right lateral flexion of L4 on L5 (Fig. 8.44).

According to most authorities, 90% of all disc lesions occur at one level and involve one nerve root. For that other 10% the following discussion is presented (Figs. 8.45 to 8.47).

Figure 8.45 is an illustration showing 4th lumbar disc compression of the 5th nerve root.

Figure 8.46 is an illustration showing the 4th lumbar disc compressing the 4th lumbar nerve root. This is unusual and has occurred in two patients who required surgery for repair, as documented by this author. A differential diagnosis we have encountered in practice is that at about 15° straight leg raise in a patient with disc protrusion into the intervertebral foramen the entire pelvis lifts off of the table instead of flexion occurring at the hip as in normal patients (Cox sign).

It is possible for a large disc protrusion to compress two nerve roots: both the one exiting at its intervertebral level as well as the nerve root originating at its level to exit at the foramen one level below (Fig. 8.47). The indication for the disc protrusion demonstrated in Figure 8.47 would be a patient who has nerve root dysesthesias in two dermatomes of the same extremity. This would indicate either two disc protrusions or a prolapse, such as is demonstrated here, impinging on two nerve roots at one level. If the former were the case, treatment of both disc protrusions would result in closed reduction of both discs. This would afford relief even in the absence of your knowledge of whether one or two disc protrusions were involved. Keep in mind that if the patient failed to show 50% relief in 3 weeks of conservative care, a neurosurgical evaluation would be sought. This would then allow discovery of such an unusual situation. As the attending physician, your duty is to be aware of this clinical possibility.

A difficult diagnostic situation is encountered when, during treatment of a 3rd lumbar disc protrusion, an L4 nerve root dermatome pattern is found. If no

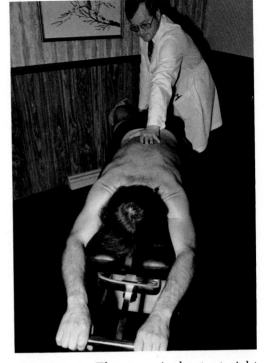

**Figure 8.44.** The arm is kept straight while applying traction to the spine and the table is right laterally flexed for a left lateral disc protrusion.

response is found in treating the 3rd lumbar disc, keep in mind the possibility of an L4 disc impingement on the intervertebral foramen. It is the author's opinion that intervertebral foramen encroachment by disc prolapse is probably a surgical case.

A thought to be entertained about the diagnosis and treatment of lumbar disc protrusion is the possibility that diseases of the female pelvis, such as urogenital infection and severe pelvic pain, might be due to nerve root compressions resulting from different types of disc degeneration (56). Herlin (56) describes a patient who had two miscarriages which, he believes, were due to a lower sacral nerve root compression which caused the lumbago and sciatica which developed afterward. He claims that there is a connection between low back pain and urogenital disorders and believes that if such a connection exists, the rationale of resecting uterine tubes and ovaries must be questioned especially as pain is not improved when

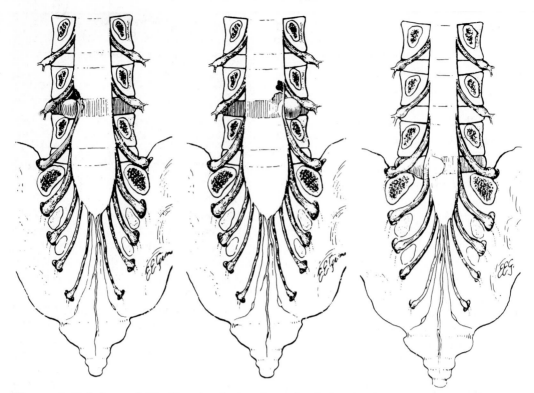

**Figure 8.45 (*above left*).** Usual relationship of 4th lumbar disc compression of L5 nerve root. The schematic illustration of the disc hernia pushing the L5 nerve root aside medially was predicted analytically and verified at operation. This patient had suffered from an intermittent, extremely painful left-sided L5 syndrome for 18 years. During periods of serious pain, the patient walked with a definite lean toward the right. Although the pain had been of long standing, the only nerve root involved in this overall picture of the disease was the left L5 nerve root. A year earlier the extensor paresis had become severely involved. Before that time, the extensor paresis had been rather variable and involved to a moderate degree. This patient had had a surgery done previously and the 4th lumbar disc exposed, but no hernia was found.

In this patient, the unnatural lean to the right indicated that the L5 nerve root was pushed medially. The patient recovered rapidly and became free of pain as he gradually regained satisfactory extensor muscle function. (Reproduced with permission from L. Herlin: *Sciatic and Pelvic Pain due to Lumbosacral Nerve Root Compression.* Springfield, IL, Charles C Thomas, 1966, p. 42.)

**Figure 8.46 (*above middle*).** Unusual lateral position of the disc prolapse extending into the intervertebral foramen to compress the L4 nerve root. This 32-year-old nurse's aide developed an acute attack of right-sided L5 syndrome 3 years prior to seeing the author. Six months prior to admission she had experienced an acute recurrence of the right-sided L5 syndrome with severe pain and extensor paresis.

During examination, the L5 syndrome was confirmed, but slight symptoms and signs from L4 were also noticed as minor radiating pain on the anterior side of the thigh. In addition, pain occurred during palpation over the muscular attachments of the adductor muscles. The Lasègue sign was positive, at a low angle, for L5. The knee jerk was normal. No sciatic scoliosis was apparent. When the patient bent to the right, distinct pain in the L5 distribution area was elicited; less pain was provoked by bending to the left. *Myelography was negative.* The diagnosis indicated a nerve root compression by a lateral disc protrusion on the right side in the 4th lumbar disc. This condition exerted a slight compression on L4 and severe compression together with a slight medial displacement on L5.

At surgery, the 4th disc level was explored and the L5 nerve root was displaced a little medially by the disc lesion. The intervertebral joint was resected in order to explore the L4 nerve root exiting the cauda equina through the intervertebral foramen. A major portion of the disc protrusion had been hidden by the intervertebral joint. Also found was the cranially displaced fragment of the nucleus pulposus that had pushed its way from the cavity and become lodged under the posterior longitudinal ligament of the spinal canal. It produced a sharp-angled cone that pinched the L5 nerve root at its angle of departure from the cauda equina.

The patient was immediately free of pain, and the extensor power returned quickly. (Reproduced with permission from L. Herlin: *Sciatic and Pelvic Pain due to Lumbosacral Nerve Root Compression.* Springfield, IL, Charles C Thomas, 1966, pp. 100–101.)

**Figure 8.47 (*opposite page, right*).** L5-S1 disc protrusion prolapse compressing both the L5 nerve root at the intervertebral foramen and the S1 nerve root at its origin at the cauda equina.

This schematic is of a 32-year-old housewife who had had two children and who had a history of intermittent low back pain and lumbago for several years. She had suffered two spontaneous miscarriages, the latest 4 months prior to admission, which had been immediately followed by the onset of left-sided sciatica.

The examination indicated mixed nerve root syndromes of a painless lateral L5 syndrome, an ordinary dominant S1 syndrome, and a left-sided S2 syndrome. The left S3 was also involved. Left S2 pain could be provoked at palpation over the inguinal region, the tuber ischii, the medial part of the fossa poplitea, and medially over the soleus muscle of the calf. S3 pain was provoked over the symphysis and the most median part of the gluteal musculature. There was no obvious scoliosis.

Diagnosis was of a large hernia in the 5th lumbar disc extending from the left lateral to the median line with its maximum bulk where the S1 nerve root runs over the disc.

Surgery confirmed the presence of a large disc hernia. The disc was evacuated and recovery was excellent.

Comment: The two miscarriages appear to have been due to a lower sacral nerve root compression which caused the onset of the lumbago with the sciatica developing later.

Herlin (56) documents other urogenital diseases due to lumbosacral nerve root compression. On page 79 (56) he discusses a situation which he had encountered in which severe pelvic pain and urogenital infection might be due to a cause similar to that of sciatica—nerve root compressions from the outside due to different types of disc degeneration. He believes that there is the possibility that whole pelvic diseased states depend upon multiple nerve root compressions of the S2 and the lower sacral nerve roots. Surgical relief of lumbosacral nerve roots resulted in normalization of such diseases as salpingitis, painful irregular menstruations, vaginal discharge, sluggish frequent urination, cystitis, prostatitis, urethritis, infertility, impotency, and vertigo. (Reproduced with permission from L. Herlin: *Sciatic and Pelvic Pain due to Lumbosacral Nerve Root Compression.* Springfield, IL, Charles C Thomas, 1966, pp. 14, 16, 19, 31, 120, 128, 168 and 169.)

oophorosalpingitis is caused by sacral
nerve root compression.

## APPLICATION OF PHYSICAL THERAPY FOLLOWING REDUCTION

Following closed reduction, positive
galvanism over the disc protrusion is performed as shown in Figure 8.48. One positive pad is placed directly over the disc
protrusion with the negative pad next to
it, and the other positive pad may be
placed on the gluteal region so as to sedate
the sciatic nerve there or placed over B54
in the popliteal space with the negative
pad opposite to it. Also, placing of the
positive pad over the Achilles tendon hastens the relief of sciatic pain. The galvanic
current is applied for 10 minutes. Following physical therapy, the patient is fitted
with a back support of 9 or 10 inches with
steel supports.

## HOME CARE FOR THE LOW BACK PAIN PATIENT

The following instructions for home
care are given to the patient:

1. *Do not sit.* Sitting is the worst thing
for a disc protrusion as it forces it to protrude.

2. Alternate hot moist heat for 10 minutes with 5 minutes of ice. Put the heat
on 4 times and the cold on 3 times, beginning and ending with heat.

3. Wear a back brace 24 hours a day
(early in treatment).

4. If constipation develops (the bowels
often become tight), treat accordingly.

5. Have someone rub an analgesic into
the low back every 4 hours.

6. Take manganese sulfate tablets (up
to 1000 mg/day). (Discat is a formula containing manganese sulfate and the trace
minerals found in the disc.)

7. In accordance with state laws, pain
formulas are prescribed as needed.

Treatment is rendered daily at the office. There should be some relief from
pain within 5 days. This will not be complete relief, but the patient will know he
is improving. In the treatment of medial
disc protrusion, relief may be slower, but
regardless, the patient should have great

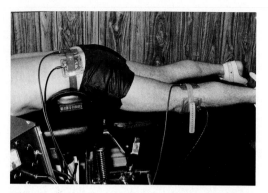

**Figure 8.48.**  Positive galvanism being applied.

relief from pain within 2 or 3 weeks. If
the relief is not what is expected, consultation with a neurosurgeon is indicated
due to the possibility of a disc prolapse
and the presence of a free fragment within
the spinal cord.

## Summary of Closed Reduction of Disc Protrusion

The closed reduction technic for the
disc protrusion is summarized below.
Careful study will allow you to apply this
technic with the use of the Cox table;
seeing a presentation, however, will
greatly enhance utilization of the technic
and the table.

1. Have the patient lie supine on the
table, as described earlier, and test for
tolerance to traction.

2. Plane traction is applied by opening
the caudal section of the table. Place your
fingertips on the patient's spinous processes and the paravertebral musculature
at the involved level. When you feel traction at that level or a slight tautening of
the muscles around the spinous processes,
discontinue opening of the caudal section.
Traction can also be accomplished by
having the patient grasp the armrest at
the head of the table while his ankles are
in the cuffs and pull himself cephalad,
which saves time.

3. Maintain contact on the spinous process of the vertebra directly above the disc
protrusion. For example, if you are treating a 4th lumbar disc protrusion, maintain
contact on the spinous process at L4 and
press down on the spinous process while

exerting pressure cephalad against the inferior portion of the 4th lumbar spinous process.

4. Now release the caudal section of the table, apply gentle traction by pressing down on the table, and ask the patient if he feels pain. The patient may feel discomfort; if so, stop and maintain contact for a slow count of 8 or 10 or for approximately 20 seconds. The push-pull pumping action of the caudal section of the table while the patient is under traction creates a milking action on the disc and assists in speeding recovery.

5. Repeat the above procedure to the patient's tolerance. You may feel a clicking release as you traction. This usually represents an instant relief from pain for the patient. If it is not felt, however, continue with treatment.

6. Repeat the above procedure one more time to the patient's tolerance or until you feel that a good traction has been applied to the involved segment. Three traction sessions of 20 seconds each are the rule.

7. After closed reduction, slowly return the caudal section of the table to its closed position, then release the ankle straps until this section of the table is closed, as this can cause a sharp pain in the patient's low back.

8. Treat the adductors, gluteals, and acupressure points, if necessary. The acupressure points for control of sciatic pain are illustrated on this page. Use of these points has been beneficial; treatment can be administered by pressure, galvanism, or needle acupuncture as state law allows.

9. Apply physical therapy.

10. Apply the belt to the patient before he rises from the table.

11. Give the patient instructions for home care and review them with him.

## Summary for Placing Articulations through their Normal Ranges of Motion

If the patient has only low back pain, or if you have treated him for a disc protrusion and gotten rid of his leg pain, manipulate the facets through their normal ranges of motion.

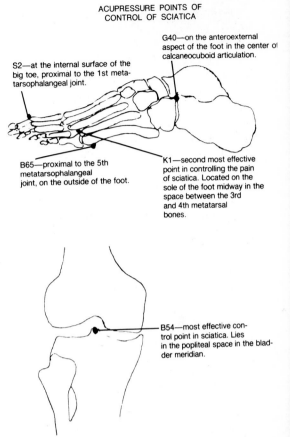

ACUPRESSURE POINTS OF CONTROL OF SCIATICA

G40—on the anteroexternal aspect of the foot in the center of calcaneocuboid articulation.

S2—at the internal surface of the big toe, proximal to the 1st metatarsophalangeal joint.

B65—proximal to the 5th metatarsophalangeal joint, on the outside of the foot.

K1—second most effective point in controlling the pain of sciatica. Located on the sole of the foot midway in the space between the 3rd and 4th metatarsal bones.

B54—most effective control point in sciatica. Lies in the popliteal space in the bladder meridian.

## CLINICAL RESEARCH FINDINGS ON DISC TREATMENT

Results of treatment of the first 100 patients with disc protrusion and sciatica seen by us at the Chiropractic Associates Diagnostic and Treatment Center, Fort Wayne, Indiana, are presented below. (Please review Tables 1.1 and 1.2 for the raw data.) The statistics leading to these results were gathered prior to 1975.

Patients with lateral disc protrusion with coronal facets responded most favorably to closed (chiropractic) reduction, whereas patients with medial disc protrusion with sagittal facets responded least favorably, requiring surgery most often. Thus, medial disc protrusion is the most difficult to treat and requires surgical intervention more often than does lateral disc protrusion.

Shapiro (57) reviewed reports on 3000 cases of single lumbar disc herniation in which he found that 43% occurred at L5-S1, 47% occurred at L4-L5, and 10% occurred at higher levels. Multiple prolapses occurred in 10% of the cases. Lecuire et al. (58) reviewed the results of 641 cases of lumbar disc herniation that went to surgery and found that 47% occurred at L5-S1, 39% occurred at L4-L5, and 2% occurred at L3-L4. Our results (see Table 8.2) show that of 69 cases of disc lesion, 48% occurred at L5-S1, 39% occurred at L4-L5, 9% occurred at L3-L4, and 4% occurred at multiple levels.

Table 8.3 breaks down our results even further into the position of the lesion in relation to the nerve root compressed. The majority (52%) of disc protrusions were lateral; 26% were medial; and the remainder were central (6%) or mixed (4%).

Table 8.4 shows the distribution of these cases of disc protrusion by level and position. Note that at L5-S1 the lateral disc protrusions were more common, while at the L4-L5 they were approximately equal in distribution. Central disc protrusion occurred in 50% at L4-L5 and in 50% at L5-S1. The occurrence of multilevel disc protrusions can be gleaned from the correlative diagnosis chart (Table 8.2). One case occurred in a patient with myelographi-

**Table 8.2.**
**Level of Lesion in 69 Cases of Disc Herniation Treated in 1975**

| Level | No. | % |
|---|---|---|
| L3-L4 | 6 | 9 |
| L4-L5 | 27 | 39 |
| L5-S1 | 33 | 48 |
| Two or more levels | 3 | 4 |
|   L3-L4 ⎫<br>  L4-L5 ⎬<br>  L5-S1 ⎭ | 1 | |
|   L4-L5 ⎫<br>  L5-S1 ⎭ | 2 | |

**Table 8.3.**
**Position of Protrusion (in Relation to the Nerve Root Compressed) in 69 Cases of Disc Herniation Treated in 1975**

| | No. | % |
|---|---|---|
| Medial | 26 | 38 |
| Lateral | 36 | 52 |
| Central | 4 | 6 |
| Mixed | 3 | 4 |

**Table 8.4.**
**Level of Protrusion in Relation to Position in 69 Cases of Disc Herniation Treated in 1975**

| Level | Medial | | Lateral | | Central | |
|---|---|---|---|---|---|---|
| | No. | % | No. | % | No. | % |
| L5-S1 (33)[a] | 12 | 36 | 19 | 58 | 2 | 6 |
| L4-L5 (27) | 13 | 48 | 12 | 44 | 2 | 8 |
| L3-L4 (6) | 1 | 17 | 5 | 83 | 0 | 0 |
| Multilevel (3) | See Table 8.2; one case was myelographically proven | | | | | |

[a] Numbers in parentheses are total number of cases at each level.

**Table 8.5.**
**Results in 69 Cases of Disc Herniation Treated in 1975**

| Result | Lateral | | Medial | | Central | | Multiple | |
|---|---|---|---|---|---|---|---|---|
| | No. | % | No. | % | No. | % | No. | % |
| Excellent | 31 | 86 | 22 | 84 | 3 | 75 | 1 | 33.3 |
| Good | 3 | 8 | 4 | 15 | | | 1 | 33.3 |
| Surgery | 2 | 6 | | | | | 1 | 33.3 |
| Unknown | | | | | 1 | 25 | | |

**Table 8.6.**
**Results (in Relation to Facet Facings Involved) in 69 Cases of Disc Herniation Treated in 1975**

| Facet Facing at Site of Lesion | Result | | |
|---|---|---|---|
| | Excellent | Good | Surgery |
| Coronal | 41 | 4 | 1 |
| Sagittal | 3 | 1 | |
| Mixed | 13 | 2 | 1 |
| Unknown | | | 1 |

cally proven disc protrusion who was awaiting surgery when he came to our office for treatment.

Of these 69 cases, 33 (48%) had sciatic pain extending into the right extremity, 29 (42%) had sciatic pain extending into the left extremity, and 4 (6%) had bilateral sciatica.

Table 8.5 shows that excellent results were obtained in the majority of cases of lateral and medial disc protrusions. Poor results were obtained in cases of multilevel disc protrusion.

Table 8.6 shows the distribution of these cases by treatment result and facet facing involved. It should be noted that

46 of the 69 cases had coronal facets and less than 5% had sagittal facets at L4-L5 and L5-S1 bilaterally. On the other hand, over 65% of the cases involved the coronal facets and 23% involved mixed facets or tropism. (Remember the word tropism is derived from the Greek word *trope*, meaning turn.) Results in the other 7% were unknown.

Farfan and Sullivan (59) indicate that annular tears are related to the orientation of the facets; i.e., asymmetrical articular processes led to asymmetrical degeneration and disc protrusions tended to be on the side of the more oblique joint surface. Also, they believe that when one facet facing is coronal and the other is sagittal, loss of rotational stability occurs.

Statistics presented in Table 8.7 show that 36 cases of disc protrusion were male and 33 were female. Among the nonsurgical cases, the youngest was 20 years old and the oldest was 71 years old. The mean average age in the nonsurgical cases was 43.45 years. Of the 3 surgical cases, 2 were female and 1 was male; the average age was 55 years, with the youngest being 42 years old and the oldest being 74 years old. The average age at surgery is essentially unimportant because of the small number of cases.

Of the 69 cases, 30 involved the left extremity and 33 involved the right extremity, with 6 cases of bilateral involvement. Of the 6 cases of bilateral sciatica, 2 involved two discs and 4 had central-type protrusions. Of the 6 cases of bilateral sciatica, only one patient needed surgery. This patient (Case 7) had spondylolisthesis of the 4th lumbar vertebral body with a central-type disc lesion and had had surgical repair prior to chiropractic treatment. A second surgery was performed because of poor conservative response, and again this surgery was not successful. The author believes that in case 7 a medial disc at L5-S1 on the left side was present which was responsible for the pain following the second surgery.

In almost all 69 cases, back pain preceded sciatica (Table 8.8). According to Horal (60), 35% of low back pain sufferers develop sciatica.

Careful study of the statistical data in Table 8.7 also shows that coughing, sneezing, straining, bending, lifting, and sitting aggravate sciatica and/or low back pain. Keep in mind that the normal pressure of cerebrospinal fluid in the lateral recumbent position varies between 100 and 200 mm $H_2O$, while the pressure in the sitting position is 200 mm $H_2O$ higher than that in the recumbent position (61). This is the physiological reason the patient with a disc lesion must avoid sitting.

A rise in venous pressure following coughing, sneezing, or straining hinders absorption of cerebrospinal fluid and thus raises the fluid pressure. This is the principle behind Queckenstedt's sign in which the internal jugular vein is compressed, resulting in an increase in cerebrospinal fluid pressure.

Sciatica, as can be seen from the statistical data presented, may extend along the entire length of the sciatic nerve or any portion of the same. Remember that the disc may protrude and irritate the annulus fibrosus, creating low back pain and/or antalgic lean without radiating sciatica. This is a basis of Horal's statement (60) about the development of sciatica in low back pain sufferers.

Statistics were compiled on the incidence of back pain, sciatica, or surgery in other family members in each of the 69 cases. In 50 of the 69 cases, the family history of back pain, sciatica, or surgery was recorded. The other 19 cases were not reported on as to family incidence. Of the 50, 26 were male and 24 were female. The statistics have been divided into male and female patient categories to ascertain any differences in familial incidence. Of the 50 cases, 28 (56%) showed a familial tendency of back pain, leg pain, or surgery. The remaining 22 (44%) denied or did not know of any family incidence other than themselves.

Table 8.9 presents data on the incidence of male patients treated and on the number and percent of their family members having the same problems. Note that the only male patient requiring surgery, Case 19, had a father who had required surgery.

Table 8.10 presents data on the incidence of female patients treated and on the number and percent of their family members having the same problems. One

**Table 8.7.**
**Statistical Data on 69 Cases of Low Back Pain and Sciatica Treated in 1975**

| Case | Occupation | Age | Family History of | | | Extremity Involved[a] | Back Pain Simultaneous, Before, or After Leg Pain | Pain Aggravated by[b] | Extension of Sciatic Pain | Sex[d] |
|---|---|---|---|---|---|---|---|---|---|---|
| | | | Back Pain | Sciatica | Surgery | | | | | |
| 1 | Farmer | 62 | Mother Brother | Mother Brother | None | L | Before | C SN ST B L S | B T K C F toes | M |
| 2 | Housewife | 33 | Unknown | Unknown | Unknown | R | | C SN ST B L S | B T K | F |
| 3 | Factory | 24 | Mother Father Brother | Mother Father Brother | None | R | Before | C SN ST B L S | B | M |
| 4 | General Electric—heavy lifting | 28 | Father | Father | None | L | Before | C SN B L S | B T K C F toes | M |
| 5 | Housewife | 49 | Mother | Mother | Mother | L | Before | C SN ST S | B T K C | F |
| 6 | Bus driver | 35 | Father | Father Mother | None | R | Before | C SN ST B L S | B T | F |
| 7 | Secretary | 50 | Unknown | Unknown | Unknown | Bilateral | Simultaneous | B L S | B T K C F toes | F |
| 8 | Retired | 67 | Unknown | Unknown | Unknown | R | Before | SN ST B L S | B T K C F | M |
| 9 | Housewife | 39 | Sister Mother | Sister Mother | None | Bilateral | Before | C SN ST B L S | B T K C F toes | F |
| 10 | Steelworker | 21 | Mother | Mother | None | L | Before | C SN ST B L S | B T K C F | M |
| 11 | Unknown | 22 | Unknown | Unknown | Unknown | Bilateral | Before | C SN S | B T K C F toes | F |
| 12 | Student, secretary | 51 | Unknown | Unknown | Unknown | L | Before | Unknown | B T | F |
| 13 | Factory | 29 | Father Sister | Father Sister | Father | R | Before | SN B L S | B T K C F toes | F |
| 14 | Railroad | 55 | None | None | None | R | Before | ST B L S | B T K C F | M |
| 15 | Farmer, business | 46 | Father Sister | Father Sister | None | R | Before | C SN ST B L S | B T K C F toes | M |
| 16 | Housewife | 64 | None | None | None | Bilateral | Before | C SN ST B L S | B T K C F toes | F |
| 17 | Filling station | 47 | None | None | None | L | Before | ST B L S | B T K C F | M |
| 18 | Auto salvager | 55 | Unknown | Unknown | Unknown | L | Before | C SN ST B L S | B T K C F toes | M |

| No. | Occupation | Age | | | | Side | Onset | | | Sex |
|---|---|---|---|---|---|---|---|---|---|---|
| 19 | Attorney | 42 | Father | Father | None | R | Before | C SN ST B LS | BTKCF | M |
| 20 | Factory | 56 | Father | Father | None | R | Before | ST B S LS | BTKCF | M |
| 21 | Student | 19 | Mother | Mother | None | R | Before | C SN ST B LS | BTKCF | M |
| 22 | Railroad | 36 | Father | Father | None | L | Before | C SN ST B LS | BT | M |
| 23 | Insurance | 30 | Unknown | Unknown | Unknown | L | Before | C SN ST B LS | B | M |
| 24 | Supervisor | 44 | Sisters (2) | None | None | R | Before | C SN ST B L | BTKCF | M |
| 25 | Housewife | 51 | None | None | None | R | Before | C SN ST B LS | BTKCF | F |
| 26 | Plumber | 31 | None | None | None | R | Before | ST B LS | BT | M |
| 27 | Housewife | 45 | Mother | Mother | None | L | Before | B LS | BTKCF | F |
| 28 | Secretary | 52 | None | None | None | L | Before | C SN ST B LS | BTKC | F |
| 29 | Truck driver | 61 | Unknown | Unknown | Unknown | L | Before | C SN ST B LS | BTKCF | M |
| 30 | Veterinarian | 34 | Unknown | Unknown | Unknown | L | Before | C SN ST B LS | BTK | M |
| 31 | Housewife | 36 | Father | Father | Father | R | Before | C SN ST B LS | BTK | F |
| 32 | Engineer | 37 | Mother | Mother | None | L | Before | C SN ST B LS | BTKCF toes | M |
| 33 | Truck driver | 29 | Mother | Mother | None | R | Before | C SN ST B LS | BTKCF | M |
| 34 | Gardener | 71 | Unknown | Unknown | Unknown | L | Before | C SN ST B LS | BTKCF | M |
| 35 | Housewife | 33 | Father, Brother | Father, Brother | Father, Brother | R | Simultaneous | C SN ST B LS | BT | F |
| 36 | Cement worker | 30 | Father | Father | None | R | Before | C SN ST B LS | BTK | M |
| 37 | Secretary | 41 | None | None | None | L | Before | C SN ST B LS | BTKC | F |
| 38 | Secretary | 41 | None | None | None | R | Before | B LS | BTKC | F |
| 39 | Retired worker | 67 | Sister | Sister | None | L | Before | ST B LS | BTKCF | F |

**Table 8.7.—Continued**

| Case | Occupation | Age | Family History of | | | Extremity Involved[a] | Back Pain Simultaneous, Before, or After Leg Pain | Pain Aggravated by[b] | Extension of Sciatic Pain | Sex[d] |
|---|---|---|---|---|---|---|---|---|---|---|
| | | | Back Pain | Sciatica | Surgery | | | | | |
| 40 | Housewife | 59 | Brothers (2) Sister | Brothers (2) Sister Nephew | Brothers (2) Nephew | L | No back pain | B L S | B T K C F | F |
| 41 | Housewife | 67 | None | None | None | R | Before | SN B L S | B T K C F | F |
| 42 | Factory worker | 48 | Unknown | Unknown | Unknown | Bilateral | Simultaneous | C SN ST B L S | B T K C F | M |
| 43 | Factory worker | 37 | None | None | None | R | Before | C SN ST B L S | B T K | M |
| 44 | Housewife | 46 | None | None | None | R | Before | C SN ST B L S | B T K C | F |
| 45 | Housewife | 62 | None | None | None | L | Before | C SN ST B L S | B T K | M |
| 46 | Factory worker | 56 | None | None | None | R | Before | C SN ST B L S | B T K C F toes | F |
| 47 | Farmer, insurance agent | 60 | None | None | None | Bilateral | Before | C SN ST B L S | B T K C | M |
| 48 | Housewife | 48 | Unknown | Unknown | Unknown | R | Before | B L S | B T K C F | F |
| 49 | School teacher | 45 | Father Mother | Father Mother | None | R | Before | C SN ST B L S | B T K C F toes | F |
| 50 | Housewife | 63 | Unknown | Unknown | Unknown | R | Simultaneous | C SN ST B L S | B T K C F | F |
| 51 | Chemical Sales | 39 | None | None | None | L | Unknown | S | Back only | M |
| 52 | Waitress | 30 | None | None | None | L | Simultaneous | C SN ST B L S | B T K C F | F |
| 53 | Housewife | 62 | None | None | None | R | Before | C SN ST B L S | B T K C F toes | F |
| 54 | Factory worker | 39 | Unknown | Unknown | Unknown | R | Before | C SN ST B L S | B | M |
| 55 | Factory worker | 36 | None | None | None | L | Before | C SN ST B L S | B T K | M |
| 56 | Deliveryman | 21 | None | None | None | L | Before | ST B L S | B T K | M |
| 57 | Truck driver | 44 | Unknown | Unknown | Unknown | R | Before | C SN ST B L S | Testicles | M |

| 58 | Factory worker | 36 | Unknown | Unknown | Unknown | L | Before | C SN ST B L S | Left testicle | M |
|---|---|---|---|---|---|---|---|---|---|---|
| 59 | Clerk in fabric store | 51 | Father Mother Sister | Father Mother Sister | | L | After | C SN ST B L S | B T | F |
| 60 | Housewife | 25 | Mother | Mother | Unknown | R | Before | Standing | B T K | F |
| 61 | Works in printing shop | 61 | Unknown | Unknown | Unknown | R | Before | C SN ST B L S | B T K and groin | F |
| 62 | Housewife | 51 | Father Sister | Sister | | R | Before | S | B T K | F |
| 63 | Factory worker | 20 | Father Mother Brother | Father Mother Brother | | R | Before | C SN ST B L S | B | M |
| 64 | Unknown | 74 | Unknown | Unknown | Unknown | R | Before | Unknown | B T K C F | F |
| 65 | Clerk-typist | 39 | None | None | None | L | Simultaneous | C SN ST B L S | B T K C | F |
| 66 | Laborer | 30 | None | None | None | R | Before | C S | B | M |
| 67 | Unknown | 33 | Father | None | None | R | Before | C B L S | B | M |
| 68 | Manual laborer | 42 | Father | None | None | L | Before | C SN ST B L S | B T | M |
| 69 | Housewife | 47 | Unknown | Unknown | Unknown | L | Before | C SN ST B L S | B T K | F |

a L, left; R, right.
b C, coughing; SN, sneezing; ST, straining; B, bending; L, lifting; S, sitting.
c B, buttock; T, thigh; K, knee; C, calf; F, foot.
d M, male; F, female.

**Table 8.8.**
**Onset of Back Pain in Relation to Sciatica in 69 Cases in 1975**

| | |
|---|---|
| Before | 59 |
| After | 1 |
| Simultaneous | 6 |
| No back pain | 1 |
| Unknown | 2 |

**Table 8.9.**
**Familial Incidence of Low Back Pain, Sciatica, or Surgery in 26 Male Patients**

| | Father | | Mother | | Brother | | Sister | |
|---|---|---|---|---|---|---|---|---|
| | No. | % | No. | % | No. | % | No. | % |
| Back pain | 11 | 42 | 6 | 23 | 3 | 11.5 | 3 | 11.5 |
| Sciatica | 7 | 27 | 6 | 23 | 3 | 11.5 | 1 | 4 |
| Surgery | 1 | 4 | | | | | | |

**Table 8.10.**
**Familial Incidence of Low Back Pain, Sciatica, or Surgery in 24 Female Patients**

| | Father | | Mother | | Brother | | Sister | | Nephew | |
|---|---|---|---|---|---|---|---|---|---|---|
| | No. | % | No. | % | No. | % | No. | % | No. | % |
| Back pain | 7 | 29 | 6 | 25 | 2 | 8 | 6 | 25 | 1 | 4 |
| Sciatica | 6 | 25 | 6 | 25 | 2 | 8 | 6 | 25 | 1 | 4 |
| Surgery | 1 | 4 | 1 | 4 | 2 | 8 | 1 | 4 | 1 | 4 |

woman, Case 40, had two brothers and a nephew who required surgical repair for disc lesion as well as a sister who had both back pain and sciatica. Another woman, Case 7, had had surgery with no relief from pain, sought chiropractic treatment with no relief, and had a second surgery with poor result.

Thus, there was a stronger familial tendency to back pain and sciatica among men than among women (Tables 8.9 and 8.10), although the incidence among mothers of both men and women suffering from back pain and/or sciatica was equal. There also seems to be a higher incidence of back pain, sciatica, or surgery among sisters.

Table 8.11 presents data on the x-ray evaluation of these 69 patients. Spinal tilt primarily refers to right or left lateral flexion of the vertebral column from a given lumbar level. Sciatic scoliosis means that some vertebral body rotatory subluxation

pattern definitely could be ascertained above the level of the disc lesion. This scoliosis might have been primarily of the Lovett-positive, Lovett-negative, or excess variety. The lumbosacral angles for each case are given. Scoliosis is defined as the voluntary or reflex attempt to avoid pain; in medial disc protrusion the patient lists toward the side of the pain, whereas in lateral disc protrusion the patient lists away from the side of the pain.

The lumbosacral angle in these cases varied from as low as 5° to as high as 56°, with a mean average of 28°. In 42 of 64 cases in which the lumbosacral angle was known, it was below 30°. The lumbosacral angle has been found to be between 37° and 42° by many authorities, and the fact that this angle is decreased in the disc lesion is apparent from this statistic. This would be expected because of the loss of lumbar lordosis typically noted in cases of disc lesion. The author, therefore, has noted a decrease in lumbar lordosis in cases of disc lesion. Horal (60), Hult (62), and Splitoff (63) found that there was a decreased inclination of the lumbosacral joint to protect it from annular change. It has been noted that the facet syndrome and increased sacral angles generally elicit little sciatic pain but do elicit severe back pain. The author believes that this is the result of pressure on the nerve root as the facet of the vertebra below enters the upper third of the intervertebral foramen as well as the facet irritation of the sinuvertebral and dorsal ramus.

The incidence of developmental abnormalities in the lumbar spine which are associated with disc lesion is given in Table 8.12.

Of 6 spondylolisthesis cases, 5 were at the L5 level and 1 was at the L4 level. The case at the L4 level had an L4-L5 disc surgically repaired twice with poor result. Of the 5 cases at the L5 level, 3 involved the L5-S1 disc and 2 involved the L4-L5 disc. All 5 patients made excellent recoveries.

Of the 7 spines demonstrating transitional changes at the lumbosacral level, 6 showed unilateral pseudosacralization of L5 and 1 showed unilateral pseudosacralization of L6. Interestingly, all 6 pseudosacralizations occurred on the left side.

**Table 8.11.**
**X-ray Evaluation in 69 Cases of Low Back Pain and Sciatica Treated in 1975**

| Case | Spinal Tilt from Whichever Level Cephalad | | Sciatic Scoliosis | | Lumbosacral Angle (°) |
| | Right | Left | Right | Left | |
|---|---|---|---|---|---|
| 1 | | L5 | | | 10 |
| 2 | | L5 | | | 24 |
| 3 | L4 | | | | 15 |
| 4 | | | | | 10 |
| 5 | | L5 | | | 10 |
| 6 | | L5 | | | 36 |
| 7 | | | | Positive | 25 |
| 8 | L5 | | | | 42 |
| 9 | | | | | 40 |
| 10 | L4 | | | | 23 |
| 11 | L4 | | Positive | | 27 |
| 12 | | L4 | | Positive | 5 |
| 13 | L4 | | | | 12 |
| 14 | L5 | | | | 37 |
| 15 | L5 | | | | 34 |
| 16 | L5 | | | | 45 |
| 17 | | L5 | | | 53 |
| 18 | | L4 | Positive | | 30 |
| 19 | | L5 | Positive | | 14 |
| 20 | | L4 | | | 12 |
| 21 | L3 | | | Positive | 47 |
| 22 | | L5 | Positive | | 22 |
| 23 | | L5 | | | 25 |
| 24 | | L5 | | | 29 |
| 25 | L5 | | Positive | | 10 |
| 26 | L4 | | | | 35 |
| 27 | L5 | | | | 36 |
| 28 | | L4 | | Positive | 20 |
| 29 | | L4 | | | 22 |
| 30 | L4 | | | | 26 |
| 31 | | | | | 25 |
| 32 | | | | | 25 |
| 33 | | L4 | | Positive | 20 |
| 34 | | L5 | | | 30 |
| 35 | L4 | | Positive | | 15 |
| 36 | | L3 | | | 15 |
| 37 | | L5 | | Positive | 34 |
| 38 | | | | | 29 |
| 39 | | L5 | | | 50 |
| 40 | L4 | | | | 20 |
| 41 | | L4 | | Positive | 29 |
| 42 | L4 | | | Positive | 38 |
| 43 | L5 | | Positive | | 56 |
| 44 | | L5 | | | 25 |
| 45 | L5 | | | Positive | 15 |
| 46 | | | | | 22 |
| 47 | | L5 | | Positive | 36 |
| 48 | | L5 | | Positive | 29 |
| 49 | | L5 | Positive | | 47 |
| 50 | | | | Positive | 10 |
| 51 | L5 | | | | 20 |
| 52 | L4 | | | | 45 |
| 53 | | L4 | | | 46 |
| 54 | | L5 | | | 30 |

**Table 8.11.—*Continued***

| Case | Spinal Tilt from Whichever Level Cephalad | | Sciatic Scoliosis | | Lumbosacral Angle (°) |
|------|------|------|------|------|------|
| | Right | Left | Right | Left | |
| 55 | | L5 | | | 37 |
| 56 | | | | | Unknown |
| 57 | | L3 | | Positive | 44 |
| 58 | L3 | | Positive | | 19 |
| 59 | | L3 | Positive | | 35 |
| 60 | | L4 | Positive | | 27 |
| 61 | | | Positive | | 50 |
| 62 | | L5 | | Positive | Unkown |
| 63 | L4 | | Positive | | 23 |
| 64 | | L4 | Positive | | Unknown |
| 65 | | L5 | | | 26 |
| 66 | | L5 | Positive | | 30 |
| 67 | | L4 | | Positive | Unknown |
| 68 | Unknown | Unknown | Unknown | Unknown | Unknown |
| 69 | L3 | | | | 26 |

**Table 8.12.**
**Incidence of Developmental Abnormalities of the Lumbar Spine in 69 Cases of Low Back Pain and Sciatica Treated in 1975**

| Abnormality | No. of Patients | Level |
|------|------|------|
| Spina bifida | 4 | S1 |
| Spondylolysis | 3 | L5 |
| Spondylolisthesis | 5 | L5 |
| | 1 | L4 |
| Transitional changes | 7 | |
| Pedicle hypoplasia | 38 | |
| Hypoplastic disc | 9 | |

Transitional segments in normal spines have been found to occur in approximately 6% of the population; in this study of 69 disc lesions, the segments were found to occur in 7 cases or 10% of the patients. This shows a minimally increased incidence of a disc lesion in the transitional segments. Other authors have found no increased incidence of the disc lesion in patients with transitional segments. This author does show a slight increase in his cases. Lecuire (58) found a 13% incidence of transitional change in 641 surgical cases.

Much discussion has been given to the normal development of the pedicles at L5 and, to a lesser extent, at L4. When all pedicles in the lumbar spine on lateral lumbar projections were measured according to Finneson's technic (64), 38 of the 69 cases had underdeveloped pedicles at the L4 and the L5 levels. Of the 38 cases of pedicle hypoplasia, the L5 level was involved in all cases, with the L4 level involved in 11 cases and the L3 level involved in 2 cases. It is not the intent of the author to discuss normal pedicle development in the low back, but it can be stated that whether the pedicle was normal or abnormal, underdeveloped pedicles occurred in 55% of the cases of disc lesion.

Hypoplastic discs were found in 9 cases at the L5-S1 level, usually in conjunction with sacralization and always with accompanying underdeveloped pedicles at that level.

In Case 21, the patient also had a well-developed knife-clasp syndrome at the L5-S1 level. This patient also had a left pseudosacralization. Both developmental anomalies, as well as the disc lesion, are capable of pain production.

Cases 64 through 68 are from another clinic. The author did not view the x-rays and, therefore, cannot discuss the facet arthritis or the spondylosis in these cases. The incidence of narrowed disc space was certainly not always at the level of the disc lesion, and when reading the film, one must be careful not to place blame on the disc at the level of thinning and degenerative changes. The offending disc may have good space with no degenerative change either above or below the level of demonstrable x-ray degeneration.

Retrolisthesis was found in 11 of these cases, and in all except 3, it occurred at the 5th lumbar level. Again, these cases occurred in conjunction with underdeveloped pedicles. The incidence of retrolisthesis of the lumbar spine is not within the scope of this book; however, one does question whether underdeveloped pedicles and retrolisthesis represent the abnormal state which has been associated with them in the past. This author believes that the primary importance of underdeveloped pedicles is the narrowing of the anteroposterior diameter of the vertebral canal which leads to greater incidence of root pressure in disc protrusion. This is discussed in relation to the narrowed and trefoil vertebral canal in Chapter 7.

Table 8.13 lists the pathologies found on x-ray. Other pathological findings associated with the disc lesion were osteitis condensans ileii in Case 2; advanced aortic atherosclerosis in Case 16—a patient with angina pectoris due to angiographically proven coronary insufficiency; advanced degenerative changes in Cases 18 and 20; renal calculus in Case 24; Paget's disease of the right innominate in Case 39; a complete surgical laminectomy at L4, old healed infectious tubercular spondylitis of the left sacroiliac joint, and advanced osteoporosis in Case 61.

The data in Table 8.14 indicate that lumbar lordosis was usually decreased, spinal tilt was noted, pain on palpation at the level of the lesion with percussion was usually evident, and limitation of motion was well documented. Jugular compression was found to be negative in most cases. When there is no mark in the column, the test was negative.

The leg raise sign was often positive bilaterally. This occurred typically in the well leg raise sign accompanying medial disc protrusion. When the well leg is raised in the presence of a medial disc protrusion on the opposite side, the nerve root is stretched over the disc and results in aggravation of the sciatic nerve.

Kemp's sign is often bilaterally positive; this usually occurs in cases of central or medial disc protrusion in which some contact can be made with both nerve roots as the test is performed.

Neurological examination of the sensory changes revealed that 55 of the 69 cases had increased or decreased cutaneous sensation over the involved dermatome. Of these 55 with positive sensory changes, 43 (78%) were of decreased cutaneous sensation.

The motor changes found in the lower extremity were decreased dorsiflexion of the foot in 14 cases of L4 disc compression of the 5th lumbar nerve root and in 12 cases of plantar flexion weakness caused by 5th lumbar disc compression of the 1st sacral nerve root. Dorsiflexion of the great toe revealed weakness in 7 cases of 5th lumbar nerve root compression caused by the 4th lumbar disc. Great toe plantar flexion revealed weakness in 3 cases of 5th lumbar disc compression of the 1st sacral nerve root. Atrophy of the thigh or calf was found in only 2 of the cases. The ankle jerk was found to be diminished or absent in 18 cases of 5th lumbar disc lesions.

In comparison of the first 100 cases with the last 69, (Table 8.15), no great difference is noted between the location of the disc lesion in relation to the nerve root involved and the level of disc lesion. The big change is in the need for surgery. Although 2 of the 36 cases of lateral discs protrusion (5.5%) in the latter study did require surgery, there was a dramatic drop in the number of cases of medial disc protrusion requiring surgery, from 20.9% in the first 100 cases to none in the last 69 cases. It must be mentioned that of the 4 cases of central disc protrusion, 1 (25%) required surgical repair. Three cases of multilevel disc lesion occurred. One had excellent response, one good, and one required surgery. The multilevel disc is by far the most difficult to diagnose and treat, regardless of the approach used.

Table 8.16 shows the statistical results

**Table 8.13.**
**Incidence of Pathologies Found at X-ray**

|  |  |
|---|---|
| Schmorl's nodes | 1 |
| Widened disc space | 5 |
| Narrowed disc space | 38 |
| Limbus vertebrae | 0 |
| Discogenic spondylosis | 17 |
| Facet arthritis | 20 |
| Retrolisthesis | 11 |
| Other | 15 |

**Table 8.14.**
**Orthopedic and Neurological Evaluation in 69 Cases of Low Back Pain and Sciatica Treated in 1975**

| Case | Lumbar Lordosis[a] | Spinal Tilt[b] | Level of Pain on Palpation | | Level of Percussion Pain | Jugular Compression | ° of Flexion Possible | ° of Extension Possible | ° of Right Lateral Flexion |
|---|---|---|---|---|---|---|---|---|---|
| | | | Right | Left | | | | | |
| 1 | D | R | L4-L5 | L4-L5 | L4-L5 | Positive | 20 | 10 | 20 |
| 2 | D | L | L3-S1 | L1-S1 | | | 15 | 0 | 5 |
| 3 | D | R | L4 | L4 | | | 15 | 5 | 10 |
| 4 | D | | | L4-L5 | L5 | Negative | 60 | 30 | 20 |
| 5 | | L | | L4-L5 | L4-L5 | Negative | 60 | 20 | 20 |
| 6 | D | | L4-L5 | | | Negative | 40 | 10 | 0 |
| 7 | | | | L4 | | Negative | 90 | 30 | 20 |
| 8 | D | R | L4-L5 | | L4-L5 | Negative | 30 | 10 | 0 |
| 9 | | | L5 | L4 | L4-L5 | Negative | 90 | 30 (much pain) | 20 |
| 10 | D | R | L4-L5 | L4-L5 | | Negative | 45 | 5 | 20 |
| 11 | D | R | L4-L5 | L4-L5 | | Negative | 30 | 30 | 20 |
| 12 | D | L | L4 | L4 | L3-L4 | Negative | 5 | 0 | 5 |
| 13 | I | | L4-L5 | | L4-L5 | Negative | 60 | 10 | 20 |
| 14 | | | L4-L5 | L4-L5 | | | 70 | 10 | 15 |
| 15 | D | | L5 | | L5 | Negative | 20 | 20 | 20 |
| 16 | D | | L4-L5 | L4-L5 | L4-L5 | Negative | 80 | 20 | 20 |
| 17 | D | R | | L4-L5-S1 | L5 | Negative | 20 | 30 | 0 |
| 18 | | | | L4-L5 | | | 90 | 20 | 20 |
| 19 | D | L | L4-L5 | | L5 | Positive | 20 | 0 | 5 |
| 20 | D | R | L4 | | L4 | Negative | 30 | 0 | 5 |
| 21 | | R | | L5 | L5 | Negative | 45 | 30 | 20 |
| 22 | D | R | L5 | L5 | | | 15 | 5 | 20 |
| 23 | D | L | L5 | L5 | | | 45 | 5 | 5 |
| 24 | | L | L5-S1 | | L5 | Negative | 60 | 0 | 0 |
| 25 | – | – | L4-L5 | L4-L5 | L4-L5 | Negative | 30 | 5 | 10 |
| 26 | D | R | L4-L5 | | | Negative | | | |
| 27 | D | | | L5-S1 | L5-S1 | Negative | 30 | 10 | 10 |
| 28 | D | L | | L4-L5 | L5-S1 | Negative | 30 | 30 | 0 |
| 29 | D | L | L3-L5 | L3-L5 | | | 45 | 5 | 5 |
| 30 | N | R | L4-L5-S1 | L4-L5-S1 | | | 40 | 5 | 20 |
| 31 | | | L5-S1 | | L5 | Negative | 60 | 10 | 10 |
| 32 | | | | L5-S1 | None | Negative | 5 | 5 | 2 |
| 33 | I | L | | L4-L5 | L4-L5 | Negative | 10 | 20 | 0 |
| 34 | D | L | | L5 | | | 10 | 0 | 5 |
| 35 | D | R | L3-L4 | | L3-L4 | Negative | 10 | 0 | 20 |
| 36 | D | L | | L5 | L5 | Negative | 35 | 10 | 0 |
| 37 | D | L | | L5 | L5 | Negative | 30 | 0 | 20 |
| 38 | | | | L4-L5 | L4-L5 | Negative | 20 | 5 | 10 |
| 39 | I | | | L4-L5 | None | Negative | 60 | 10 | 10 |
| 40 | | | | L4-L5 | L4 | Positive | 60 | 20 | 20 |
| 41 | D | L | L3-L4-L5-S1 | L3-L4-L5-S1 | L4-L5 | Negative | 10 | 10 | 0 |
| 42 | D | R | L5-S1 | L5-S1 | L5-S1 | Positive | 70 | 5 | 10 |
| 43 | D | R | | L5-S1 | L5-S1 | Negative | 30 | 30 | 5 |

| ° of Left Lateral Flexion | ° of Right Rotation | ° of Left Rotation | Patrick-Fabere Sign[c] | | Kemp's Sign[c] | | ° of Positive Leg Raise (°) | | Other Pertinent Findings |
|---|---|---|---|---|---|---|---|---|---|
| | | | Right | Left | Right | Left | Right | Left | |
| 0 | 10 | 10 | − | − | + | − | | 50 | |
| 15 | 5 | 15 | | | + | + | 35 | 75 | History of urinary infections |
| 20 | | | | | + | + | 60 | | |
| 20 | 30 | 30 | − | − | − | + | Not well defined | | |
| 20 | − | − | − | − | + | − | 60 | 45 | |
| 0 | 0 | 0 | − | − | + | − | | | |
| 20 | 15 (much pain) | 15 (sciatica intensified) | − | − | − | − | | | |
| 20 | 15 | 15 | + | − | − | + | 25 | | |
| 2 | 30 | 30 | − | − | + (L5) | + (L4) | 80 | 80 | |
| 5 | | | | | − | − | 30 | 30 | |
| 5 | 30 | 10 | − | − | | | | 45 | |
| 5 | 5 | 5 | − | − | + | + | 60 | | |
| 20 | | | − | − | + | + | | | |
| 10 | | | | | | | 35 | 50 | Hypertension, angina pectoris, coronary artery insufficiency |
| 20 | 30 (pain) | 30 (pain) | + | − | − | + | 30 | 40 | |
| 20 | 30 | 30 | − | − | + | − | 60 | 45 | |
| 0 | 10 | 10 | − | − | − | + | | | |
| 20 | | | | | | | | | |
| 0 | 10 | 10 | − | − | + | − | 50 | | |
| 5 | 0 | 0 | − | − | − | + | | 60 | |
| 20 | 30 | 30 | − | − | − | − | 80 | 80 | |
| 0 | 5 | 5 | | | | + | 80 | 60 | |
| 20 | | | | | + | | 30 | | Renal calculus |
| 20 | 10 | 10 | + | − | + | − | 40 | 60 | Left carotid pulse diminished, hypertension |
| 10 | 20 | 20 | − | − | + | + | | | |
| | | | − | − | − | − | | | |
| 0 | 20 | 20 | − | − | + | − | 40 | 50 | |
| 20 | | | − | − | + | − | | 80 | |
| 15 | | | | | + | | | 45 | |
| 5 | | | | | | + | 60 | | |
| 10 | 10 | 10 | − | − | − | − | | 40 | |
| 2 | 0 | 0 | − | − | + | − | 10 | | |
| 15 | 20 | 0 | − | − | + | − | | 40 | |
| 15 | 0 | 0 | | | + | | 15 | 0 | |
| 10 | | | | | | | 40 | 0 | |
| 20 | 0 | 0 | − | − | + | − | 30 | 0 | Urinary retention |
| 10 | | | − | + | + | + | 30 | 45 | |
| 10 | 10 | 10 | + | − | − | + | | 60 | Angina pectoris |
| 20 | | | − | − | + | − | | 5 | Pain following sigmoidoscopy on September 12, 1975 |
| 20 | 30 | 30 | − | − | + | − | 60 | | |
| 0 | 10 | 10 | + | − | + | − | 30 | 60 | |
| 0 | 10 | 10 | − | − | + | + | 60 | | |
| 20 | 10 | 20 | + | − | − | + | 60 | | |

**Table 8.14.—Continued**

| Case | Lumbar Lordosis[a] | Spinal Tilt[b] | Level of Pain on Palpation Right | Left | Level of Percussion Pain | Jugular Compression | ° of Flexion Possible | ° of Extension Possible | ° of Right Lateral Flexion |
|---|---|---|---|---|---|---|---|---|---|
| 44 | D | L | L5 |  | L5 | Negative | 60 | 10 | 20 |
| 45 | D | R | L5-S1 | L5-S1 | L5-S1 | Negative | 30 | 10 | 10 |
| 46 |  |  | L5-S1 |  | L5-S1 | Negative | 90 | 20 | 20 |
| 47 | D |  | L5 | L5 | L4-L5-S1 | Negative | 40 | 30 | 10 |
| 48 |  |  | L5-S1 | L5-S1 |  |  | 90 | 10 |  |
| 49 | D |  | L5-S1 |  | L5-S1 | Positive | 60 | 30 | 20 |
| 50 | L | L | L3-L4 | L3-L4 |  |  | 0 | 0 | 20 |
| 51 | L | R | L4-L5 | L4-L5 |  |  | 90 | 20 | 20 |
| 52 |  |  |  | L4-L5 | L4-L5 | Negative | 90 | 20 | 20 |
| 53 | D | L |  | L4 | L4 | Positive | 20 | 20 | 10 |
| 54 | D | L |  | L4-L5 | L4-L5 | Negative | 10 | 5 | 5 |
| 55 | D | L | L4-L5-S1 | L4-L5-S1 |  |  | 10 | 0 | 10 |
| 56 | D | R | L5 | L3-L4-L5 |  |  | 30 | 5 |  |
| 57 | N |  | L3-L4 | L3-L4 |  |  |  |  |  |
| 58 | D | L | L3-L4 | L3-L4 |  |  |  |  |  |
| 59 | D | R | L2-L3-L4 | L2-L3-L4 | L3 |  | 50 | 5 | 15 |
| 60 | I |  | L3-L4-L5-S1 | L3-L4-L5-S1 |  |  | 60 | 10 |  |
| 61 |  | L | L1-L5 | L1-L5 |  |  | 50 | 0 | 5 |
| 62 | I | L | L5 |  |  |  |  |  |  |
| 63 | L |  |  | L3-L4-L5-S1 |  |  | 45 | 0 | 5 |
| 64 | D | L |  |  |  |  | 99 |  |  |
| 65 | D | L |  |  | L5 |  | 10 | 0 | 20 |
| 66 |  | L |  | L1-L2-L3 |  |  | 45 | 10 | 0 |
| 67 |  |  |  |  | L4 |  | 15 | 15 | 0 |
| 68 | N |  | L5-S1 | L5-S1 | L5 |  | 10 | 0 | 10 |
| 69 | N | R | L4-L5 | L4-L5 |  |  | 15 | 5 | 20 |

[a] I, increased; D, decreased.
[b] L, left; R, right.
[c] −, negative; +, positive.

**Table 8.15.**
**Comparison of the First 100 Cases Treated Prior to 1975 with the 69 Cases Treated in 1975**

|  | First 100 Cases (%) | 69 Later Cases (%) |
|---|---|---|
| Lateral | 57 | 52 |
| Medial | 43 | 38 |
| Lateral requiring surgery | 3.5 | 5.5 |
| Medial requiring surgery | 20.9 | 0[a] |
| At L3, L4 | 5 | 9 |
| At L4, L5 | 47 | 39 |
| At L5, S1 | 48 | 48 |

[a] Twenty-five percent of central disc protrusions required surgery.

**Table 8.16.**
**Results in All 169 Cases Treated**

| Position of Disc Protrusion | No. | Closed Reduction No. | % | Surgery No. | % |
|---|---|---|---|---|---|
| Lateral | 93 | 89 | 95.7 | 4 | 4.3 |
| Medial | 69 | 60 | 87 | 9 | 13 |
| Central | 4 | 3 | 75 | 1 | 25 |
| At two or more levels | 3 | 2 | 66.7 | 1 | 33.3 |

when the first 100 cases are combined with the 69 treated in 1975.

A general comment about the statistics presented in this chapter must be made by the author. Chiropractors function without the benefit of hospital privileges, which creates two problems. First, chiro-

| ° of Left Lateral Flexion | ° of Right Rotation | ° of Left Rotation | Patrick-Fabere Sign^c | | Kemp's Sign^c | | ° of Positive Leg Raise (°) | | Other Pertinent Findings |
|---|---|---|---|---|---|---|---|---|---|
| | | | Right | Left | Right | Left | Right | Left | |
| 20 | 30 | 30 | − | − | + | − | | 35 | |
| 0 | 10 | 10 | − | − | − | + | 60 | 60 | |
| 15 | | | + | + | + | + | | | Prostatic hypertrophy with a history of prostatitis not responding to antibiotics |
| 20 | 20 | 20 | + | − | + | − | | | |
| | | | | | + | | | | |
| 20 | 10 | 10 | + | | + | − | 40 | | |
| 20 | 25 | 30 | | | | + | 0 | 0 | |
| 10 | 20 | 15 | | | | + | 0 | 0 | |
| 20 | 30 | 30 | + | + | + | + | | | |
| 10 | 20 | 20 | + | − | + | − | 30 | | |
| 20 | 10 | 10 | + | − | + | − | 20 | | |
| 0 | 0 | 0 | − | − | − | + | 75 | | |
| | | | | | | + | 80 | 0 | |
| | | | | | − | | | | |
| 15 | 20 | 20 | | | + | | | 85 | |
| | | | | | | + | | | |
| 15 | | | | | + | | | | |
| 10 | | | | | + | + | 45 | 45 | |
| | | | | | + | − | 55 | | |
| 0 | 0 | 0 | − | − | − | + | | 40 | |
| 20 | 30 | 30 | − | − | + | − | 75 | 60 | |
| 20 | 0 | 30 | − | − | + | − | 70 | 70 | |
| 20 | | | | | | − | 75 | 40 | |
| 5 | | | | | | + | 75 | | |
| 10 | | | | | | + | | | |

practors do not have the advantage of constant nursing care for their patients, and second, patients must be ambulatory enought to get to and from the chiropractor's office. If chiropractors could treat a significant number of those patients whose condition is severe enough to normally require hospitalization, possibly the high percentage of good results from chiropractic treatment would drop. At present, the statistics are limited to those patients who are able to get to the chiropractor's office; for these patients, the results have been favorable.

## Comments on Interesting Cases from the Statistics

In Case 4, a 28-year-old white man had had a biopsy of the kidneys performed on August 20, 1974, and a myelogram performed on December 9, 1974. Following this, he was told that he had involvement of the 3rd, 4th and 5th discs and that surgical repair was indicated at all three segments. This patient was first examined by the author on January 27, 1975. The myelograms he brought did indeed reveal disc involvement at the three levels indicated. Treatment from January 27, 1975, to February 27, 1975, yielded complete relief from the back and sciatic complaints as well as a urinary problem. He returned to his job as a die caster at that time. It is interesting to note the response of patients to treatment. In this case, after five treatment sessions, the patient had subjectively 75% less leg pain and 50% less back pain. Five more treatments rendered 100% relief of both back and leg pain. The patient was given a total of 14 treatment sessions.

In Case 1, a 62-year-old white man with left leg S1 dermatome sciatica had received chiropractic adjustments of the side posture attitude for 2 months prior to his first visit to the author's office. As has been indicated before, it has been more difficult to treat patients who have received torsion-type adjustments before undergoing traction-type reduction. It took the author 3 months in Case 1 as opposed to 1 month in Case 4 to achieve the same response to treatment. It has been this author's experience that slow treatment results usually follow the use of side-posture torsion adjustments. In Case 1, the patient had also recently undergone repair for an inguinal rupture with disc lesion, but the author had found no distinct correlation between these two conditions.

In Case 7, the patient had undergone surgery on January 30, 1973, for removal of a 4th lumbar disc with 10% spondylolisthesis at that level. Prior to surgery the patient had sciatica, bilaterally, into the buttocks. Following surgery, the patient developed pain radiating into both extremities of the entire sciatic nerve. Another surgery was recommended; however, she sought consultation at this author's clinic on February 3, 1975, before having this second surgery. The author's opinion was that the patient had a central L4-L5 disc protrusion as well as correlative evidence of an L5-S1 left medial disc protrusion. The patient was treated for 2 months with a poor response. Consultation with numerous orthopedic and neurological surgeons resulted in a decision to do a fusion at the L4-L5 level along with disc removal.

The surgery was performed in mid-1975. During this time, the patient developed marked constipation and the necessity of a rectocele repair also became evident. It should be noted that spondylolisthesis in the presence of disc lesion should have every opportunity of conservative management before surgical repair is first attempted. Surgical repair, with or without fusion, is somewhat controversial, as some eminent authorities believe that in the presence of spondylolisthesis the disc should be surgically removed. The patient should also undertake strenuous exercise as soon as possible, with no limitations of mobility (15). Others conclude that the spondylolisthesis should be accompanied by fusion (65). Either way the author believes that surgery for a disc lesion in the

presence of spondylolisthesis should definitely be a last resort. In Case 7, the author believes that attention was given to the L4-L5 spondylolisthesis with a disc problem, while the suspected L5-S1 left medial disc lesion was ignored at surgery. No opportunity was given to explore treatment of the suspected L5-S1 disc lesion following surgery. This case had an unfortunate result due primarily to an initial surgery which, at best, might have been avoided.

The patient in case 9 was referred from out of state and underwent treatment once or twice each day from March 18, 1975, to March 29, 1975. A very involved medical history preceded this patient. She had a history of cystitis with the back problem. Surgical history revealed hysterectomy at age 27. The patient's back problem started in January 1970, after a fall. She had been seen by orthopedists, osteopaths, neurosurgeons, and chiropractors. Myelography had been performed, which was not positive. Various forms of physical therapy, injections, and manipulations had been attempted. Thirteen treatment sessions at the author's clinic resulted in absence of positive leg raise sign, negative Kemp's sign, as well as a subjective statement of an approximately 80% relief of back and leg pain. At the end of 10 days treatment, the patient maintained discomfort in the left lateral thigh. On the initial examination the patient revealed disc height at the L4 level, and, on standing, a tilt view of 14° of 8.5 mm left and 8 mm right. Ten days later the disc space, under the same conditions, was 19 mm bilaterally. The L5-S1 disc space, initially 9 mm in height, reached 12 mm 10 days later. These films were taken in the upright posture. Upon returning home the patient did not receive continued treatment and the future response of her problem is not known. The first response was extremely favorable and the author believes that, had treatment continued, it would have yielded the desired response.

The patient in Case 15 had a history of 2 years of right leg pain with back pain. Repeated injuries during that time had intensified the problem. Chiropractic adjustments had given him relief, but the pain continued to increase until side-posture adjustments no longer helped him.

He was then referred to the author's clinic. At that time he was taking Darvon for pain. The patient mentioned that an extremely cold feeling in both lower extremities accompanied the pain. The patient felt a 60% subjective symptom relief after the first treatment. Subsequent treatments did not reveal increased relief and continued traction treatment sessions were required to maintain this relief. Consultation with surgeons did not result in surgery. Medial disc protrusion has statistically proven to be difficult to handle, even in the presence of coronal facets as were exhibited by the patient. It must be pointed out that this patient continued to participate in strenuous business and social activities, resulting in less relief.

Case 16 involved a central disc lesion creating bilateral 5th lumbar dermatome sciatica. This patient had had extensive atherosclerosis and cardiac catheterizations. She was receiving 1600 units of vitamin E per day for treatment of this disc lesion, administered by the referring doctor and not by this author, resulting in relief of her angina. Extensive degenerative change of the 5th lumbar disc indicated previous disease at that level, but there was no objective involvement at this time. The central disc lesion, as seen in this case, is the most difficult disc lesion to treat. As is typical of this patient, many discs do not tolerate side posture or torsion manipulation. They respond best to traction reduction.

In Case 19, the patient had received routine chiropractic adjustments prior to referral to the author's office. The patient's back pain and sciatica required narcotic control. Complete absence of the leg raise sign was noted. Traction reduction produced no pain in this man's low back, indicative of prolapse and free fragmentation of the disc as opposed to a disc protrusion with an intact annulus fibrosus. As pointed out elsewhere, a patient not yielding effective response after 3 weeks conservative treatment is referred for surgical consultation. Because of this patient's extreme pain, he was referred at the end of 10 days. Surgical repair was performed with excellent results.

The patient in Case 20 had received 2 months of torsion-type adjustments prior to consulting with the author. On his first visit to the author's office, he received an 80% subjective relief of pain. The patient returned to work in 10 days. As is done with all cases of disc lesion, he continued with periodic treatment for 3 months to ensure adequate healing of the disc before he returned to full normal duties.

The reader will note the absence of knee jerk test results in this survey. This absence is due to the fact that alterations of this deep reflex are so rarely observed that they are believed to be insignificant for this test. Only in the presence of a 4th lumbar nerve root involvement would the physician find this reflex altered, implying that a 3rd lumbar disc was involved. Relative infrequency of this involvement is noted in the cases presented here.

The patient in Case 24 complained of low back pain and sciatica beginning May 3, 1975; he had missed work starting May 20, 1975, until his first visit at the author's clinic on July 10, 1975. The patient had received chiropractic manipulation during this period and was finally referred to this clinic by his attending chiropractic physician. On initial examination, the patient stated he had no urinary problem. The first treatment session revealed objective findings of a negative Kemp's sign and a straight leg raise. After the initial treatment, the patient stated that he slept well for the first night in 3 months and felt 100% relieved. He returned to work July 24, 1975. The follow-up treatment was not remarkable, but on September 15, 1975, the patient returned, complaining that he passed a kidney stone on September 1, 1975. He mentioned a history of prostate infection for which antibiotics had been prescribed. Following passing of this stone, he developed back and leg pain once again which was relieved during two treatment sessions. An interesting point is that he has had no more urinary difficulty since being treated for the disc protrusion. Again, note the correlation between urogenital problems and disc lesion.

In Case 27, the reader will notice that Kemp's sign was positive when the patient bent away from the side of the pain with a lateral disc lesion on the left. The author has observed that, in the case of prolapse or when a free fragment is present, the Kemp's sign sometimes may be altered, as in this case. Therefore, when Kemp's sign is reversed from what is expected in protrusion, prolapse is suspected. This patient was first seen on July 29, 1975. The first treatment resulted in relief of the sciatic pain with the low back pain remaining. Two weeks treatment resulted in the return of all normal motion and orthopedic signs. The patient was allowed to resume all normal activities on September 18, 1975, and was advised to resist rotation movements of the lumbar spine, such as raking leaves and running a push vacuum sweeper.

The patient in Case 31 had a history of back pain of 10 years duration and leg pain for the past 2 or 3 years. She had been treated by her family chiropractor, although her pain had increased. Interestingly, this patient, with a 5th lumbar disc lying medial to the right S1 nerve root, developed some left leg sciatica during the course of her treatment. This was perceived to be in the medial disc which might be termed central in variety, since it is capable of contacting both right and left 1st sacral nerve roots, if it is large enough. When the opposite leg becomes involved, it is generally found to yield quickly to treatment. Also, all of the lumbar facets in this patient were sagittal in facing. This patient is the only one in whom this has been found by the author. The patient was first seen August 14, 1975. After seven treatment sessions, the patient felt no pain, with absent leg raise sign, negative Kemp's signs, and all motions returned to normal. On November 20, 1975, this patient complained of some mild left leg S1 dermatome sciatica. This pain was relieved following two treatment sessions. Of interest, the hemorrhoid problem experienced by the patient subsided following treatment. The neurological reason for this will be discussed later.

Case 33 of an extremely overweight man is typical of many cases of disc protrusion in that he had extremely tight hamstring muscles. The reader should remember that tight hamstring muscles prevent flexion of the pelvis on the femoral heads, resulting in hypermobility of the lumbar spine, especially on flexion motion. This aggravation of the fibrocartilage and its supportive ligaments leads to and aggravates disc protrusion. The author always stretches hamstring muscles during treatment and places the patient on exercises to do the same. This man took the author's suggestion, changing his occupation from truck driving to garage work in an effort to prevent sitting which aggravates the disc lesion. He was also placed on a weight-reducing diet. It should also be noted that a history of constipation and duodenal ulcer was relieved along with the disc lesion.

The patient in Case 38 could not walk due to leg pain which occurred after an automobile wreck in 1970. Also, she had had a bout with polio in 1961. She had visited the Mayo Clinic for consultation after the wreck and had returned home, seeking chiropractic care. She had been in the hospital for traction treatment frequently during April and August of 1975 for the low back pain and right leg pain. Her attending doctor referred her to this clinic on October 14, 1975. Her right leg measured two inches shorter than her left leg in the prone recumbent posture, but this deficiency was not noted on standing x-ray evaluation. Treatment sessions resulted in objective findings of the return of normal motion and of the absence of Kemp's sign. The muscle strength of the lower extremities improved. The patient's subjective symptoms, in this author's opinion, did not improve to the same extent as her objective findings. In November 1975, a neurosurgeon was consulted and no surgery was recommended. Some form of litigation was involved with this case and, as has been stated by another authority in this book, these cases sometimes do not yield results as quickly as non-litigation cases (66).

Case 40 involved a patient with intense 5th dermatome sciatica of a severe nature with complete absence of back pain. An explanation for this combination of back pain and sciatica, or one without the other, has been given elsewhere. The sciatica began following a sigmoidoscopic examination on September 12, 1975. Note the familial involvement of disc lesion for this patient. She was referred to the author by her attending chiropractor on October 21, 1975, and after three treatment sessions, the patient experienced a 50% subjective relief of leg pain. Her Kemp's sign was negative, as was the leg raise sign. By November 6, 1975, the patient felt that she was walking better than she had for several years. A history of stubborn constipation was also relieved, and she was able to stop taking Valium and Darvon for pain.

The patient in Case 41 had a complete laminectomy at the 4th lumbar level with complete removal of the L3-L4 disc and alleged fusion afterward. The pain continued, so she sought care on October 16, 1975, primarily for right 5th lumbar dermatome sciatica, with little back pain. On November 24, 1975, the motions of her low back had returned to normal, the Kemp's sign was negative, and the leg raise was negative. The author lists the patient's response as "good" because some posterior knee pain persisted. Otherwise, it would be an "excellent" result, since the patient now has almost complete relief from pain. It might be pointed out that the author has had only one patient (Case 7) who had already undergone back surgery with poor result and who has not responded well to this form of treatment.

Case 47 involved a patient who had had an 18-year history of low back pain and alternating bilateral sciatica in differing dermatome patterns. This patient was seen on November 24, 1975, and was suffering primarily from bilateral L5 dermatome sciatica. The right great toe was extremely numb and cold. It was this author's opinion that the marked degenerative change in the 5th lumbar disc was responsible for the first sacral dermatome sciatica noticed in the past. The first treatment resulted in such relief from back pain that the patient was able to sleep well for the first time in several years. His leg pain was also gone, with his Kemp's sign still positive to a mild degree on the right side. The leg raise sign was negative. By December 30, 1975, the patient had regained normal mobility of the low back and a normal lumbar lordosis without antalgic lean. Of note was the absence of prostatic involvement experienced by the patient for several years. It is interesting to point out that this patient had received lumbar torsion-type adjustments from a chiropractor prior to this author's treatment. The torsion-type adjustments

tended to aggravate his back. This is important to consider in establishing a course of treatment for this type of patient.

The patient in Case 52 had had a previous bout of sciatica 3 years prior to this one. This time, one treatment gave complete relief of all symptoms.

In Case 55, the reader should note that the Kemp's sign is reversed. Although the patient had a left medial 5th lumbar disc, the Kemp's sign was negative to the left and positive to the right. The only comment to be made is that every clinical sign is not always perfect. It is probably safe to state that all signs that could point to a disc lesion are not present in a given patient. It is the careful correlation of those signs that leads to a correct diagnosis.

Cases 64 through 67 are from the office of John R. Bernzott, D.C. of Connersville, Indiana, who used the same method of treating disc lesions. Case 64 was of particular interest in that Dr. Bernzott had treated the patient with side-posture lumbar roll adjustments, with no results, prior to his taking a class to utilize the technique described in this chapter. Even after traction manipulation the patient failed to respond within 3 weeks and was referred to a surgeon. The diagnosis was a right lateral 4th lumbar disc prolapse. The surgeons noted that traction manipulation, when applied, failed to cause pain in this patient's low back. Following operative removal of the 4th lumbar disc, the surgeon found that Dr. Bernzott's diagnosis, without the use of myelography, was correct. The surgeon invited Dr. Bernzott to visit with him and discuss this diagnostic approach to the disc lesion.

The patient in Case 43 had been given side-posture adjustments resulting in a worsening of his low back pain and sciatica. The treating physician referred him to this clinic. The right medial disc responded very well to treatment. It should be noted that there was a minimal amount of pain during traction which led the author to diagnose the condition as a prolapse rather than as a protrusion.

Case 46 was of a 56-year-old woman with a history of 20 years of low back pain which resulted in right leg 5th lumbar dermatome sciatica. The chronicity of the condition led to weakness of the quadriceps, hamstrings, and gluteal muscles so that the patient could not climb steps. Her equilibrium was bad and she experienced dizziness. Her response to treatment has been labeled "good." She was relieved of the sciatica, regained the ability to climb steps, and her dizziness subsided. She does continue to have treatment every 2 weeks. The author believes that the chronic back condition so debilitated the patient that treatment will be necessary for a longer period of time.

The patient in Case 22 injured his back while climbing out of his attic 9 days prior to his first visit at the author's clinic. He experienced back and leg pain of such intensity that he was taken to a hospital and placed in traction. He developed bilateral S1 dermatome sciatica. He was advised to have surgery but refused. One treatment session in the author's clinic resulted in loss of antalgic posture and sciatic pain. This patient had a 10% spondylolisthesis at L5 which was at the same level of disc involvement.

### Stoddard's Osteopathic Technic (67)

"The treatment of intervertebral disc herniation should start long before it occurs. We should manipulate and mobilize osteopathic spinal lesions long before they lead to these degenerative changes and not leave them to take their course. If on examination of the spine we find areas of restricted mobility or even single lesions, our duty is to release the restricted joints and insure normality as far as is within our power.

"I am of the firm opinion that a herniated disc can sometimes be replaced by manipulation, but when a true prolapse of the disc occurs, I am convinced that it is impossible to replace the nuclear material by manipulation. At that stage all that can be achieved by manipulation is the empirical attempt to shift the position of nerve root and prolapsed nuclear material so that less pressure occurs on the nerve root.

"By herniation of a disc I envision a bulging of the annulus sufficient to press on and irritate the posterior longitudinal ligament and dura mater without a complete rupture of the annulus and the posterior longitudinal ligament. If there is

sufficient outer annular fibers and posterior ligaments to hold the herniation from protruding right through them I think it ought to be possible to reposition the nuclear material—not that such a state of affairs is desirable, it is a highly vulnerable condition—but clinically at least such cases are rewarding in that the patient obtains a dramatic relief of symptoms, even though at a later date he may well have a relapse. After all, a track has been formed in the circular fibers of the annulus and such a tract does not repair well, if at all, because cartilage once torn is not repaired with cartilage but merely with fibrous tissue. At best we can hope for fibrous tissue repair and provide additional support either by improving the muscles surrounding the joint or by using artificial external supports.

"When nuclear material has escaped into the spinal canal and has become wedged between the nerve root and the intervertebral foramen, manipulation can sometimes alter the site of pressure or shift the prolapsed material to another site where there is less irritation of the nerve roots. If the technics are designed to achieve this and they are sufficiently gentle to avoid further damage, they are well worth attempting because in roughly half of the cases the attempts succeed. If the attempts are successful, the patient has still to observe caution; the hope is that the prolapsed material will in time shrink and cause less trouble. In the meantime a laminectomy has been avoided. If the attempt is unsuccessful and the technic is designed to avoid further damage, the patient is no worse off and, if necessary, can still take advantage of surgical procedures" (67).

Stoddard's guide to the prognosis of the effect of manipulation on the disc lesion is based on straight leg raising tests. If the test is positive at 30° or less, the prospects of success are distinctly limited. The smaller the angle, the less likely is manipulation to be successful, and the lower the level of disc lesion, the less chance of success. A probable reason for this observation is that the lowest intervertebral foramen has the smallest hole and the largest nerve root. There is, therefore, less opportunity for maneuver and alteration of position.

Given a patient with a disc prolapse at the L4-L5 level, and a straight leg raise that is positive at 45°, the chances of success by manipulation are more than 50%, and by success I do not mean complete relief of pain but a substantial reduction of pain and a reduction of physical signs.

Stoddard's technic of stretching the sciatic nerve involves placing the patient on his side while stretching the lower extremity over the side of the table. The idea is to make sure that the articular facets are at least mobile and that adhesions are released on the nonpainful side. The technic is applied on both sides. Stoddard believes that this procedure alters the position of the nerve root and the prolapsed disc. According to Stoddard, during application of the flexion and extension technic with use of the McManis table, "*the lower leaf of the table ought not be pressed far down into too much flexion in case gapping of the joint causes a herniation of the disc*" (67) (italics added).

The technic is useful on both the thoracic and the lumbar spine, but here you must rely on patient cooperation and on the patient's ability to grip the top of the table firmly and yet relax the spine. Such controlled relaxation is not easy by any means but should be possible by the average cooperative patient.

A combination of movements can be obtained by using the lower leaf of the McManis table to open to two of its ranges, but such combined movements are complex, are not easy to control, and are rarely indicated anyway. The goal is to place the pivot of movement just below the level of the lesion and, while articulating all levels of the lower thoracic and lumbar joints, to pay special attention to those joints at which there is a *restricted range of movement*.

## CASE STUDIES OF PATIENTS WITH DISC LESIONS

**Case 1** is of a 40-year-old white man who had right low back and lower extremity pain in the 5th lumbar dermatome. He was referred to us by his insurance carrier and treating chiropractor. He had been treated for several months without relief and was wearing a transcutaneous electrical nerve stimulator (TENS) unit when first seen.

Straight leg raise is positive at 40° on the right. Range of motion is 30° on flexion, and 15° on extension. No muscle weakness of the lower extremity is noted. There is hypoesthesia on the right at L5. Among the deep reflexes the ankle jerk is 2+. Doppler examination reveals normal circulation of the lower extremities.

X-rays reveal:

1. Left lateral flexion subluxation of L4 on L5 (Fig. 8.49).
2. L5-S1 disc degeneration with minimal L5 anterolisthesis on the sacrum (Figs. 8.50 and 8.51). This would be pseudospondylolisthesis due to discal degeneration, since the pars interarticularis is ossified on the oblique view.
3. A soft tissue density can be seen on the CT scan (Fig. 8.52), which is projected to the right in the neural canal causing significant encroachment of the neural canal. This was believed to be a probable herniated nucleus pulposus on the right at the L4-L5 level.

Diagnosis is of an L4-L5 right nuclear protrusion compressing the right L5 nerve root.

With the authorization of the insurance carrier, the patient was treated numerous times a day at the outset of care with the understanding that if the patient did not receive at least a 50% improvement in the first 3 weeks, a neurosurgical consultation would be obtained. The treatment consisted of Cox flexion distraction, positive galvanism to the L4-L5 disc

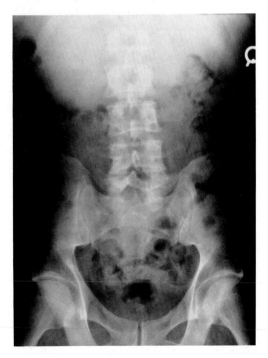

**Figure 8.49.** Posteroanterior view.

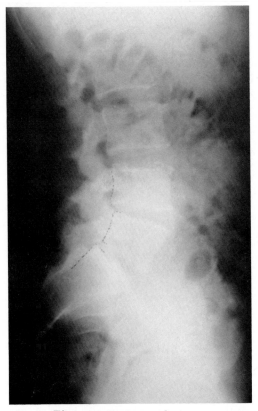

**Figure 8.50.** Lateral view.

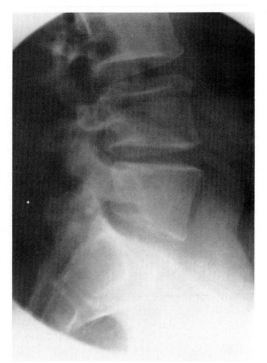

**Figure 8.51.** Lateral spot film.

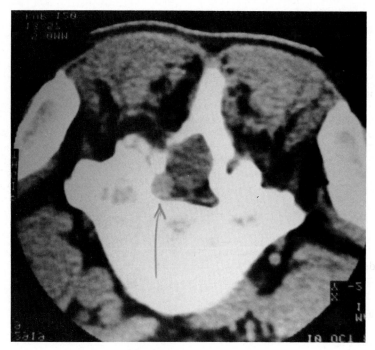

**Figure 8.52.** CT scan.

and to B54, alternating hot and cold fomentations, a back brace, exercises, avoidance of sitting, and nutritional supplements of Discat and the vitamin B complex. Arch supports for pes planus were prescribed. This is the standard care given to patients with disc protrusion as discussed in this chapter.

After 3 weeks of treatment the patient experienced a 50% objective and subjective relief from pain. He no longer used the TENS unit. Treatment was then reduced to 3 days/week for 3 weeks, then 2 days/week for 3 weeks, and then 1 visit weekly for the remainder of the time until 3 months of care had been completed. He was then referred back to his referring chiropractor for follow-up care, and a letter outlining his care was sent.

At the end of 3 months, the leg pain was gone and 75% of the low back pain was relieved.

**Case 2** is of a 34-year-old white man who in April of 1978 jumped on a steel grate on his right leg, causing right hip pain. (Since then, he has also experienced pain in his right leg at night.) He saw a chiropractor who treated him without relief. In May 1978, he was hospitalized and had a myelogram that was negative. Another myelogram, in November 1978, was also negative. In November 1979, an epidural venogram that showed a swollen ligamentum flavum was performed. Due to persistent pain a third myelogram was done in 1980 and was negative. In November 1980, Mayo Clinic saw him and said that they could not help him. In June 1982, after kneeling down to tie his shoes, the patient felt low back and right leg pain. He was hospitalized and a fourth myelogram and a CT scan were performed. He was given an epidural venogram that revealed a filling defect at the right L5-S1 level. The patient now decided to consult our clinic.

On examination, Déjérine's triad is positive and the straight leg raise is positive at 50° on the right. Range of motion is 90° on flexion, 20° on extension, 20° on right lateral flexion, 15° on left lateral flexion, 20° on right rotation, and 20° on left rotation. The test for Bechterew's sign along with the Valsalva maneuver is positive for low back and right leg pain. The hamstring muscles are short. Muscle weakness on right plantar flexion and hypoesthesia of the right S1 dermatome are also noted. Deep reflexes are active and equal.

X-rays reveal:

1. An unstable facet syndrome at L5-S1 (Fig. 8.53).

2. Eisenstein's measurement for stenosis (Fig. 8.54).

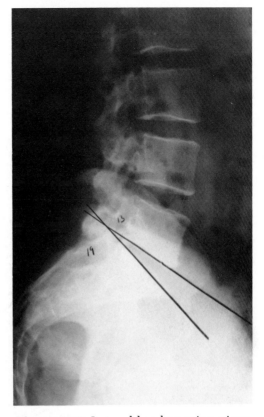

**Figure 8.53.** Lateral lumbar spine view.

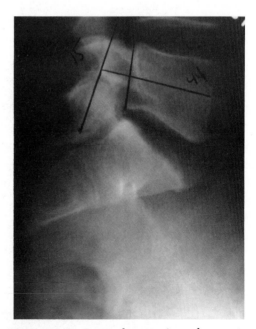

**Figure 8.54.** Lateral spot view shows stenosis.

3. Normal myelograms (Figs. 8.55 and 8.56).

4. A filling defect in the right L5-S1 area on the epidural venogram (Figs. 8.57 and 8.58).

Diagnosis is of an unstable facet syndrome at L5-S1 and an L5-S1 right nuclear protrusion.

Treatment consisted of Cox flexion distraction manipulation, but because of patient failure to follow directions well, relief from pain took longer than it should have. Nevertheless, after 3 months of care the patient experienced a more than 90% subjective relief from low back pain and total relief from right leg pain. Therapy for a disc and facet syndrome was applied.

**Case 3** is of a 68-year-old white man with right leg pain. The pain had started 4 months

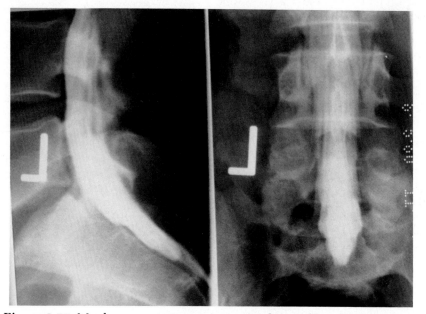

**Figure 8.55.** Myelogram, posteroanterior (*right*) and lateral (*left*) views.

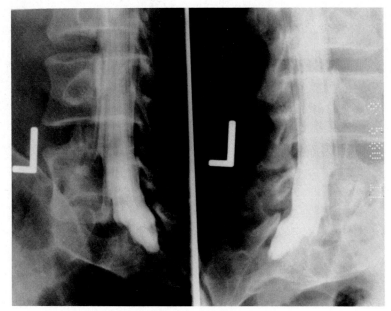

**Figure 8.56.** Myelogram, oblique views.

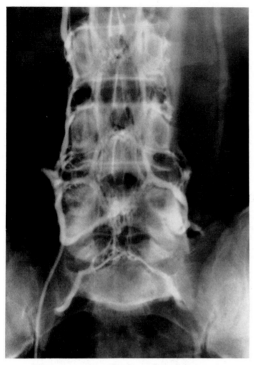

**Figure 8.57.** Epidural venogram.

ago for no known reason, and the patient had no history of back pain. He is a retired dentist and had leaned over a dental chair for 40 years in a right lean posture. He has been to a chiropractor for the past 6 weeks but had experienced no relief from pain.

On examination, Déjérine's triad is positive for leg pain. Range of motion is 30° on flexion, 5° on extension, 20° on right lateral flexion, 5° on left lateral flexion, 10° on right rotation, and 10° on left rotation. Straight leg raise is positive at 25° on the left with a positive Braggard's sign. Deep reflexes are 2+ bilaterally. Sensory examination reveals hypoesthesia of the left L5-S1 dermatomes. There is a right lean of the lumbar spine and a loss of lumbar lordosis (see Figs. 8.59 to 8.66).

X-rays reveal:

1. A right lateral lean of the lumbar spine (Fig. 8.59) with a right lateral flexion of L5 on the sacrum (Fig. 8.62). Note that L4 and L5 fail to laterally flex left on lateral bending (Figs. 8.60 and 8.61), but the functional spinal units above do laterally flex left.

2. A severe facet syndrome of L5 on the sacrum with a sacral angle and lumbar lordosis angle of 46° (Fig. 8.63). Note the large anterolateral lipping and spurring at the L3-L4 level with attempts at pathological arthrodesis (see Figs. 8.65 and 8.66).

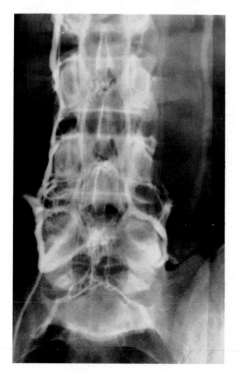

**Figure 8.58.** Epidural venogram.

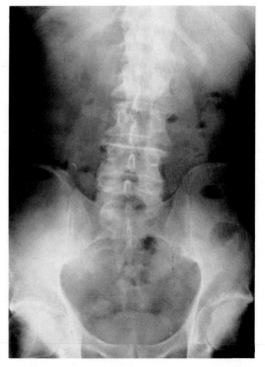

**Figure 8.59.** Posteroanterior view.

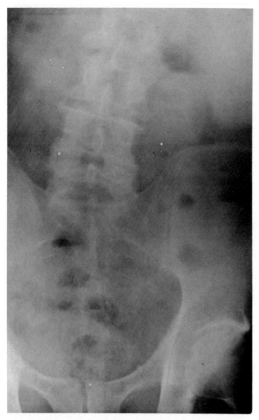

**Figure 8.60.** Right lateral bending view.

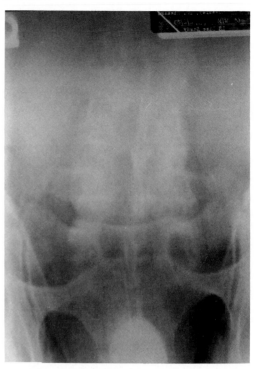

**Figure 8.62.** Posteroanterior tilt view.

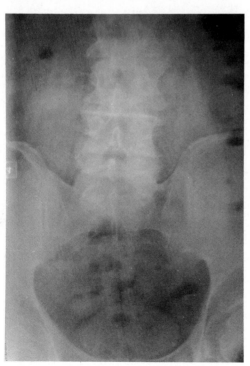

**Figure 8.61.** Left lateral bending view.

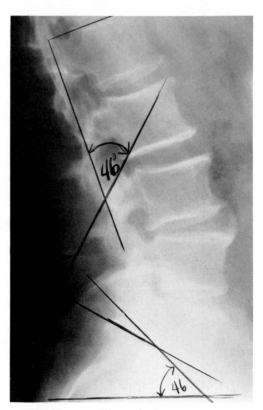

**Figure 8.63.** Lateral view.

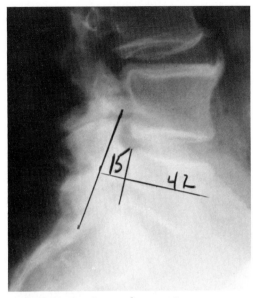

**Figure 8.64.** Lateral spot view.

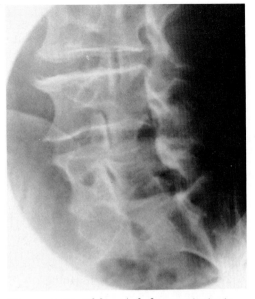

**Figure 8.66.** Oblique (left anterior) view.

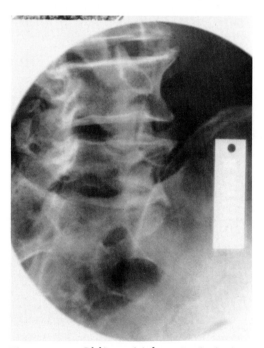

**Figure 8.65.** Oblique (right anterior) view.

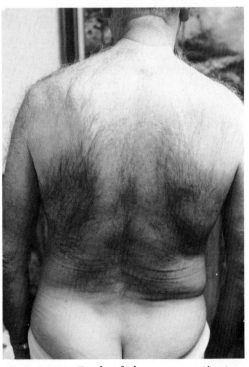

**Figure 8.67.** Back of the same patient as in Figures 8.59 through 8.66.

3. A normal Eisenstein measurement for no stenosis (Fig. 8.64).

4. A right lean of the spine with a low right shoulder and a sharp body angle at the waist on the right compared with that on the left (Fig. 8.67).

Diagnosis is of an L4-L5 left lateral nuclear protrusion or possible prolapse, an L5-S1 facet syndrome, and an L3-L4 discogenic spondylosis with arthrodesis.

Treatment consisted of Cox flexion distraction manipulation, as described earlier, which was applied for 3 weeks with 2 visits daily. No relief from pain was obtained and a neurosurgical consultation was sought. Myelography revealed a large prolapse of the L4-L5 disc. Surgical removal of the L4-L5 disc prolapse relieved the left leg pain, and the patient was discharged on the fourth postoperative day.

**Case 4** is of a 31-year-old married woman who experienced right anterior thigh numbness with a feeling "like rubber bands snapping." Her feeling of numbness started 4 years ago following the birth of twins. It eases when she turns on her left side but returns when she lies on her right side and is worse on standing for long periods or on bending and lifting.

On examination, range of motion of the thoracolumbar spine is within normal limits. The straight leg raise is negative. Patrick's sign is negative. Muscle strengths are all normal. Knee and ankle jerk deep reflexes are active and equal to 2+. Sensory examination reveals hypoesthesia of the right anterior lateral thigh. The patient has weak abdominal muscles and is obese. Tenderness over the inguinal ligament and anterior ilium and thigh is found on palpation.

X-rays reveal a short femoral head on the left compared with that on the right and a facet syndrome of L5 on S1 (Figs. 8.68, 8.69, and 8.70).

Clinical diagnosis is of meralgia paraesthetica. The lateral femoral cutaneous nerve can be compressed in the abdomen or the inguinal

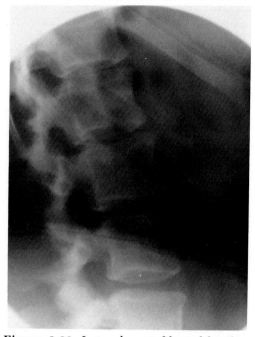

**Figure 8.69.** Lateral spot film of lumbar spine.

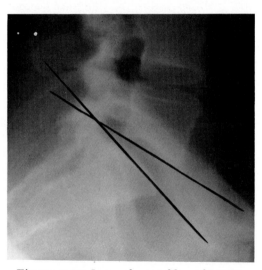

**Figure 8.70.** Lateral spot film of L5-S1.

area by scar tissue or a pendulous abdomen. In this case, the latter was the cause.

The patient was advised to wear a girdle for support and was given exercises to do for abdominal strengthening. Flexion distraction manipulation was applied to the lumbar spine, especially at the L1, L2, L3, and L4 levels.

The recommendation that she wear an abdominal support while exercising to lose

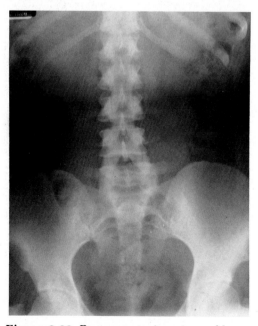

**Figure 8.68.** Posteroanterior view of lumbar spine and pelvis.

weight and firm the abdominal muscles was made so that pressure would be taken off the lateral femoral cutaneous nerve during exercise. One visit for manipulation gave her total relief from the meralgia pain—an amazing result for both patient and doctor!

**Case 5** is of a 35-year-old white man who has low back and left leg pain. Six weeks prior to his first visit, the patient had developed low back pain after cutting firewood. The leg pain started sometime later. Four years previously, he had jumped off a pipe and landed sideways, with his weight on his left leg. He had worked 4 or 5 days and then went to the hospital for a week of bed rest. He then visited a chiropractor who relieved him of his pain after a month of treatment. Since then, he has had low back pain off and on, and 6 months ago his left great toe became numb and he couldn't lift his left foot.

For the last 6 weeks he has been receiving chiropractic rotation adjustments of the lumbar spine. No x-rays or examination was given and the patient was told his "hip was out." On a scale of 1 to 9, the patient rates his pain at 9 and has experienced pain at night.

On examination, the patient has obvious left limp. Déjérine's triad is positive. Leg pain extends to the left great toe. Vital signs are all within normal limits. Range of motion reveals 10° on flexion, 5° on extension, 10° on right lateral flexion, 10° on left lateral flexion, 10° on right rotation, and 10° on left rotation. Straight leg raise is positive at 25° on the left, creating leg pain. Braggard's sign is positive. The test for Bechterew's sign with the Valsalva maneuver is positive for low back and left leg pain. The test for Lindner's sign creates low back pain. There is no spinal tilt and there is normal lumbar lordosis. Toe walk is normal. An inability to heel walk on the left is noted. On muscle strength testing, left dorsiflexion of the foot and great toe and eversion of left foot are impossible against gravity without any resistance. The left knee jerk is +1. Left hypoesthesia at the L5 dermatome is noted on sensory examination.

X-rays reveal:

1. Good pelvic alignment, no marked lean of the lumbar spine, and a bone architecture that is normal (Fig. 8.71).
2. A Lovett-positive curvature with the spinous processes rotated left into the concavity (Fig. 8.72).
3. Marked inferiority of the right hemipelvis compared to the left hemipelvis (Fig. 8.73). There is no lateral flexion of L4 on L5, and most of the right lateral flexion actually is

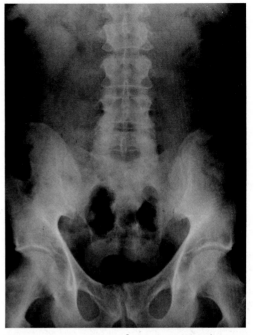

**Figure 8.71.** Neutral posteroanterior upright view.

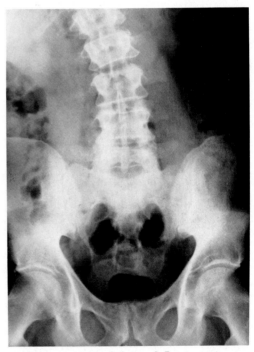

**Figure 8.72.** Left lateral flexion view.

the pelvis dropping inferior to spare movement of the lumbar spine.

4. A lumbar lordosis of 39° (normal 46° ± 3°) and a sacral angle of 42° (Fig. 8.74). There

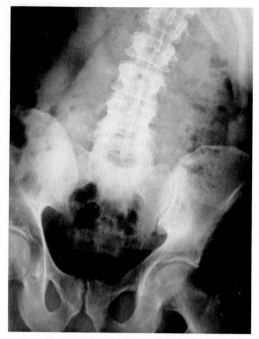

**Figure 8.73.** Right lateral flexion view.

is marked narrowing of the L4-L5 disc space (Fig. 8.75) with posteriority of L4 on L5 and discogenic spondylosis at the L4-L5 level.

Clinical impression is of an L4-L5 disc protrusion or prolapse resulting in L5 nerve root compression.

Based on the muscle atrophy, deep reflex loss of the patellar reflex, loss of sensory sensation of the left L5 dermatome, weakness of dorsiflexion of the foot and great toe on the left, and the overall persistent pain of a worsening nature, the consideration of surgery for a nuclear prolapse and referral to a neurosurgeon were made.

The following were found at myelography: a large filling defect at the left L4-L5 disc level (Fig. 8.76), an anterior indentation of the dye-filled column posterior to the L4-L5 disc space (Fig. 8.77), a large L4-L5 filling defect on the left (Figs. 8.78, 8.79, and 8.80).

On operation, a huge free fragment of disc was found in the epidural space on the left under the dural sac and L5 nerve root. This was removed in a single piece and measured 5 x 1.5 cm. After this was removed the dural sac and nerve root collapsed. There was also a very hard, old looking sequestrated disc under the posterolongitudinal ligament. The interspace was narrowed but would admit a 2 mm series of punches and curettes.

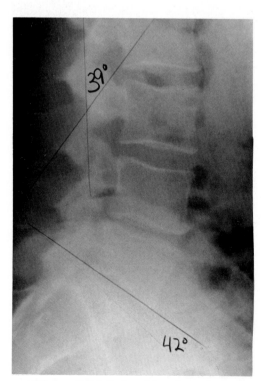

**Figure 8.74.** Lateral lumbar view.

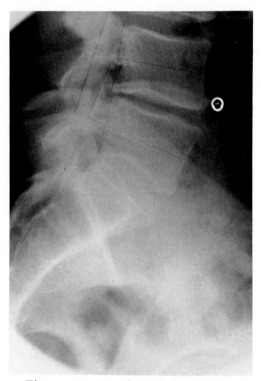

**Figure 8.75.** Lumbosacral spot view.

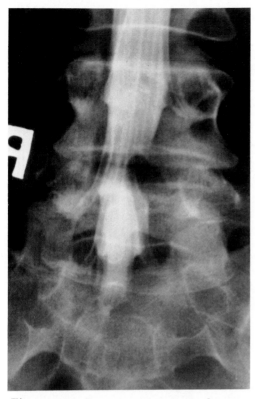

**Figure 8.76.** Posteroanterior myelogram.

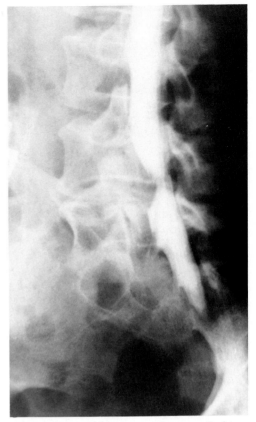

**Figure 8.78.** Oblique myelogram (left anterior).

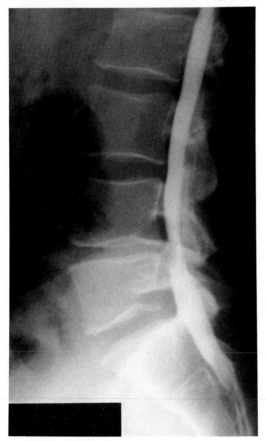

**Figure 8.77.** Lateral myelogram.

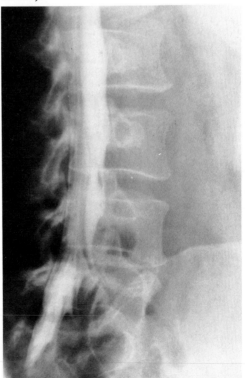

**Figure 8.79.** Oblique myelogram (right anterior).

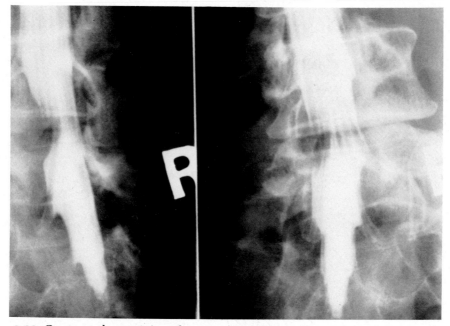

**Figure 8.80.** Contrast these views of a normal (*right*) and an indented (*left*) L4-L5 dye-filled column.

The patient was given a general anesthetic and was placed prone on the Harrington laminectomy frame. Care was taken to pad all pressure points. There were good peripheral pulses. The back was prepped and draped in the routine manner. A midline incision was made from L4 to the sacrum and was carried down through the subcutaneous tissue and fascia. The muscles were stripped subperiosteally on the left from the sacrum, L5, and L4.

A partial hemilaminectomy was done to L4 with Kerrison and Leksell rongeurs. The ligamentum flavum was removed dorsally by sharp dissection laterally with a Kerrison ronguer. The dural sac and L5 nerve root were identified. The free fragment of disc was very readily found and removed. Lateral bone onto the facet was removed. The sequestrated disc on the posterior longitudinal ligament had to be curetted with a series of up-and-down cutting curettes. The intervertebral nucleus pulposus was removed with straight and up-cutting rongeurs. The disc was very degenerated. The cartilaginous end plates were scraped. At the end of the procedure the nerve root was completely decompressed. The L4 nerve root could be palpated and there was no fragment against that. The L5 nerve root was completely free.

The wound was irrigated with a solution of Bacitracin in normal saline and then closed in layers with Dexon and staples on the skin.

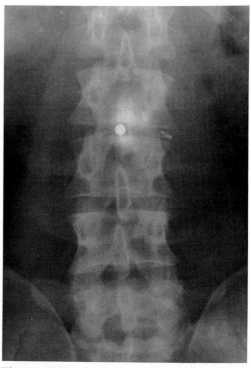

**Figure 8.81.** Anterposterior view shows lead from a shotgun blast within the nucleus pulposus of the L2-L3 disc.

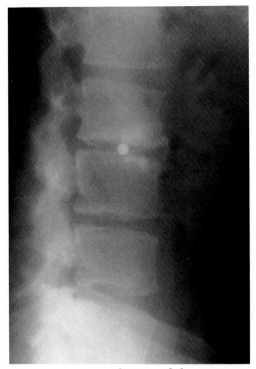

**Figure 8.82.** Lateral view of the same patient as in Figure 8.81.

Blood loss was less than 50 cc. There were no apparent complications. The patient tolerated the procedure well.

The patient was told that the chances of return of dorsiflexion of the foot were uncertain and could not be guaranteed. The patient understood this and was very happy with the relief of his leg and back pain. This author finds that muscle weakness requires immediate surgical consideration if return of function is reasonably expected. Long-term muscle weakness may not return any more with surgery than with conservative care, however. Medicolegally it can be difficult to defend prolonged conservative care in the face of loss of dorsiflexion of the foot.

Figures 8.81 and 8.82 provide a humerous conclusion to this chapter. Much has been written about possible prosthesis application for the intervertebral disc. It seems the patient presented in Figures 8.81 and 8.82 had sought to escape from confinement in prison and his captors felt otherwise. What more perfect aim could have been taken to allow such perfect placement of an artificial nucleus pulposus?

## References

1. Dommisse GF, Grabe RP: The failures of surgery for lumbar disc disorders. In Helfet AJ, Gruebel-Lee DM (eds): *Disorders of the Lumbar Spine.* Philadelphia, JB Lippincott, 1978, pp 202, 203.
2. Hirschberg GG: Treating lumbar disc lesion by prolonged continuous reduction of intradiscal pressure. *Tex Med* 70:58–68, 1974.
3. Neugebauer J: Re-establishing of the intervertebral disc by decompression. *Med Welt* 27:19, 1976.
4. Tien-You F: Lumbar intervertebral disc protrusion, new method of management and its theoretical basis. *Chin Med J [Engl]* 2(3):183–194, 1976.
5. Tsung-Min L, et al: Verticle suspension traction with manipulation in lumbar intervertebral disc protrusion. *Chin Med J* 3(6):407–412, 1977.
6. Burton C: Gravity is now a useful tool in low back pain treatment. *Fam Treat Ctr* 7:4, 1977.
7. Tkachenko SS: Closed one-stage reduction of acute prolapse of the intervertebral disc. *Ortop Traumatal Protez* 34:46–47, 1973.
8. Mathews JA, Yates DAH: Treatment of sciatica. *Lancet* 1:352, 1974.
9. Pomosov DV: Treatment of slipped discs by a closed reduction method. 76-7 *Voen Med Zh* 7: July 1976.
10. Edwards JP, et al: A comparison of chiropractic technics as they relate to the intervertebral disc syndrome. *Dig Chiro Econ* 92–101, November/December 1977.
11. Potter GE: A study of 744 cases of neck and back pain treated with spinal manipulation. *J Can Chiro Assoc* 154–156, December 1977.
12. Sharubina I: Effectiveness of using medical gymnastics together with traction in a swimming pool in the overall treatment of discogenic radiculitis. *Vopr Kurortol Fizioter Lech Fiz Kult* 38:536–557, 1973.
13. Gupta RC, Ramarao SV: Epidurography in reduction of lumbar disc prolapse by traction. *Arch Phys Med Rehabil* 59: July 1978.
14. Lind G: *Auto-Traction, Treatment of Low Back Pain and Sciatica, An Electromyographic, Radiographic and Clinical Study.* Linkoping, 1974.
15. Anonymous: Treatment of lumbar disc protrusion by automatic chiropractic traction instrument. Translated at the National College, 1982. (Available from library of author, JM Cox.)
16. Raney FL: The effects of flexion, extension, valsalva maneuver and abdominal compression of the large volume myelographic column. International Society for Study of the Lumbar Spine, June 5–8, 1978.
17. Eagle R: A pain in the back. *New Scientist* 170–173, October 18, 1979.
18. Hukins DWL, Hickey DS: Relation between the structure of the annulus fibrosus and the function and failure of the intervertebral disc. *Spine* 6(2):110, 1980.
19. Nachemson AL: The lumbar spine, an orthopaedic challenge. *Spine* 1(1):59–69, 1976.
20. Tindall GT: Clinical aspects of lumbar intervertebral disk disease. *J Med Assoc Ga* 70:247–253, 1981.
21. Malec J, Cayner JJ, Harvey RF, Timming RC: Pain management: long term follow-up of inpatient program. *Arch Phys Med Rehabil* 62:369–372, 1981.
22. Trief P: Chronic back pain, a tripartite model of

outcome. *Arch Phys Med Rehabil* 64(1):53–56, 1983.

23. Chrisman OD, Mittnock T, Snook GA: A study of the results following rotatory manipulation in the lumbar intervertebral disc syndrome. *J Bone Joint Surg* 46A:517–524, 1964.

24. Mensor MC: Non-operative treatment, including manipulation, for lumbar intervertebral disc syndrome. *J Bone Joint Surg* 37A:925–936, 1955.

25. Colonna PC, Friedenberg ZB: The disc syndrome, results of the conservative care of patients with positive myelograms. *J Bone Joint Surg* 31A:614–618, 1949.

26. Wilson JN, Ilfeld FW: Manipulation of the herniated intervertebral disc. *Am J Surg* 83:173, 175, 1952.

27. Bernini PM, Simeone FA: Reflex dystrophy. *Spine* 6(2):180–184, 1980.

28. Bogduk N: The anatomy of the lumbar intervertebral disc syndrome. *Med J Aust* 1:878, 1976.

29. Farfan HF: *Mechanical Disorders of the Low Back.* Philadelphia, Lea & Febiger, 1973, p 24.

30. Helfet AJ, Grubel-Lee DM: *Disorders of the Lumbar Spine.* Philadelphia, JB Lippincott, 1978, p 46.

31. Tsukada K: Histologische Studien über die Zwischenwirbelscheibe des Menschen. *Altersvanderugen Mitt Akad Kioto* 25:1–29, 207–209, 1932.

32. Malinsky J: The ontogenetic development of nerve transmissions in the intervertebral disc of man. *Acta Anat* 38:96, 1959

33. Hirsch C, Inglemark BG, Miller M: The anatomical basis for low back pain. Studies on the presence of sensory nerve endings in ligamentous, capsular and intervertebral disc structures in the human lumbar spine. *Acta Orthop Scand* 1:33, 1963–1964.

33a. Yoshizawa H, O'Brien J, Smith WT, Trumper M: The neuropathology of intervertebral discs removed for low-back pain. *J Pathol* 132:95–104, 1980.

34. Sunderland S: Anatomical paravertebral influence on the intervertebral foramen. In: *The Research Status of Spinal Manipulative Therapy.* Bethesda, MD, National Institute of Neurological and Communicative Disorders and Stroke, NINCDS Monograph No 15, DHEW No. 76-998, 1975, p 135.

35. Edgar MA, Ghadially JA: Innervation of the lumbar spine. *Clin Orthop* 115:35–41, 1976

36. Lazorthes G, Poulhes J, Espagno J: Etude sur les nerfs sinu-vertebraux lumbaires le nerf de roofe existe-t-il? *CR Assoc Anat* 34:317, 1948.

37. Shinohara H: A study on lumbar disc lesions. *J Jpn Orthop Assoc* 44:553, 1970.

38. Macnab I: Common vertebral joint problems. In GP Grieve (ed): *Mobilisation of the Spine,* ed 3. London, Churchill Livingstone, 1979, p 63.

39. Farfan HF: A reorientation in the surgical approach to the degenerative lumbar intervertebral disc. *Orthop Clin North Am* 8(1):9–12, 1977.

40. Schultz AB: Mechanical factors in the etiology of idiopathic low back disorders. In: *American Academy of Orthopaedic Surgeons Symposium on Idiopathic Low Back Pain.* St Louis, CV Mosby, 1982, pp 206–207.

41. Spurling R, Grantham E: Neurologic picture of herniations of the nucleus pulposus in the lower part of the lumbar region. *Arch Surg* 40:375–388, 1940.

42. Falconer M, McGeorge M, Begg A: Observations on the cause and mechanism of symptom-production in sciatica and low-back pain. *J Neurol Neurosurg Psychiatry* 11:13–26, 1948.

43. Hirsch C: An attempt to diagnose the level of a disc lesion clinically by disc puncture. *Acta Orthop Scand* 18:132–140, 1948.

44. Wiberg G: Back pain in relation to the nerve supply of the intervertebral disc. *Acta Orthop Scand* 19:211–221, 1941.

44a. Smyth M, Wright V: Sciatica and the intervertebral disc. *J Bone Joint Surg* 40A:1401–1417, 1958.

45. Lindblom K: Technique and results of diagnostic disc puncture and injection (discography) in the lumbar region. *Acta Orthop Scand* 20:315–326, 1950.

46. Cloward R, Buzaid L: Discography technique, indications and evaluation of the normal and abnormal intervertebral disc. *AJR* 68:552–564, 1952.

47. Collis J, Gardner W: Lumbar discography: an analysis of one thousand cases. *J Neurosurg* 19:452–461, 1962.

48. Holt E: Fallacy of cervical discography. *JAMA* 188:799–801, 1964.

49. Hudgins W: Diagnostic accuracy of lumbar discography. *Spine* 2:307–309, 1977.

50. Kellgren J: Observations on referral pain arising from muscle. *Clin Sci* 3:175–190, 1938.

50a. Sinclair D, Feindel W, Weddell G, Falconer M: The intervertebral ligaments as a source of segmental pain. *J Bone Joint Surg* 30B:515–521, 1948.

51. LaMotte RH: Nociceptors in skin, joint, muscle and bone. In: *American Academy of Orthopaedic Surgeons Symposium on Idiopathic Low Back Pain.* St Louis, CV Mosby, 1982, pp 417 and 427.

52. Torkildsen A: Lesions of the cervical spine roots as a source of pain simulating sciatica. *Acta Psychiatr Neurol Scand* 31:333–444, 1956.

53. Murphy F: Sources of pain in disc disease. *Clin Neurosurg* 15:343–351, 1968.

54. Cyriax J: *Textbook of Orthopaedic Medicine,* ed 3, vol 1: *Diagnosis of Soft Tissue Lesions.* Baltimore, Williams & Wilkins, 1969, pp 450–457.

55. Kessler RM: Acute symptomatic disc prolapse: clinical manifestations and therapeutic considerations. *Phys Ther* 59(8):985, 1979.

56. Herlin L: *Sciatic and Pelvic Pain due to Lumbosacral Nerve Root Compression.* Springfield, IL, Charles C Thomas, 1966, pp 79, 80, and 83.

57. Shapiro R: *Myelography,* ed 2. Chicago, Year Book Medical Publishers, 1968, p 323.

58. Lecuire J: 641 Operations for sciatic neuralgia due to discal hernia, a computerized statistical study of the results. *Neurochirurgie* 19:501–512, 1973.

59. Farfan HF, Sullivan JD: The relationship of facet orientation to intervertebral disc failure. *Can J Surg* 10:179–185, 1967.

60. Horal J: The clinical appearance of low back disorders. *Acta Orthop Scand Suppl* 118:7–109, 1969.

61. Keele CA, Neil E: *Samson Wright's Applied Phys-*

*iology*, ed 10. London, Oxford University Press, 1961, p 51.

62. Hult L: The Munkfors investigation. *Acta Orthop Scand Suppl* p 16, 1954.

63. Splitoff C: Roentgenographic comparison of patients with and without backache. *JAMA* 152:1610, 1953.

64. Finneson BE: *Low Back Pain*, Philadelphia, JB Lippincott 1973, p 257.

65. Scoville WB, Corkill G: Lumbar spondylolisthesis with ruptured disc. *J Neurosurg* 40:530, 1974.

66. Blau L, Kent L: Conservative and surgical aspects of disc lesion management. Follow-up review of 244 cases. *West J Med* 120:356–357, 1974.

67. Stoddard A: *Manual of Osteopathic Technic.* New York, Harper & Row, 1969.

# CHAPTER 9

*Through education I learn to do by choice
what other men do by constraints of fear.*
                              **—Aristotle**

# The Facet Syndrome

Two studies done by Cox et al. (1, 2) reveal that 26% of patients with low back pain have facet syndrome either alone or in conjunction with other findings. The exact amount of low back pain caused by the facet syndrome needs further documentation, however. A close look at the stresses exerted on the lumbosacral articulation from facet syndrome should, therefore, be of great importance to the chiropractic physician treating this condition. On the radiograph of a patient with suspected facet syndrome (Fig. 9.1), lines should be drawn under the plate of the superior vertebra and above the plate of the inferior segment, posteriorly to their intersection; these lines should cross within or anterior to the articular facets.

The line drawn posteriorly from the inferior plate of the superior body is called Macnab's line (Fig. 9.2). In the patient with the facet syndrome or hyperextension of L5 on the sacrum, the tip of the superior facet of the vertebra below falls above Macnab's line (3). Normally, the facet tip is below this line. The facet being above Macnab's line must, therefore, be found in recumbent and upright films to confirm that the patient has facet syndrome (Figs. 9.3 and 9.4).

Hellems and Keats (4) found the normal sacral angle to be 41° (Fig. 9.5). At this degree of sacral inclination, 80% of the superimposed body weight is carried upon the vertebral bodies and the sacral promontory. Although only 20% of the weight is carried upon the articular facets, this weight constitutes 10 times more pressure per square inch on the facets than the weight carried upon the knee with a person in the upright posture. This should give some idea of the strain produced on the articular facets.

Increase of the sacral angle shifts weight bearing posteriorly onto the posterior elements and facets (Fig. 9.6). The articular facets were never created to stand this shearing stress. As the sacral base inclines farther, a hyperextension subluxation of the upper motion segment and/or hyperflexion subluxation of the lower motion segment must take place. Look at Figure 9.7; in this figure you see a 65° sacral base angle with facet syndrome.

## STABILITY IN THE FACET SYNDROME AND AN INDICATION OF RESPONSE TO MANIPULATION

Although the articular facets are well supplied with nerve fibers from the dorsal ramus of the spinal nerve, discussion continues as to the role that the articular facet plays in the etiology of low back and lower extremity pain. Van Akkerveeken determined a measurement for stability or instability of the lumbar spine from use of lateral lumbar films in order to determine damage to the posterior longitudinal ligament and the annulus fibrosus. This measurement is illustrated in Figure 9.8.

According to Van Akkerveeken (5), in a normal lumbar spine in full extension, with the annulus fibers and longitudinal ligaments intact, a line drawn along the posterior longitudinal ligament shows a fairly smooth arch. If the annulus fibers are cut, there is a definite posterior sliding of each vertebra posteriorly upon the vertebra below. If lines are drawn along the inferior plate of the vertebra above and along the superior plate of the vertebra below and the intersection of these lines is called *point a*, there should be less than a 3-mm difference in length between the

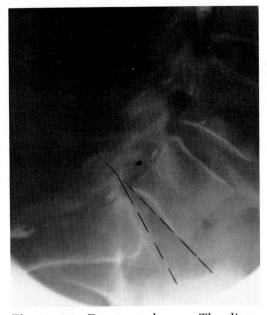

**Figure 9.1.** Facet syndrome. The lines drawn as an extension of the body plates intersect within or anterior to the articular facets.

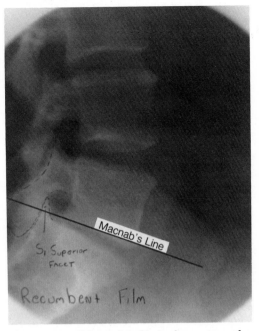

**Figure 9.3.** Macnab's line shown on the recumbent view. The sacral facet extends above the line.

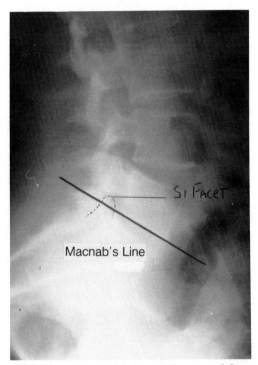

**Figure 9.2.** Macnab's line. The sacral facet falls above the line drawn to extend posteriorly from the 5th lumbar inferior body plate.

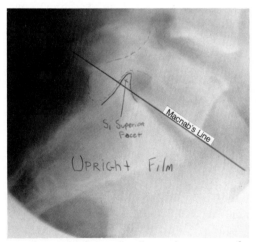

**Figure 9.4.** Macnab's line shown on the upright view. As in the recumbent view, the 1st sacral facet lies above the line.

line drawn from *point a* to the posterior margin of the superior vertebra and the line drawn from *point a* to the posterior margin of the inferior vertebra. If the difference is 3 mm or more, instability is present, meaning that there is damage to the annular fibers and/or the posterior

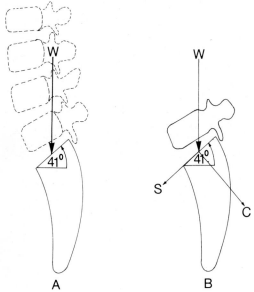

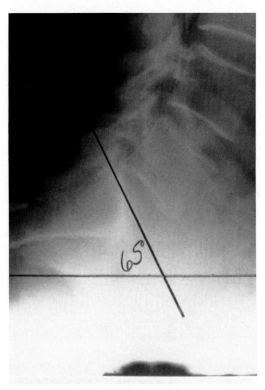

**Figure 9.5.** Position of the normal sacrum during erect standing. A, the superincumbent weight (W) passing through the posterior edge of the lumbosacral joint. B, the compression (C) and shearing (S) components of the superincumbent weight. (Reproduced with permission from B. LeVeau: *Biomechanics of Human Motion.* Philadelphia, W. B. Saunders, 1977, p. 94.)

**Figure 9.7.** Increased sacral angle and hyperextension of L5 on the sacrum.

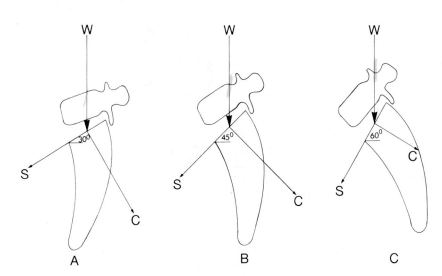

**Figure 9.6.** Change in the compression (C) and shearing (S) force components with change in the sacral angle. W, weight. (Reproduced with permission from B. LeVeau: *Biomechanics of Human Motion.* Philadelphia, W. B. Saunders, 1977, p. 95.)

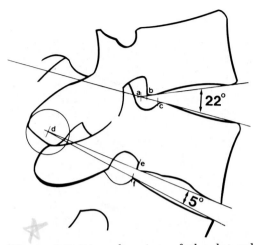

**Figure 9.8.** Line drawing of the lateral aspect of lumbar segment in full extension, illustrating radiologic instability and methods of measuring it (degrees of tilt and length of parallel displacement). The lower segment is stable; *de = df* in length. At the upper segment, radiologic instability is demonstrated; in this case, *line ab* is 3 mm shorter than *line ac* (see text for explanation). (Reproduced with permission from P. F. Van Akkerveeken, J. P. O'Brien, and W. M. Park: Experimentally Induced Hypermobility in the Lumbar Spine. *Spine* 4(3):238, 1979.)

longitudinal ligament. We utilize this measurement as a prognostic aid to determine the response of a patient to treatment as well as to predict future difficulty in the lumbosacral spine.

It has also been shown that the greater the discal angle, the more severe the facet syndrome. The discal angle (*edf*) shown in Figure 9.8 is 5°, a sign of stability and no facet syndrome. The other angle (*bac*) is 22°, a sign of severe facet syndrome. This author believes that any discal angle over 15° is a sign of severe facet syndrome (Fig. 9.9).

Figure 9.10 demonstrates the use of Van Akkerveeken's line measurement to determine stability. The spine shown in Figure 9.10 is stable. Figure 9.11 demonstrates the use of this measurement in a patient with an unstable spine. A line is drawn from the point of intersection (A) to the posterior border of the 5th lumbar

body above (B) and to the posterior border of the sacrum below (C). The distance from A to B measures 16 mm; the distance from A to C measures 22 mm. By Van Akkerveeken's measurement, therefore, the lumbosacral articulation is unstable, showing that the annulus and posterior longitudinal ligament are damaged.

The facet syndrome has been accused of causing much low back pain; a review of our present knowledge about the sensitivity of the articular bed of the facet, therefore, is in order.

Increasingly in the literature, articles are appearing concerning the nerve innervation of the articular facets. There are important anatomical relationships in the lumbosacral region of the adult, which are traceable to embryonic development. In their discussion of the pain relationships evolving from biomechanical faults of the lumbosacral complex, Carmichael and Burkhart (6) state that the paraxial mesoderm that condenses alongside the notochord becomes segmented into somites. Each somite then differentiates into a scleratome (which contributes to vertebrae formation), a myotome (which forms axial and appendicular muscle), and a dermatome (which forms the dermis). The developing neural tube innervates each somite and its derivatives so that the nerve pattern becomes segmental.

Each scleratome divides transversely and each hemiscleratome reaggregates with a hemiscleratome adjacent to it, becoming the centrum that forms most of the vertebral body. These divisions and reaggregations determine important anatomical relationships in the adult: (a) the spinal nerve, which originally would have run through the scleratome, now runs between the vertebrae, and (b) the myotome forms muscle that spans adjacent vertebral segments, thus establishing the patterns for back muscles.

The notochord, surrounded by the centrum, undergoes mucoid degeneration and usually disappears completely except for the nucleus pulposus of the intervertebral disc.

The centrum eventually forms part of the membranous vertebral column. Each vertebra undergoes chondrification and

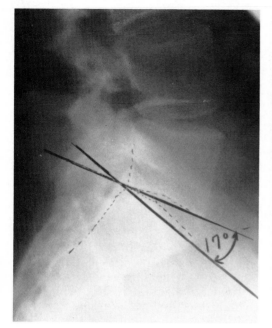

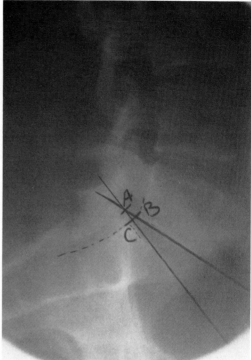

**Figure 9.9.** Lines are drawn to determine whether there is facet syndrome. Note that the angle is 17°. The greater this angle becomes, the greater the severity of the facet syndrome due to hyperextension of L5 and/or due to hyperflexion of the sacrum. The closer this angle is to 5°, the more stable the articulation.

**Figure 9.10.** Van Akkerveeken's lines are drawn and show stability of the annulus fibrosus and posterior longitudinal ligament.

ossification, a process completed several years after birth. The costal elements form a substantial part of the transverse process of the adult lumbar vertebra and the major portion of the lateral part of the sacrum.

Thus by the process reviewed above, the individual vertebrae are formed and the overall shape of the vertebral column is established. The five lumbar vertebrae typically are massive and show some differentiation. Generally, the vertebral foramen (which determines the shape of the spinal canal) becomes more triangular at L5 as the pedicles shorten, but the distance between the foramina shows little change.

## STRUCTURAL FACTORS OF THE LUMBOSACRAL REGION

The joint between L5 and S1 is the single most common site of problems in the vertebral column because of, but not

limited to, the following anatomic reasons: (a) this joint bears more weight than any other vertebral joint, (b) the center of gravity passes directly through these vertebrae, (c) a transition occurs here between the mobile presacral vertebrae and the relatively stable pelvic girdle, and (d) there is a change in the angle that exists between these two vertebrae.

In 1976, Mooney and Robertson (7) pointed out that Ghormley had coined the phrase *facet syndrome* in 1933 and that lesions of the intervertebral disc could not explain all low back and leg pain complaints. From his review of surgical literature, Sprangfort (8) found that only 42.6% of surgical patients obtained complete relief of back and leg pain following surgery.

Mooney and Robertson (7) also discovered that the injection of an irritant fluid into the facet joint caused referred pain patterns indistinguishable from pain complaints frequently associated with the disc

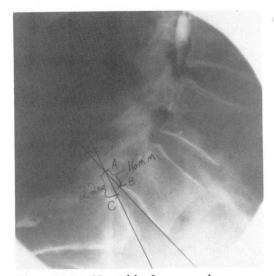

**Figure 9.11.** Unstable facet syndrome, as *line AB* is more than 3-mm longer than *line AC.*

syndrome. Even straight leg raising and diminished reflex signs were obliterated by precise local anesthetic injection into the facet joint. Injection of steroids and local anesthetic into the facet joint in a group of 100 consecutive patients suggested that this treatment alone achieved long-term relief in one fifth of the patients with lumbago and sciatica and partial relief in another one third of these patients. This author would point out, however, that far less than half of the patients received long-term relief from pain from use of this technic. The point to be emphasized here is that the physician must be clinically careful to realize that a combination of therapy may be necessary to bring maximum relief of the patient's complaints.

## FACET PAIN PATTERNS

In June of 1976, Lora and Long (9) wrote that the results of stimulation in and around the facets yielded interesting pain patterns. Typical radicular radiation is not generated by stimulation of the nerves in and around the facet, but widespread referral of sensation even into the leg is possible. This referral of sensation, however, characteristically has a diffuse non-

radicular character, is difficult for the patient to localize, and has not gone below the knee in any patient.

Stimulation of the L5-S1 facet characteristically produces sensation or reproduces pain in the coccyx, which is usually unilaterally, in the hip, which is usually described by the patient as being in the hip joint, and diffusely down the posterior thigh. Stimulation may occasionally travel circumferentially around the body along the course of the inguinal ligament into the groin.

Stimulation at the L4-L5 facets characteristically produces a local sensation at the level of the electrode, which radiates diffusely into the posterior hip and thigh. Coccygeal radiation of sensation is less commonly observed with L4-L5 stimulation than with L5-S1 stimulation, but it does occur. Stimulation at L3-L4 characteristically produces radiation upward into the thoracic area. Pain or sensation radiates around the flank and into the groin and anterior thigh much more diffusely with L3-L4 stimulation than with L5-S1 stimulation. Coccygeal sensations in the perineum are produced more commonly with L3-L4 stimulation than with L4-L5 stimulation but less commonly with L3-L4 stimulation than with L5-S1 stimulation. It appears that radiation of pain, at least as judged by stimulation of the posterior ramus by use of this technic, may be much more diffuse than is generally supposed. Although hip, thigh, and groin radiations are well known from studies of patients with disc protrusion, the observation that stimulation characteristically reproduces pain in the coccygeal area or produces sensation in this region is not as well known. *It certainly seems possible that coccydynia is, in fact, another manifestation of lumbar degenerative disc disease.*

Stimulation at the T12, L1, L2, and L3 levels does not produce leg or coccygeal sensations. Radiation of sensations is limited to the upper back, to thoracic and cervical regions, and around the course of the T12, L1, and L2 nerve roots in a diffuse fashion on the anterior abdominal wall.

This author would note that these are scleratogenous type pains that do not cause any sensory or motor deficits in the lower extremity. These pains never radiate below the knee and are usually isolated to the buttock and upper thigh. When motor and sensory changes are noted down the lower extremity, a disc lesion should be suspected. Figure 9.12 shows the distribution of sensations from L4-L5 and L5-S1 facet irritation.

McCall et al. (10) studied the referral of induced pain from the posterior lumbar elements in order to (a) trace the exact area of pain referral from the L1-L2 and the L4-L5 levels and (b) compare the distribution and intensity of the pain produced by intra-articular versus pericapsular provocation. In their study, normal subjects were given injections of 0.4 ml of 6% saline. Pain started within 25 seconds of each injection, with the episode usually lasting 5 minutes. At both the L1-L2 and the L4-L5 levels, injection into the joint interior (intra-articular provocation) produced less intense pain than did pericapsular injection.

The upper lumbar level was more sensitive than was the lower lumbar level. The distribution of referred pain from either intra-articular or pericapsular injection was the same, but the intensity was worse with the pericapsular injection than with intra-articular injection.

In general, injection into the upper lumbar level referred pain to the flank region, whereas injection at the L4-L5 level referred pain to the buttocks. Thigh pain never extended beyond the knee. No contralateral pain was noted. No demonstra-tion of significant leg pain was produced in these normal subjects.

There is an absence of nerve endings in the articular cartilage and synovium. The fibrous capsule of the synovial joint, however, is innervated.

McCall et al. (10) question the existence of scleratomes because of the considerable overlap of pain patterns between upper and lower lumbar spine facets.

From the results of the above study, one can see that irritation of the articular facets at L4-L5 and L5-S1 can result in pain in the coccyx, perineum, groin, buttock, and flank and into the posterior thigh, radiating as far as the knee. Our therapeutic interest in the facet is the maintenance of its ability to maintain its normal ranges of motion and thereby render it as free of subluxation as possible.

## CASE STUDIES

**Case 1** is of a patient who suffers with bilateral cramp-like feelings in the legs after he walks a given distance. At age 47, he has noted impotency within the last couple of months. He had undergone a myelogram (note the dye in the subarachnoid space in Figure 9.13) and was told that nothing had showed up. (This author would interject that the findings on myelography are seldom helpful, as Cyriax (13) has noted. Furthermore, numerous authors (13–24) believe that myelography is not really necessary for the diagnosis of a disc lesion and that a careful clinical history and examination is more accurate.)

This patient not only has the facet syndrome but also has stenosis. The anteroposterior di-

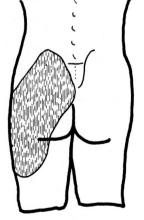 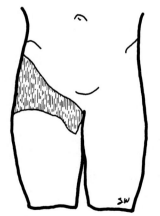

**Figure 9.12.** Distribution of sensations from L4-L5 and L5-S1 facet irritation.

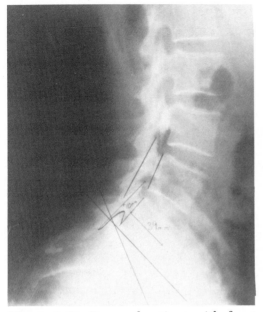

**Figure 9.13.** X-ray of patient with facet syndrome and stenosis.

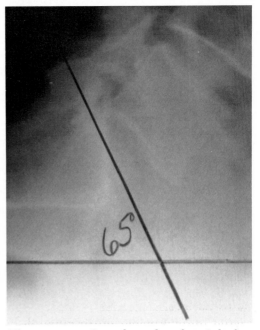

**Figure 9.14.** Sacral angle of 65° before treatment.

ameter of the vertebral body is 39 mm, and the spinal canal, as measured by Eisenstein's technic, is 10 mm. According to Verbiest (11), any sagittal diameter of the canal less than 12 mm is stenotic. Other authors, as noted in Buehler's article (12), believe that any diameter less than 13 mm (or even 15 mm) is stenotic.

Treatment resulted in the gradual relief of the low back pain and the leg discomforts over a 3-month period. The stenosis could not be altered, but note that the sacral angle has been reduced from 65° to 58° (Figs. 9.14 and 9.15). This author has found that a 5° reduction of the sacral angle by flexion distraction manipulation renders maximum relief of the patient's symptoms. Note also a reduction of the facet syndrome and relief of the stress on the articular facets.

**Case 2** is of a 65-year-old white salesman who had had low back pain for 12 days. He had experienced an immediate sharp low back pain on lifting a bag of salt, had visited a chiropractor, and had felt better after 3 visits. He had returned to work but had had a recurrence of the low back pain. Since his doctor was on vacation, he was referred to us. He also suffered from constipation.

On examination, Déjérine's triad is positive for low back pain. The straight leg raise is bilaterally positive for low back pain. Range of motion is 10° on flexion, 5° on extension, 10° on right lateral flexion, 10° on left lateral flex-

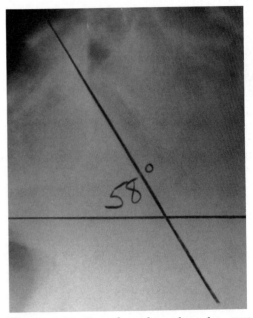

**Figure 9.15.** Sacral angle reduced to 58° following distraction manipulation.

ion, 10° on right rotation, and 10° on left rotation. No motor or sensory changes are noted. Circulation in the lower extremities is good. No other pertinent positive orthopedic signs are noted.

X-rays reveal:

1. Loss of lumbar lordosis (Fig. 9.17) and an inferior left hemipelvis (Fig. 9.16).

2. A stable facet syndrome at L5-S1 (Fig. 9.18). Note that Van Akkerveeken's measurement ($ab = 9$ mm, $ac = 12$ mm) reveals 3-mm difference between $ab$ and $ac$ and, therefore, a stable facet syndrome.

3. Stenosis at L5 (Fig. 9.19), as indicated by Eisenstein's measurement (see Chapter 7, "Stenosis," for a review).

4. Adynamic ileus (Figs. 9.16 and 9.17). Note also distension of the large and the small bowel.

5. A 9-mm short leg following relief of low back pain (Fig. 9.20). (Remember that short leg is determined following relief of all low back pain so as to get a true reading without antalgic fault.)

This patient has:

1. Stable facet syndrome at L5 with probable L5-S1 annular sprain.

2. Short left leg.

3. Stenosis (suspected) at the L5 level. If there were signs of intermittent claudication, a CT scan could be ordered.

This patient was kept in the office for a half day of care consisting of mild galvanic and tetanizing currents to the paravertebral musculature followed by goading of acupuncture points B24 to B54. Flexion distraction was gently instituted and was increased with patient tolerance. Kinesiology consisted of ad-

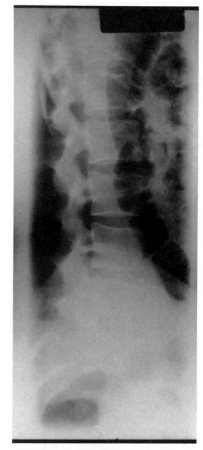

**Figure 9.17.** Lateral lumbar projection. Note the loss of lumbar lordosis.

ductor muscle origin and insertion goading, gluteus medius and minimus origin and insertion goading, and pressure into the gluteus maximus belly. Cathartics and an enema were ordered for use at home. Finally, a 9-mm lift was added to the left shoe and a Cox lumbar brace was fitted.

The patient was advised to use hot and cold alternating packs on his low back, do Cox exercises 1, 2, and 3, and avoid sitting.

He experienced a 50% relief from pain on the first day and a 100% relief from pain after 5 days of treatment. He was seen twice daily for the first two days.

**Case 3** is of a 54-year-old married woman who had had low back pain for 2 weeks. She was taking pain pills prescribed by her family doctor, which did not help. Sitting, lying, standing, and bending all aggravated the pain.

On examination, range of motion is 30° on flexion, 10° on extension, 10° on left lateral flexion, 10° on right lateral flexion, 20° on right rotation, and 20° on left rotation. Straight

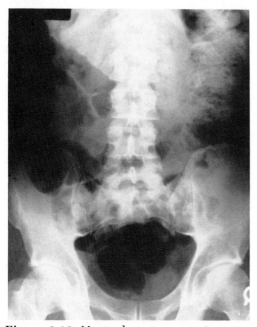

**Figure 9.16.** Neutral posteroanterior projection. Note the adynamic ileus.

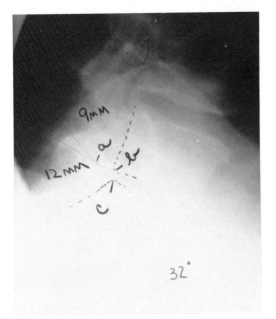

**Figure 9.18.** Lateral spot view for Van Akkerveeken's measurement.

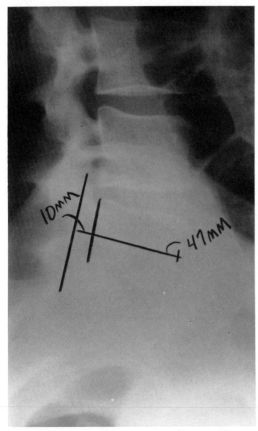

**Figure 9.19.** Markings, according to Eisenstein's technic, indicating stenosis.

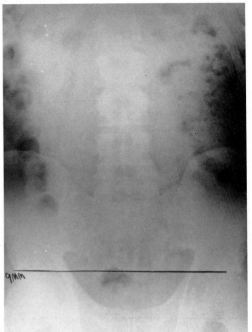

**Figure 9.20.** X-ray showing 9-mm short leg following relief of all low back pain. A 9-mm lift was used under the left shoe for correction, as was described in Chapter 4 for correction of short leg.

leg raise is positive on the right at 45°. No motor or sensory changes are noted.

X-rays reveal:

1. The intercrestal line cutting the L5 body (Fig. 9.21). The transverse processes of L5 are less developed than those of L3. As MacGibbon and Farfan (25) point out, this places the L5-S1 disc in greatest stress.

2. Facet syndrome at L5-S1 (Fig. 9.22), which is unstable as determined by Van Akkerveeken's measurement.

3. Disc thinning at L5-S1 (Fig. 9.22).

This patient has a facet syndrome at L5-S1, which is unstable, and discogenic spondyloarthrosis at L5-S1.

Treatment consisted of Cox flexion distraction (with the use of a Dutchman roll) for facet syndrome, as discussed in this chapter; goading of acupressure points B24 to B49; and application of sinusoidal current to the paravertebral muscles. The patient was advised to do Cox exercises 1, 2, 3, 5, 6, 7, and 8 at home (see exercise sheet for numbers), apply alternating heat and cold before the exercises, avoid sitting, and take Discat, calcium (nonphosphorous), and B vitamins.

The patient was treated daily until there was a 50% improvement and then was treated

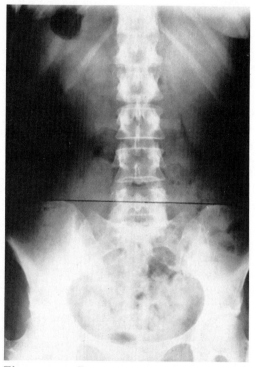

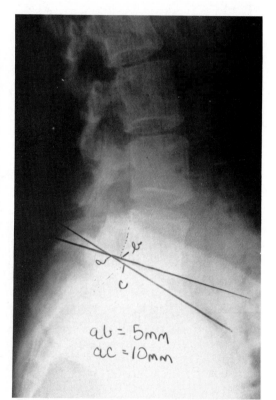

**Figure 9.21.** Posteroanterior neutral view of the lumbar spine and pelvis. Note the intercrestal line cuts the L5 body.

**Figure 9.22.** Lateral view showing an unstable facet syndrome and L5-S1 disc degeneration.

twice weekly until maximum relief was obtained. She obtained 50% relief from pain in 3 weeks of care and stopped treatment.

**Case 4** is of a 28-year-old white man who has low back and left leg pain. This man is 6 feet tall, weighs 176 lb, and has a mesomorphic build. On November 23, 1981, while lifting 3 tires at work, he felt a sudden weakness in his low back and could hardly walk. His company sent him to a chiropractor. He returned to work February 1982. He was then seen by a neurosurgeon who said that no surgery was necessary. By November 1982, the pain had become so bad that he stopped work. His job was inspecting tires by bending forward to look inside the tire.

On examination, range of motion is 90° on flexion, 22° on extension, 20° on right lateral flexion, 20° on left lateral flexion, 30° on right rotation, and 30° on left rotation. The test for Kemp's sign is negative. No motor changes are noted in the lower extremities. The patient has hypoesthesia of the left S1 dermatome. Doppler examination reveals adequate circulation. There is hamstring shortness.

X-rays reveal:

1. Normal lateral motion as shown on neutral and lateral ending studies (Figs. 9.23, 9.24, and 9.25) of the lumbar spine and on tilt views of L5-S1 (Figs. 9.26, 9.27, and 9.28).
2. Facet syndrome at L5-S1 (Fig. 9.29), which is stable as determined by Van Akkerveeken's measurement (see Fig. 9.8).
3. Stenosis at L5 (Fig. 9.30). Eisenstein's measurement (see Chapter 7) reveals that the body is 45 mm and the vertebral canal is 13 mm (10.4 mm with correction factor for magnification error of 80%).

This patient has a facet syndrome at L5-S1, which is stable; stenosis at L5; and probable nuclear bulge at L5-S1.

The patient's insurance company requested that, following our examination, we treat this man according to our recommendation, i.e., to provide 3 weeks of daily care, up to 3 or 4 treatments daily, while the patient attended Low Back Pain School. Treatment consisted of facet syndrome care, application of hot and cold packs, sinusoidal currents, and performance of Cox exercises (1 to 8), especially the hamstring stretching exercise. With no signs of intermittent claudication, we felt that the stenosis was not a problem to be concerned with at this time.

At Low Back Pain School, the patient learned proper lifting and the avoidance of rotation of the lumbar spine, i.e., how to pick up objects from the floor so as to avoid lumbar flexion or rotation, how to lift objects by keeping them close to the body, and how to reduce intradiscal pressure by avoiding prolonged sitting. He was given a book written for lay people in which the basic anatomy and mechanics of the low back are explained.

At the end of 3 weeks of care, the patient was totally relieved of his low back and left leg pain and was referred back to his own chiropractor.

**Case 5** is of a 29-year-old white woman who has mild low back pain on lifting and bending as a delivery person and truck driver. She had been hospitalized for the pain and had had the following studies performed which were all normal: upper and lower gastrointestinal barium studies, gallbladder study, ultrasound, ultrasound of the uterus, lumbar spine and pelvic x-rays, thoracic spine x-rays, and chest x-rays.

On examination, range of motion is normal. The straight leg raise is negative, except for tight hamstrings. Deep reflexes are active and equal. No sensory changes are noted. There is pain on palpation at L4-L5 and L5-S1 into the buttocks and gluteus medius.

X-rays reveal:

1. A 6-mm shortness of the left femoral head and hemipelvis (Fig. 9.31). The facets at L5-S1 are bilaterally sagittal.
2. Normal lateral bending studies (Figs. 9.32 and 9.33).
3. Hyperextension of L4 on L5 and L5 on S1 as shown on the lateral view (Fig. 9.34). Minimal spurring of the L4 anterosuperior body plate also is noted.
4. Results with a 6-mm heel lift in place under the left foot (Fig. 9.35). The lumbar spine is straightened.

Treatment consisted of addition of a 6-mm lift to the left shoe to straighten the lumbar spine. Cox distraction manipulation was performed with the use of a Dutchman roll. The patient was instructed on sagittal facet instability, and Low Back Wellness School instruction was given on how to lift, bend, and carry with minimal strain to this unstable low back.

The patient experienced the absence of back pain after 1 visit.

**Case 6** is of a 54-year-old white woman who has had right low back pain radiating down the right buttock, posterior thigh, and calf to the ankle for 2 weeks.

On examination, a spinal curve to the left with left low hemipelvis is noted. Straight leg raise is positive on the right at 50°. Range of

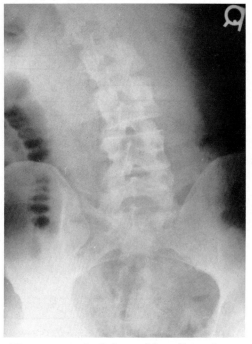

**Figure 9.23.** Left lateral bending view.

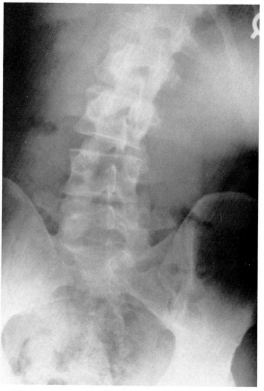

**Figure 9.25.** Right lateral bending view.

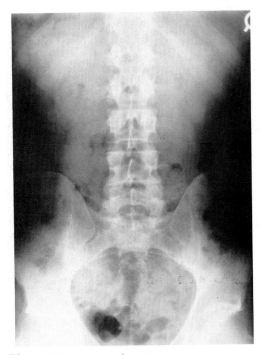

**Figure 9.24.** Neutral posteroanterior view.

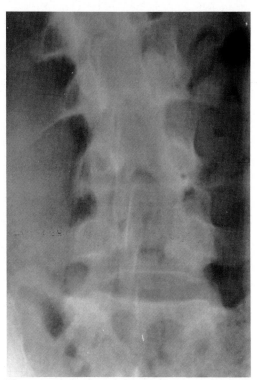

motion is 90° on flexion, 10° on extension, 20°
on right lateral bending, 5° on left lateral bending, 30° on right rotation, and 10° on left
rotation. The test for Kemp's sign is positive

**Figure 9.26.** Special posteroanterior tilt
view of L5-S1 in left lateral bending.

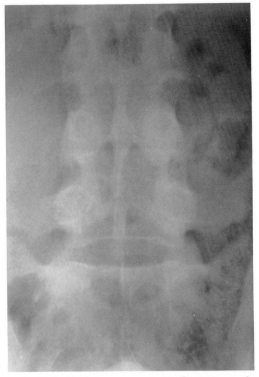

**Figure 9.27.** Posteroanterior tilt view with the patient in the neutral upright posture.

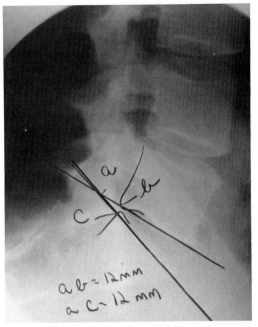

**Figure 9.29.** Lateral spot view showing stable facet syndrome.

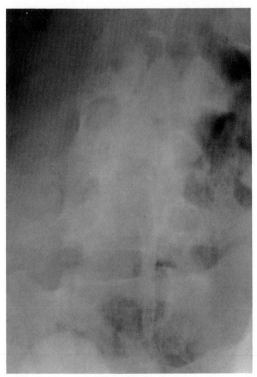

**Figure 9.28.** Special posteroanterior tilt view of L5-S1 in right lateral bending.

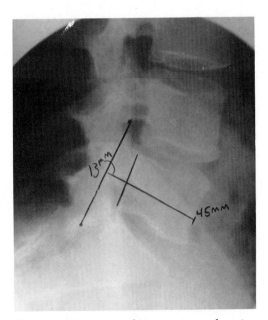

**Figure 9.30.** Lateral spot view showing stenosis, as determined by Eisenstein's measurement.

on the left. There is pain on palpation at L5-S1 into the right buttock and posterior thigh. The deep reflexes are active and equal.

X-rays reveal:

1. A 22-mm short left femoral head with a

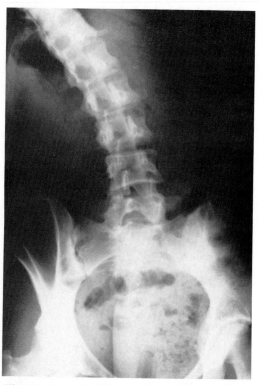

**Figure 9.32.** Left lateral bending view.

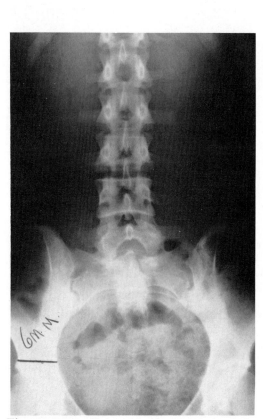

**Figure 9.31.** X-ray showing 6-mm left short femoral head.

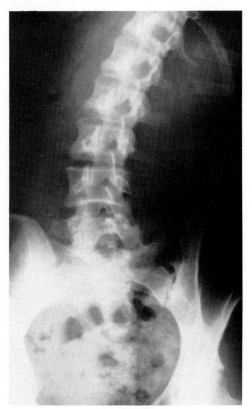

**Figure 9.33.** Right lateral bending view.

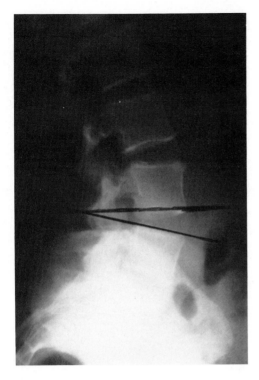

**Figure 9.34.** Lateral view showing hyperextension of L4 on L5.

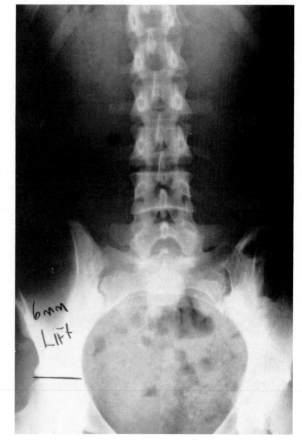

**Figure 9.35.** X-ray of straightened lumbar spine with a 6-mm lift correction to the left shoe.

low hemipelvis and a left nonrotatory lean of the lumbar spine (Fig. 9.37).

2. Good left lateral bending (Fig. 9.36) but hypomobility of L4 to laterally flex on L5 on right lateral bending (Fig. 9.38).

3. Stable facet syndrome of L5 on S1 and an impending facet syndrome of L4 on L5 (Fig. 9.39). Minimal spur formation of the anterolateral superior vertebral body plate of L3 is also noted.

4. Overcorrection for a short left leg with a 19 mm heel and sole lift (Fig. 9.40).

5. Overcorrection for a short left leg with a 13-mm heel and sole lift (Fig. 9.41).

6. A straightened lumbar spine with a 9-mm heel and sole lift (Fig. 9.42).

Treatment consisted of reduction of the facet syndrome as shown on page 256. A 9-mm heel lift and 4-mm sole lift were placed under the left shoe.

This patient obtained complete relief of low back pain.

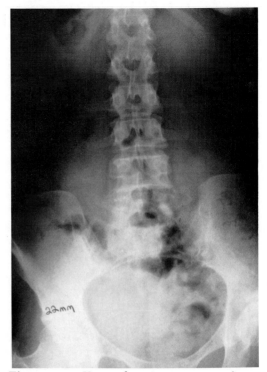

**Figure 9.37.** X-ray showing a 22-mm short left inferior head and hemipelvis in comparison to the right inferior head and hemipelvis.

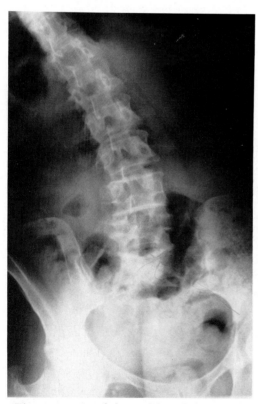

**Figure 9.36.** Left lateral bending view.

**Figure 9.38.** Right lateral bending view showing the hypomobility of L4 to laterally flex on L5 to the right.

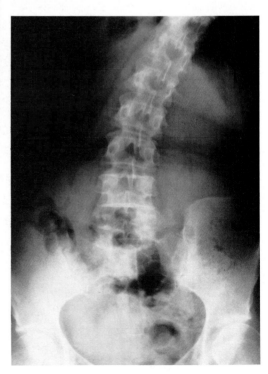

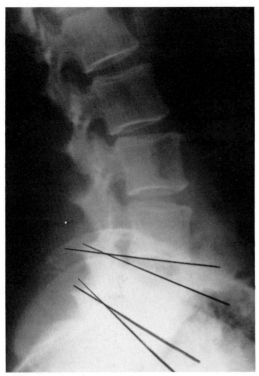

**Figure 9.39.** X-ray showing a stable facet syndrome of L4 on L5 and L5 on S1.

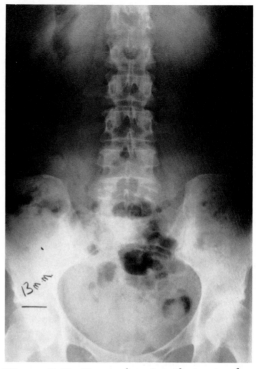

**Figure 9.41.** X-ray showing that use of a 13-mm lift still overcorrects for the left short leg.

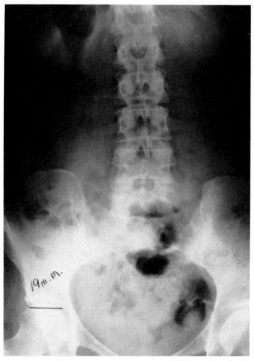

**Figure 9.40.** Posteroanterior Chamberlain view showing overcorrection for the left short leg with use of a 19-mm heel and sole lift.

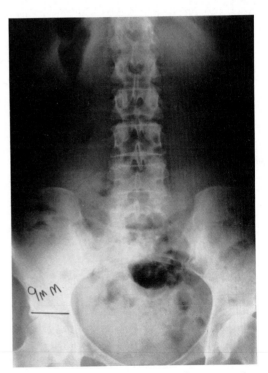

**Figure 9.42.** X-ray showing that use of a 9-mm lift balances the pelvis.

*Comment:* Case 6 emphasizes the importance of x-rays for leveling the pelvis properly. Also, the proper straightening of the lumbar spine is brought about by the proper lift. Use lifts while taking x-rays for determination of short leg!

## TREATMENT OF THE FACET SYNDROME

Whether the facet syndrome is stable or unstable, its treatment is very similar to the treatment for spondylolisthesis.

Figure 9.43 is an x-ray of a patient with facet syndrome (the same patient as is shown being treated in Figures 9.44 to 9.46).

A Dutchman roll, as shown in Figure 9.44, is placed under the abdomen so as to establish a slight kyphosis at the L5-S1 segment. This serves to bring the superior facet of sacrum caudally out of the upper third of the intervertebral foramen at L5-S1. Remember that in the treatment of facet syndrome above the spondylolisthetic segment, we are interested in bringing the superior facet of the spondylolisthesis vertebra downward out of the intervertebral foramen, whereas in the treatment of facet syndrome alone, we are interested in tractioning the superior facet

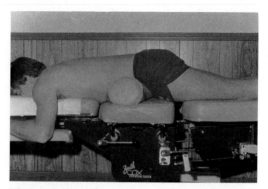

**Figure 9.44.** The patient lies on the Cox distraction table, with a hyperflexion Dutchman roll placed under the abdomen.

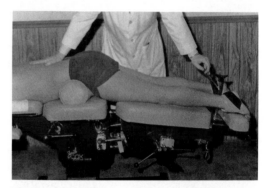

**Figure 9.45.** The contact hand thenar eminence lifts the spinous process of L5 cephalad while distraction is applied downward on the caudal section of the Cox table.

of the vertebra below the facet syndrome downward from the upper area of the intervertebral foramen. Therefore, in the treatment of facet syndrome the thenar contact is maintained on the spinous process of the facet syndrome segment involved, i.e., L5 if it is at the L5-S1 level, whereas in the treatment of spondylolisthesis the thenar contact is maintained on the spinous process above at L4, which is shown in Figures 9.45 and 9.46.

At this time, no more downward force should be applied to the caudal section of the table than can be pressed with one finger. The force is maintained for 3 sessions of 20 seconds each while a gentle push-pull or pumping action with the caudal section of the table is applied. *Remember to use gentle distraction!*

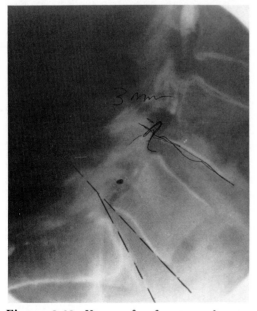

**Figure 9.43.** X-ray of a facet syndrome. Note the intersection of the body plate lines anterior to the sacral facets.

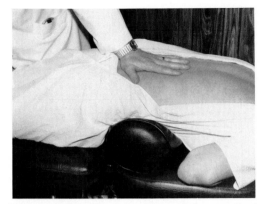

**Figure 9.46.** Close up view of the contact hand on the spinous process of L5. Keep the traction arm straight with the spine and do not angle the force of distraction.

A belt support is used in the treatment of severe cases. All patients are sent to Low Back Wellness School, especially if the facet syndrome is unstable. Cox exercises 1, 2, 3, 6, 7, and 9 are prescribed for patients with the facet syndrome (see the Cox exercises in Chapter 8).

## References

1. Cox JM, Fromelt KA, Shreiner S: Chiropractic statistical survey of 100 consecutive low back pain patients. *J Manipul Physiolog Ther* 6(3):117–128, 1982.
2. Cox JM, Shreiner S: Chiropractic manipulation in low back pain and sciatica: statistical data on the diagnosis, treatment and response of 576 consecutive cases. *J Manipul Physiolog Ther* 7(1):1–11, 1984.
3. Macnab I: *Backache.* Baltimore, Williams & Wilkins, 1977, p 200.
4. Hellems HK, Keats TE: Measurement of the normal lumbosacral angle. *AJR* 113:642–645, 1971.
5. Van Akkerveeken PF, O'Brien JP, Park WM: Experimentally induced hypermobility in the lumbar spine. *Spine* 4(3):236–241, 1979.
6. Carmichael S, Burkhart S: Clinical anatomy of the lumbosacral complex. *J Phys Ther* 59:966, 1979.
7. Mooney V, Robertson J: The facet syndrome. *Clin Orthop* 115:149–156, 1976.
8. Sprangfort EV: Lumbar disc herniation. *Acta Orthop Scand [Suppl]* 142: 1972.
9. Lora J, Long D: So-called facet denervation in the management of intractable back pain. *Spine* 1(2):121–126, 1976.
10. McCall I, Park W, O'Brien J: Induced pain referral from posterior lumbar elements in normal subjects. *Spine* 4(5):441–446, 1979.
11. Verbiest H: Fallacies of the present definition, nomenclature, and classification of stenosis of the lumbar vertebral canal. *Spine* 1(4):219, 1976.
12. Buehler M: Spinal stenosis. *Chiropractic Econ* 22:32, 1979.
13. Cyriax J: Dural pain. *Lancet* 1:920, 1978.
14. Gainer J, et al: The herniated lumbar disc. *Am Fam Pract* 127–131, September 1974.
15. Semmes E: *Ruptures of the Lumbar Intervertebral Disc.* Springfield, IL, Charles C Thomas, 1964, p 17.
16. Herlin L: *Sciatic and Pelvic Pain due to Lumbo-Sacral Nerve Root Compression.* Springfield, IL, Charles C Thomas, 1966, p 19.
17. Barbour JR: Sciatica and such conditions of the back as accompany it. *Med J Aust* 1:285–291, 1952.
18. Boult GF, Kiernam MK, Childe AE: The importance of minor myelographic deformities in the diagnosis of posterior protrusion of the lumbar intervertebral disc. *AJR* 66:752–763, 1951.
19. Leader SA, Russel MJ: The value of Pantopaque myelography in the diagnosis of herniation of the nucleus pulposus in the lumbar sacral spine. A report of 500 cases. *AJR* 69:231–241, 1953.
20. MacCarthy WC Jr, Lane FW Jr: Pitfalls of myelography. *Radiology* 65:663–670, 1955.
21. Norlen G: Ischias und Discushernie. Klinische und Chirurgishe Geischlspunlcte. *Ergeb Inn Med Kinderheilkd* 2:264–280, 1950.
22. O'Connell JCA: Sciatica and the mechanism of the protrusion of the clinical syndrome in protrusions of the lumbar intervertebral discs. *Br J Surg* 30:315–327, 1943.
23. Semmes RB: Ruptured lumbar intervertebral discs, their recognition and surgical relief. *Clin Neurosurg* 8:78–92, 1962.
24. Helfet AJ, Gruebel-Lee DM: *Disorders of the Lumbar Spine.* Philadelphia, JB Lippincott, 1978, p 116.
25. MacGibbon B, Farfan H: A radiologic survey of various configurations of the lumbar spine. *Spine* 4(3):258–266, 1979.

*People can be divided into 3 groups: (1) those who make things happen, (2) those who watch things happen, and (3) those who wonder what happened. The work of the world does not wait to be done by perfect people.*

*—Anonymous*

# Scoliosis

REUBEN F. STEVENS, D.C.

## HISTORICAL NOTES ON SCOLIOSIS

The word scoliosis is from the Greek and credit for its first usage is given to Galen (131–201 A.D.). He was the great anatomist of his time, writing nine books on anatomy (*encheirsis*). While his writings have provided many excellent descriptions, his work was faulty and inaccurate, as it was based largely on the dissection of apes and swines (1). It is possible, as some suggest, that he gained his knowledge and use of terms from the writings of Hippocrates (460–370 B.C.) who preceded him.

Early attempts at correction of the abnormal curves of the spine centered around exercises, crude traction devices and, occasionally, braces made by blacksmiths who normally made armor.

When, in 1895, Wilhelm Konrad Roentgen discovered roentgen rays, new light and understanding was shed on the problem of the curved spine. His early films, which may be seen at the museum at Munich, possess amazing clarity, especially of the full spine.

By the turn of the century, surgical fusion of the spine was used by Hibbs as a treatment for tuberculosis of the spine. It was natural that this technic be extended to the treatment of scoliosis and in 1914 he performed the first fusion for scoliosis. Others also adopted this technic, which was in vogue until about 1940, when its use began to wane due to many failures.

The progress in treatment of scoliosis seemed to be at a standstill until 1946 when Blount and Schmidt devised a traction brace with lateral pressure pads. This became known as the Milwaukee brace. This brace, used as a nonsurgical procedure or as a presurgical procedure with the additional Harrington rod instrumentation, has been a significant step forward in the management of advanced scoliosis.

During the period following the discovery of x-rays, the chiropractic profession, paralleling that of medicine, attempted to understand and mitigate the scoliotic spine. Much of this work by early investigators has been well studied and reported by Barge, who discusses the contribution of such men as Hugh B. Logan, Willard Carver, Clarence Gonstead, William Coggins, and Otto Reinert (2). In addition, Barge has added his own flavor and understanding to what he terms the "disc block" subluxation and its relationship to the development of scoliosis.

Today, with the emphasis on research at the college level, the chiropractic profession has the opportunity to collect and evaluate the effectiveness of the various technics employed in the management of ths complex condition.

## ETIOLOGY AND ANATOMICAL CLASSIFICATION

Spinal curves fall into two broad classifications: those associated with specific diseases (a partial list is given in Table 10.1) and those that occur independent of disease processes (outlined in Table 10.2).

Today, there is a worldwide ongoing search for the cause of scoliosis, especially those scolioses classified as idiopathic.

**Table 10.1.**
**Scoliosis Associated with Disease Processes**

| Age | Name of Disease | Type of Scoliosis and Location | Important Features |
|---|---|---|---|
| Any—rare since vaccine | Polio | Asymmetrical paralysis and secondary curve or symmetrical with collapsing spine | Results in severe curves up to 200°, often with cor pulmonale |
| Birth | Cerebral palsy | Usually structural, some postural | Incidence reported to be from 15% to 25%; thoracolumbar and lumbar predominant; medical treatment consists of bracing and, later, fusion |
| Any—most frequent in the 20–40 age group | Syringomyelia | Resembles idiopathic | Early neurological changes are subtle and must be looked for: impairment or loss of pain and temperature sensitivity, preservation of sensation of touch, muscular weakness |
| Childhood to puberty | Muscular dystrophy (Duchenne) | Lordosis while ambulatory | Type of muscular weakness and development of waddling gait lead to diagnosis; nonoperative treatment is preferred |
| Hereditary, symptoms at any age | Neurofibromatosis | Kyphoscoliosis or resembling idiopathic type | Skin manifestations: café au lait spots, which are tan, macular, and melanotic, are found on 90% of patients and are considered diagnostic if only six or more are found |
| Hereditary, symptoms early | Marfan's syndrome | Similar to idiopathic type | Curves often occur early; lens dislocation makes early wearing of glasses necessary; long slender fingers (arachnodactyly) pectus carinatum, and pes planus; pain in curve is common |

These account for about 70% of the cases that will be seen by the average physician. In patients with this condition, researchers have found elevated levels of copper in hair samples (3), abnormal distribution patterns of glycosaminoglycans in the intervertebral disc (4), abnormalities of the deltoid muscles on the concave side of the curves (5), and different rates of maturity in girls with idiopathic scoliosis than in a control group. Increasing evidence points toward a genetic cause which is presently the most widely accepted theory (6).

Whatever may be the factor which initiates the abnormal curving of the spine, once it is out of balance, certain physical forces and laws come into play. They perpetuate and aggrevate the problem or, in some instances, in the hands of a skilled practitioner, can be used to mitigate the consequences. Gravity has its way with all of us but especially with someone with a scoliotic spine.

Cailliet (7) explains the reaction to gravity by Wolff's principle: "The form of a bone being given, the bone elements place or displace themselves in the direction of functional forces and increase or decrease their masses to reflect the amount of the functional forces."

Barge (2) frequently speaks of the Heuter-Volkman rule which states that pres-

**Table 10.2.**
**Scoliosis Not Associated with Specific Diseases**

| Age of Onset | Type of Scoliosis | Main Features | Important Consideration |
|---|---|---|---|
| Birth | Vertebral open | With neurological defect (myelomeningocele) | Treatment—surgery |
| Birth | Vertebral closed | With neurological defect (diastematomyelia) | Present in approximately 5% of cases of congenital scoliosis |
| Birth | Vertebral | No neurological defect (hemivertebra, unilateral unsegmented bar) | Does not respond to any kind of bracing; in unsegmented bar may result in severe curves; surgical correction is the only treatment |
| Birth | Extravertebral | Congenital rib fusions | Surgical correction |
| 5–10 years and later | Postural | Nonstructural, usually slight | Usually nonprogressive or slightly progressive |
| 5 years to maximum growth | Compensatory | Nonstructural, leg length unequal | Usually nonprogressive or slightly progressive |
| Young adult to adult | Sciatic or discogenic | Transient structural signs of nerve root irritation | Disappears on correction of sciatic or disc problem |
| Young adult to adult | Inflammatory | Secondary to infection, perinephric abscess | Abnormal laboratory findings, temperature, etc. |
| 1–3 years | Infantile idiopathic[a] | Structural, secondary curves nonstructural | (1) conservative treatment with curves to 25° (2) Milwaukee brace with curves to 25°–45° |
| 3–10 years | Juvenile idiopathic[a] | Structural, secondary curves nonstructural | Treatment is same as infantile; if curve reaches 60°, use surgery |
| 10 years to maturity | Adolescent idiopathic[a] | Structural, secondary curves nonstructural | (1) conservative treatment with curves to 20° (2) conservative treatment and brace with curves to 45° (3) recommend surgery with curves of 45° to 50° or more |

[a] These three groups account for 70% of curvatures seen in the general population.

sure increase on a growth plate will retard its growth rate, while a pressure decrease will either increase its growth rate or allow for normal growth to take place. He also stresses the migration of the nucleus of the disc from its central position to a lateral position, forming what he describes as a "disc block subluxation."

Depending upon the duration of the curve, its structural nature, and the age of the patient, certain other anatomical changes take place. All soft tissues on the concave side of the curve are shortened and thickened, especially in the thoracic region if the costovertebral ligaments are involved. The muscles are shortened, with the exception of the multifidus which has been found to be shorter on the convex side of the curve due to spinous and transverse process rotation. The bony changes consist of shortening and thickening of the lamina and pedicles on the concave side and some consequent narrowing of the vertebral canal on the convex side. Direct cord pressure is, however, very rare. From the above it can be inferred that in the adult with scoliosis, certain irreversible changes have taken place and correction is rendered more difficult or impossible. Therefore, in order to be most effective, the management of scoliosis consists of early recognition, early definition, and early treatment.

A word should be said about the terminology used to describe spinal curves. The terminology committee of the Scoliosis Research Society has defined a glossary of terms which give uniformity in communication between physicians. This glossary may be seen in its complete form by referring to any one of the reference texts on scoliosis. Sufficient for our discussion is the distinction between non-structural and structural curves.

A nonstructural curve is a curve that has no structural component and that corrects or overcorrects on recumbent side-bending roentgenograms. A nonstructural curve has normal flexibility. A good example of a nonstructural curve is one seen in the lumbar spine of a patient with inequality of leg length. When the leg length is corrected by a lift, the curve disappears (Figs. 10.1 and 10.2).

A structural curve is a lateral curve of that segment of the spine lacking normal

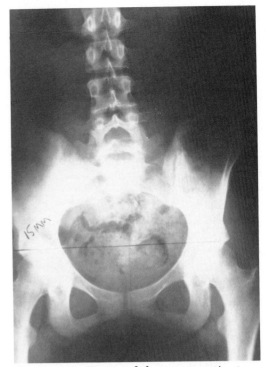

**Figure 10.2.** X-ray of the same patient as in Figure 10.1. The patient has been fitted with a 15-mm lift which has leveled the pelvis and provided relief of scoliosis.

flexibility. This is identified on x-rays by a failure to correct on lateral bending.

A major curve is always the largest curve and is usually a structural curve. A compensatory curve is the curve above or below a major curve and is usually non-structural, but it may become structural as time passes. It usually aids in the maintenance of body balance.

Lastly, curves are classified according to the position of the spine involved. Some patterns seem to occur more frequently than others. The reader is encouraged to consult a textbook on scoliosis for a complete review of the types and their frequency.

## EVALUATION OF PATIENT

### History

Recognition of scoliosis may come from the examination by the primary care physician during the routine work-up for some other presenting complaint. Sometimes patients are referred by the school

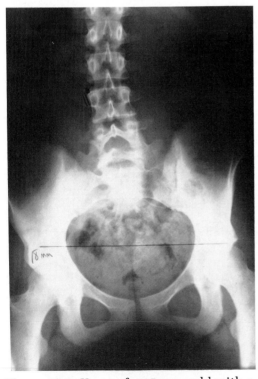

**Figure 10.1.** X-ray of a 15-year-old with a left 18-mm short leg and a levoscoliosis.

nurse, with a presumptive finding detected during a school scoliosis examination program. In either case, some basic information is needed.

The age and sex of the patient need to be recorded. The age gives a clue to a broad grouping of types of curves and possible sequences. The chronological age will be compared with the bone age and the skeletal maturity information obtained from later x-rays. It is important to note when the curve was first recognized if it differs from the presenting date. Sometimes school health records or gym class records of height are helpful in this matter. From this information, an idea regarding rate of progress may be assumed. This author found a girl with a double curve, 30° right thoracic and 30° left lumbar, who measured 63 inches tall on first examination with a previous undetected scoliosis. School height records stated the girl measured 64 inches 1 year earlier, at age 12. It could be assumed from this assessment that there had, indeed, been a very rapidly progressive curve development if, during her growth spurt, the child had lost 1 inch in height (8)! At times, however, a determination of the progressiveness of curve must await subsequent x-rays.

Developmental factors, such an approximate date of the appearance of pubic hair and voice change in boys and the appearance of pubic hair, breast enlargement, and menarche onset, if present, in girls, should be recorded. In girls, the adolescent growth spurt begins slightly before the appearance of secondary sexual characteristics at age 10 or 11 and menarche at about age 13 or 14, which corresponds to approximately two thirds of the way through the growth spurt. In boys, the adolescent spurt occurs slightly after the appearance of secondary sexual characteristics. The spurt ends at about age 14 or 15 in girls and at about age 16 or 17 in boys.

The "spurt" is just that and growth can be very rapid compared with the linear growth which preceded it. Also, usually the growth spurt involves mainly the trunk of the body; the legs continue to grow in a linear fashion. Lastly, if by chance the patient's height is known at age 2, multiplication of this figure by 2 will give you a close approximation of the expected adult height. Genetic factors should be recorded, such as the height of the father and mother and sisters and brothers. These data help give some idea of expected growth and maximum height. Inquire as to the presence of scoliosis in other family members, as the incidence is so high that the Scoliosis Research Society has considered including the term familial instead of idiopathic in the description of scoliosis.

## Physical Examination

The examination should be conducted with boys in underpants and girls in underpants and gowned. With all patients, insist that one or both parents or a responsible adult family member be present, as this enables the examiner to point out obvious findings as the examination proceeds and eliminates unnecessary duplication of reporting.

One may begin from the head down or from the feet up, but the entire body must be examined. With the feet-up approach, one would look for such things as unilateral or bilateral pes planus. The turning of one foot in or out might suggest hip joint pathology. The knees should be examined for genu valgum or genu varum; the height of the ilium, for pelvic unleveling; the scapulae, for levelness or winging; and the shoulder, for evenness and occipital leveling.

There are many grids available which make these observations easy. Also, plumb line analysis is a simple but effective way to measure and demonstrate spinal imbalance.

Next, the rotational abnormalities should be investigated by having the patient flex forward to 90°, with the arms hanging down and with the knees fully extended. The eye of the examiner may quickly detect a rib hump or lumbar rotation.

Recording these findings as exactly as possible is important, as they will form a reference point for future comparison. One device, the Scoliometer, which was developed by Dr. Sabia, is helpful. Rotation in the thoracic and lumbar spine can be measured in millimeters or centimeters, and shoulder unevenness, in degrees of deviation. This is far superior to such generalized statements as "moderate thoracic rotation," etc.

Leg length should be measured by tape measure. The landmarks used are the anterior superior iliac spine to the medial malleolus for actual leg length and the umbilicus to medial malleolus for apparent leg length. (Apparent leg length deficiency may exist due to pelvic obliquity when actual leg lengths are equal.) The figures obtained should be later confirmed by x-ray.

One should also observe the skin for café au lait spots which are tan, macular, and melanotic and are found on 90% of patients with scoliosis due to neurofibromatosis (these spots are considered diagnostic of neurofibromatosis only if six or more are present). One should also look for hairy patches in the lumbar region, which may suggest congenital malformations. Table 10.2 contains many of the more frequently observed findings. In addition to observed findings, the skin should be examined for sensitivity to heat and cold, and routine reflexes should be elicited.

If a curve exists, some idea of the flexibility can be obtained by observation of the patient in standing, sitting, and prone postures. Lateral bending and manual traction tests also help.

## Roentgenographic Examination

Mindful of the importance of limiting the exposure of these often young patients to radiation, one must proceed to the x-ray examination if physical findings indicate that a curvature exists. Studies have shown that a single anteroposterior spine exposure can result in a skin-absorbed dose of 174 mrem (9). It has been suggested that the dose to the mammary glands in females can be reduced by a factor of 5 if posteroanterior, instead of anteroposterior, projections are used (10). Genetic screening should be observed to the greatest degree possible without sacrificing important information from the examination.

The views to be used must be determined on an individual basis. If only a scoliosis screening is being done, a single standing anteroposterior view taken on a 14- x 36-inch film at 72 inches would be sufficient. If significant scoliosis has been established by the previous examination, however, a more complete study is advisable. This would include a recumbent anteroposterior view taken at 40 inches, upright anteroposterior and lateral views, and right and left lateral bending views (Figs. 10.3 through 10.6). All upright views are taken at 72 inches. If spondylolisthesis is suspected (see Figures 10.7 to 10.9), oblique lumbar views are ordered (not shown in figures). An additional weight-bearing view with the tube level with the femoral heads may be used to check leg length measurements. A sacral base projection, as recommended by Barge (2), is an excellent way to check for anomalous development or unleveling of the sacrum. This projection is taken with the patient in the weight-bearing posture and with the tube tilted to correspond to the sacral base angle determined from the previous lateral lumbar film. A single film of the left wrist and hand is made for comparison with the Greulich and Pyle atlas to determine the bone age of the patient (6, 13).

All radiographs should be marked with the patients name, the doctor or clinic name, the date taken, and the patient's age in years and months, (e.g., 13 + 4), and the position taken. Target film distance should also be included so others may reproduce the technic on reexamination.

Today, there is only one accepted way in which to measure and report the findings. This is known as the Cobb method (6, 13). A horizontal line is drawn at the superior border of the superior end vertebrae. Another line is drawn at the inferior border of the body of the inferior end vertebrae. The "end vertebrae" are those with the greatest inclinations toward the convexity of the curves. Perpendicular lines are drawn from these horizontal lines, and the angle formed by their intersection is measured. This angle is considered the curve angle.

The degree of vertebral rotation needs to be measured (6, 13). The generally ac-

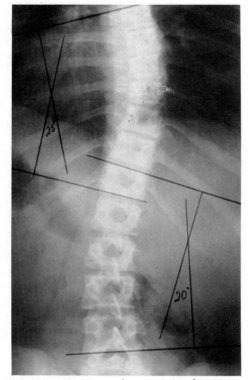

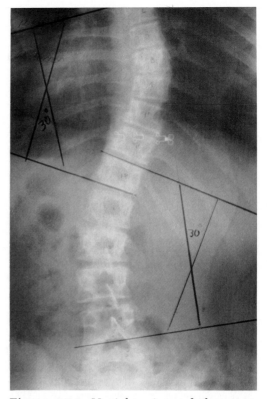

**Figure 10.3.** Recumbent view showing a 20° left lumbar and a 25° right thoracic curve.

**Figure 10.4.** Upright view of the same patient as in Figure 10.3.

cepted way is to observe, from the convex side of the curve, the migration of the pedicle toward the midline. When there is no rotation, the pedicles are evenly spaced. In a 1+ rotation the pedicles are moved slightly toward the midline, in a 2+ rotation the pedicle is moved two thirds of the way toward the midline, in a 3+ rotation the pedicle is in the midline, and in a 4+ rotation the pedicle is moved past the midline.

Some idea of the degree of skeletal maturity may be obtained by examining the degree of excursion of the iliac apophyses, as described by Risser (6, 13). Generally, this is reported as Risser 1 through 4, with the iliac crests being divided into fourths from lateral to medial. A Risser 5 is complete fusion of the iliac crest. Sometimes the epiphyses of the thoracic and lumbar vertebrae can be observed on good films. If the vertebral ephiphyses are mottled in appearance, the patient has not yet completed growth. All of the above may be

observed by the individual practitioner. Few will have a Gruelich and Pyle atlas. It is, therefore, good practice to send all films for review to a consulting roentgenologist.

## Correlative Report

Now one has obtained sufficient information to form an opinion as to the nature of the problem. From this can come a realistic prognosis and a determination of the best form of treatment.

Certain features help to distinguish and classify the scoliosis. Questions that must be answered are, What is the age of the patient? Does the curve appear to be congenital or acquired and, if acquired, at what age? Does the patient have any other disease process which would explain the presence or development of scoliosis? If not, can the scoliosis be typed as idiopathic? Are the curves structural or nonstructural or are both present in the same

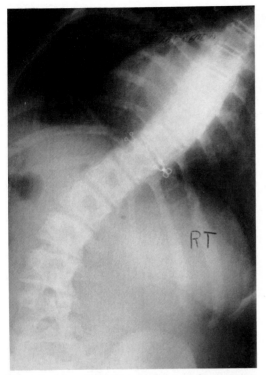

**Figure 10.5.** Upright right bending view of the same patient as in Figure 10.3.

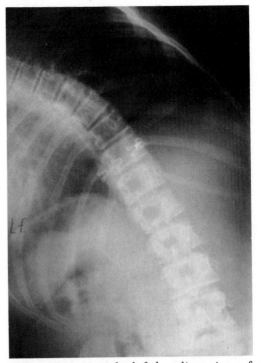

**Figure 10.6.** Upright left bending view of the same patient as in Figure 10.3.

patient? Is the curve progressive? The later question may have to await a second follow-up examination performed usually 3 or 4 months after the first examination.

## TREATMENT PROCEDURES

Today, in the best centers, a team approach is recommended for the treatment of scoliosis. If the primary care practitioner feels comfortable with his knowledge and understanding of the problem, he should begin treatment of the type indicated. There are both medical and chiropractic orthopedists who have taken a special interest and training in scoliosis management who may be consulted. Most large cities have at least one hospital with a scoliosis clinic. There are orthotic consultants skilled in the fitting of braces and other appliances. Psychological counseling is available. For the more complex and/or progressive spinal curves, an interdisciplinary approach seems the most advisable.

From the chiropractic point of view, the manipulative procedure would be the first step in the treatment of scoliosis. Distraction involving spinal traction, derotation, and lateral bending has been used, especially in Europe, as a presurgical procedure to give a greater degree of flexibility to structural curves, thus allowing a more complete surgical correction. At some centers, a postsurgical cast is used to help maintain the correction obtained by surgery.

Manipulation of the spine using the Chiro-Manis instrument and technic allows the practitioner a means with which to apply these same forces, namely, elongation, derotation, and lateral flexion, as a kinetic treatment mode rather than as a static casting technic. This is demonstrated in Figure 10.10, A to C.

The adjustive counter pressure hand is placed at the upper limit of the scoliotic curve and slowly worked downward, distracting each disc space gently, to patient tolerance, and putting the facets through their normal ranges of motion. Occasionally only one ankle cuff is used (opposite

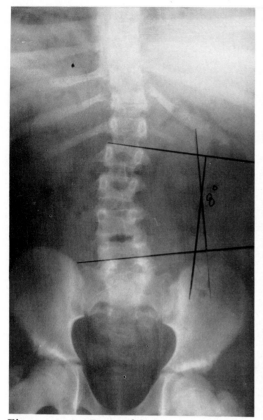

**Figure 10.7.** Recumbent view showing olisthetic scoliosis with spondylolisthesis.

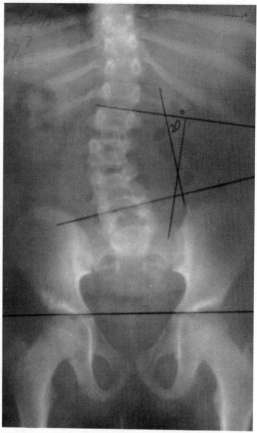

**Figure 10.8.** Upright view of the same patient as in Figure 10.7.

to the side of lateral bending) which augments the spinal straightening effect. The therapy is applied only as much as patient tolerance allows, with care taken not to overcome tissue integrity by vigorous manipulation.

The technic so described would be a low-velocity technic in contrast to the high-velocity technic of spinal articular adjusting. Both have a place in the hands of those who are skilled in their use. It should be noted, however, that in applying elongation, derotation, and lateral flexion a number of the mechanical components of the problem are addressed simultaneously (Fig. 10, A to C). Shortened muscles and ligaments are being stretched, disc compression forces are being reversed, and facet range of motion is being normalized.

Adjunctive to the manipulative technic

is the treatment of the pelvic unleveling due to a short leg or other causes. The procedure is described in Chapter 4.

The addition of other procedures used in the office depends on the practitioner's skills and experience as well as on the availability of equipment. A good procedure preparatory to manipulation is the application of moist heat and massage to the muscles of the back. Postmanipulatively, the application of electrical stimulation of the muscles on the convex side of the curve may be used. This may be done with the patient in the supine or the prone posture but not in the sitting or the standing posture. In the vertical postures, the righting reflexes offset the benefits of the stimulation. Proper application is demonstrated in Figure 10.11. The retaining of the patient for the time needed for

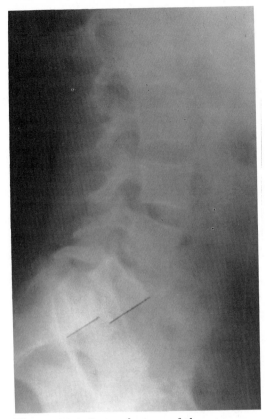

**Figure 10.9.** Lateral view of the same patient as in Figure 10.7.

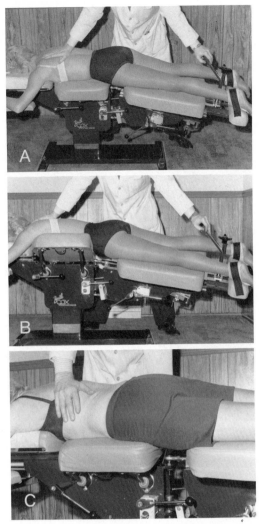

**Figure 10.10.** *A.* A patient receiving manipulation in left derotation and left lateral bending with distraction applied to a left thoracolumbar scoliosis. *B.* A patient receiving manipulation for derotation of a right thoracic curve and left lumbar curve with distraction and range of motion manipulation applied simultaneously. *C.* A patient receiving derotation applied to the articulations of a levoscoliosis of the thoracolumbar spine.

the application of the procedure enhances the effectiveness of the preceding manipulation.

Recently published reports indicate that the lateral electrical surface stimulation technic as used by Axelgaard and Brown (11) of Rancho Los Amigos Hospital is effective in arresting the progression of a large number of cases of progressive idiopathic adolescent scoliosis. The technic makes use of an electrical muscle stimulator (ScoliTron by Neuromedics, Inc.) which is used by the patient at night. Surface electrodes are placed on the posterior or midaxillary line above and below the curve apex. Correct electrode placement is crucial for successful treatment, and the placement which gives the longest mechanical lever arm and provides the greatest corrective movement is chosen.

The reported arrest of progression in 95% of the patients treated by this method who complied with all treatment protocols is exciting. Recently, the ScoliTron has received Food and Drug Administration approval, and one would assume that

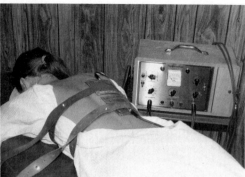

**Figure 10.11.** Sinusoidal current stimulation to the right of a scoliosis.

in some cases, its use will become a viable alternative to bracing.

Exercises have been given a bad reputation in the management of scoliosis. When used as part of a comprehensive program, however, they have their place. Obviously, muscle imbalance exists in patients with scoliosis and to argue whether it is primary or secondary is not the point of this discussion.

Generally, the exercises prescribed should affect the muscles that involve motions which would aid in straightening the curved spine. Look at the lateral flexion x-rays and observe which movements seem to straighten the curve. Then correlate these with the corresponding muscle action which produced them. This is a far better way to arrive at proper exercise prescription than trying to memorize or list specific exercises for each and every type curve that may be encountered.

Some exercises, however, are of a general nature and are used to overcome the effects of gravity and to promote flexibility. These are illustrated in Figures 10.12 through 10.17.

Not shown is the traction exercise which is accomplished by hanging from a parallel bar by the hands for 100 seconds each morning and evening. This may be accomplished by doing 10 repetitions of 10 seconds each or any combination equal to 100. Obviously, this would have its greatest effect on the thoracic spine. For the lumbar spine, use of one of the popular inversion gravity units will have an effect similar to that on the thoracic spine. A unilateral traction exercise which can be performed with the aid of an assistant is demonstrated in Figure 10.18.

Many other exercises using the inversion traction device may be prescribed for the patient with spinal curvature; they should, however, be specific to the individual problem. Young people seem to like to do exercises when a special apparatus is involved. This helps motivate compliance with an otherwise dull routine.

## Braces in the Treatment of Scoliosis

No discussion of scoliosis management is complete without including bracing. It is difficult for parents to decide whether their son or daughter should wear a brace. If the other conservative measures have not brought about arrest of curve progression, however, such action may be necessary and should be advised.

There is a general consensus that curves which have reached 20° or more and are progressing at a rate of at least 1° or more per month should have a trial in a proper brace. The main purpose of the brace is to stop progression. Sometimes a decrease in the curve angle is seen during the use of the brace. Active exercises are possible and recommended while a brace is being worn, and thus both active and passive effects are achieved. Some studies have indicated, however, that much of what is gained is found to have been lost at 5-year follow-up studies.

Moe et al. (12) suggest that curves which measure 40° or less at spinal maturation show little progression later. In general, short curves progress less than curves of greater length. Curves of more than 50° should not be treated with a Milwaukee brace, nor should curves be treated in those who have reached skeletal maturity.

Curves of 20° or less may receive other conservative measures and be watched for evidence of progression. Significant changes which would favor the recommendation of bracing would be (a) an increase in the degree of curve, (b) progression of a curve by 1° or more per month, and (c) a decrease in curve flexibility. Contraindications to bracing would be (a) the develoment of an abnormally flat thoracic spine, seen on the lateral view (these may be made worse by the brace), and (b) approaching bone maturity.

The Milwaukee brace was developed by Blount and Schmidt in 1945. In the correction and stabilization of scoliosis, it works by exerting both active and passive forces on the curve. The passive forces are supplied by the properly fitted brace, whereas the active forces are supplied by exercises performed while in the brace. (See Figures 10.19 through 10.22 of a patient in a Milwaukee brace.) Depending on certain factors, the brace is worn 22 hours a day until bone maturity is reached.

A frequently used brace for lumbar and very low thoracolumbar curves is the TLSO (thoracolumbosacral orthosis). The greater the flexibility of the curve, the more effective the brace. (See Figures 10.23 and 10.24.) This type of support is usually made of polypropylene with Velcro-fastened straps. It is lightweight, can be worn under ordinary clothing and, with proper wardrobe selection, is hardly noticed.

In summary, one would seldom use a brace for curves of less than 20°. Evidence of progression beyond this point, the type of curve, and its location are all considerations. The patient's age and bone maturity are vital, as bracing is of no value after bone maturity has been reached. Patients with curves of 50° or more are candidates for surgical repair, not for bracing.

One of the major causes of the failure with bracing, as well as with exercise and other conservative management procedures, is noncompliance on the part of the patient. It requires both physician and parents to constantly motivate the child and reinforce the reasons that it must be done. The treating physician must develop a good supportive role with the young patient and use not only his scientific knowledge but also his leadership abilities. Truly, the treatment of these problems is an art as well as a science.

Lastly, Turek (13) warns of an acute and often fatal syndrome of persistent vomiting which can occur in a patient wearing a brace which may press the superior mesenteric artery against the duodenum. If a patient wearing such a device develops the syndrome, prompt removal of the apparatus is mandatory before electrolyte imbalances develop. This syndrome may rapidly progress to a full-fledged abdominal obstruction and to death.

## Surgical Correction

The three most commonly mentioned reasons for surgical intervention are (a) cosmetic appearance, (b) prevention of the development of arthrosis and pain later in life, and (c) prevention of the development of cor pulmonale.

With the improvement in surgical technics, it does not seem proper to allow a curve to progress beyond 50°, especially in the thoracic spine. There seems to be some difference of opinion, however, as to whether adults with scoliosis have any greater incidence of back pain than those without scoliosis.

Cor pulmonale becomes a problem when there is sufficient distortion of the rib cage and subsequent lung fields to produce a pulmonary hypertension and right-side heart enlargement. In general, this is more apt to occur in curves of more than 100°. In the past, these were more frequently encountered in postpoliomyelitis and in some idiopathic infantile and neuromuscular conditions. Various respiratory tests, as well as means of evaluating cardiac dysfunction, are available. These tests are generally involved in presurgical evaluation and are of little consequence to the general practitioner, however.

Surgical fusion may be accomplished with or without the aid of additional instrumentation. Harrington rod technics have gained a solid place in the treatment of scoliosis. Dwyer instrumentation has been found to be most useful in thoracolumbar and lumbar curves. The actual technic and procedure involved in their use is well illustrated in the book, *Scoliosis and Other Spinal Deformities*, by Moe et al. (12).

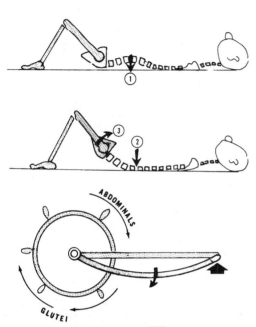

**Figure 10.12.** "Pelvic tilting" exercise. Exercises to decrease the lumbar lordosis are done in sequence. With hips and knees flexed, the low back (1) is pressed against the floor and held there (2). The pelvis (3) is then slowly raised. This action, which is performed by the abdominal, hamstring, and gluteal muscles, decreases the lordosis and gives the patient the "feeling" of pelvis motion. (Reproduced with permission from R. Cailliet: Exercises for Scoliosis. In J. V. Basmajian (editor): *Therapeutic Exercise*, edition 3. Baltimore, Williams & Wilkins, 1978, chap. 20.)

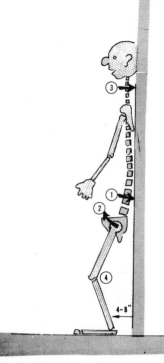

**Figure 10.13.** Erect position for pelvic tilting. With the patient leaning against a wall, the low back (1) is pressed to the wall. The pelvis is "tilted" anteriorly (2) decreasing the lumbar lordosis. The neck is also pressed to the wall (3), decreasing the cervical lordosis and elongating the spine. The knees are flexed and the feet placed 4 to 8 inches from the wall. As this exercise becomes easier, the feet are placed closer to the wall and the knees are extended. (Reproduced with permission from R. Cailliet: Exercises for Scoliosis. In J. V. Basmajian (editor): *Therapeutic Exercise*, edition 3. Baltimore, Williams & Wilkins, 1978, chap. 20.)

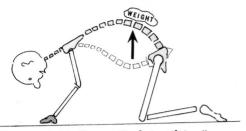

**Figure 10.14.** Prone "pelvic tilting" exercise. In patients who experience difficulty in "tilting their pelvis," the quadriped position is assumed. The low back is arched and lowered, with or without a superimposed weight. Thus, pelvic tilting is accomplished, as is greater flexibility of the lumbar spine. (Reproduced with permission from R. Cailliet: Exercises for Scoliosis. In J. V. Basmajian (editor): *Therapeutic Exercise*, edition 3. Baltimore, Williams & Wilkins, 1978, chap. 20.)

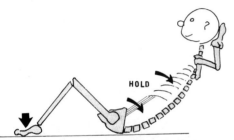

**Figure 10.15.** Isometric abdominal exercise to develop endurance and the "feeling" of abdominal contraction. The patient, who is in a full sit-up position, leans back, then sustains that position. Gradually, the reclining degree is increased, as is the duration of the sustained position. (Reproduced with permission from R. Cailliet: Exercises for Scoliosis. In J. V. Basmajian (editor): *Therapeutic Exercise*, edition 3. Baltimore, Williams & Wilkins, 1978, chap. 20.)

**Figure 10.17.** Elongation, derotation, and lateral flexion exercises. In the *above position* with the patient sitting on his feet, the lumbar region of the spine is immobilized. The overhead extended arms permit the fingers to "walk" to the left (or to the right). This exercise lateral stretches and derotates the thoracic spine. (Reproduced with permission from R. Cailliet: Exercises for Scoliosis. In J. V. Basmajian (editor): *Therapeutic Exercise*, edition 3. Baltimore, Williams & Wilkins, 1978, chap. 20.)

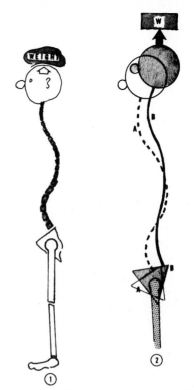

**Figure 10.16.** Distraction exercise for posture. By attempting to elevate a weight placed on the head (1), all the curves of the vertebral column approach the center of gravity; (2) the cervical and lumbar lordosis (A) are decreased (B) as the pelvis "tilts" (A to B). (Reproduced with permission from R. Cailliet: Exercises for Scoliosis. In J. V. Basmajian (editor): *Therapeutic Exercise*, edition 3. Baltimore, Williams & Wilkins, 1978, chap. 20.)

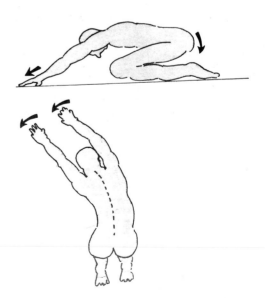

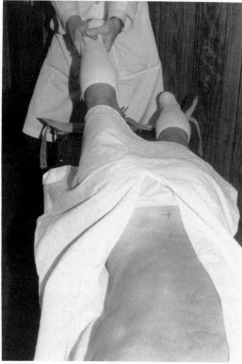

**Figure 10.18.** While traction is applied to the right lower extremity, the patient contracts the right paravertebral muscles and repeats this 15 to 20 times in the morning and the evening. This exercise is used for a lumbar or thoracolumbar curve with convexity to the right.

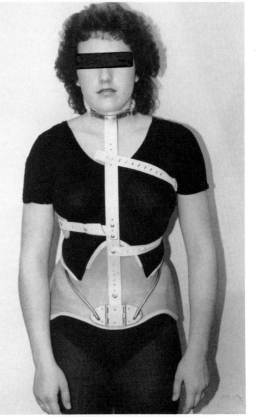

**Figure 10.19.** Milwaukee brace as worn by patient whose x-rays may be seen in Figures 10.3, 10.4, 10.5, and 10.6.

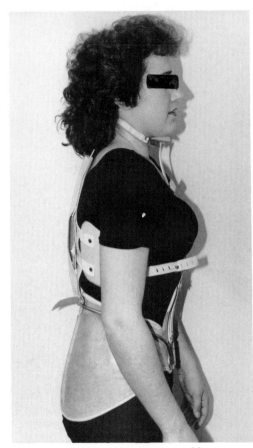

**Figure 10.20.** Lateral view of brace.

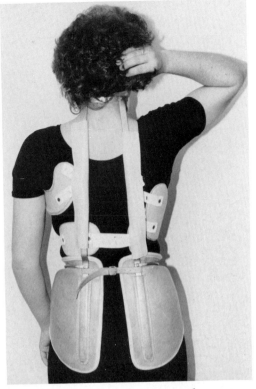

**Figure 10.21.** Note thoracic pad arrangement.

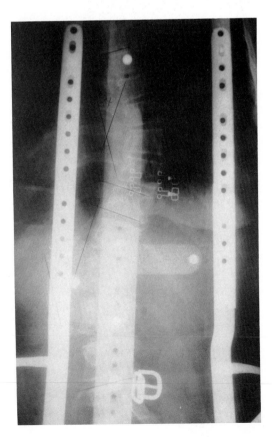

**Figure 10.22.** X-ray of the same patient as in Figure 10.19 while she is wearing the brace.

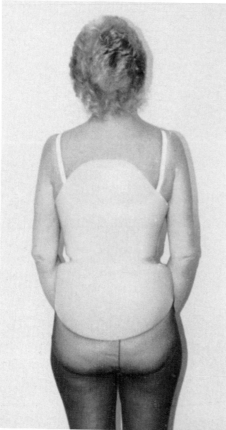

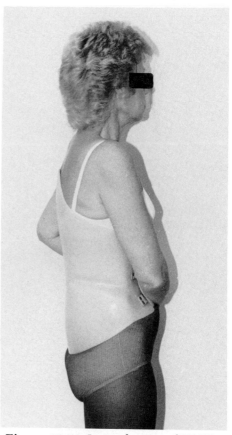

**Figure 10.23.** TLSO worn by model for demonstration.

**Figure 10.24.** Lateral view of TLSO.

## References

1. Garrison FH: *History of Medicine.* Philadelphia, WB Saunders, 1929, reprinted 1966.
2. Barge FA: *Scoliosis.* Davenport, IA, Baldwine Printing, 1982, vol III.
3. Pratt W, Phippen W: Elevated hair copper level in idiopathic scoliosis. *Spine* 5(3):230–233, 1980.
4. Ghosh P, Bushell GR, Taylor TKF, Pearce RH, Grimmer BJ: Distribution of glycosaminoglycans across the normal and the scoliotic disc. *Spine* 5(4):310–317, 1980.
5. Yarom R, Wolf E, Rubin GC: Deltoid pathology in idiopathic scoliosis. *Spine* 7(5):463–470, 1982.
6. Keim HA: Scoliosis, clinical symposia. *Ciba Found Symp* 24(1):4–7, 15–19, 1972.
7. Cailliet R: *Scoliosis: Diagnosis and Management.* Philadelphia, FA Davis, 1975, p 62.
8. Stevens RF: Treatment of adolescent scoliosis, a case study. Presented at the Academy of Chiropractic Orthopedists, Congress VI, Palm Springs, CA, May 6, 1982.
9. Nottage WM, Waugh TR, McMaster WC: Radiation exposure during scoliosis screening radiography. *Spine* 6(5):356–359, 1981.
10. Hellstrom G, Irstram L, Nachemson A: Reduction of radiation dose in radiologic examination of patients with scoliosis. *Spine* 8(1):28–30, 1983.
11. Axelgaard J, Brown JC: Lateral electrical surface stimulation for the treatment of progressive idiopathic scoliosis. *Spine* 8(3):242–260, 1983.
12. Moe JH, Bradford DS, Winter RB, Lonstein JE: *Scoliosis and Other Spinal Deformities.* Philadelphia, WB Saunders, 1978.
13. Turek SL: *Orthopaedics—Principles and Their Applications,* ed 3. Philadelphia, JB Lippincott, 1977, pp 1425–1427.

It is easy to learn something about everything, but difficult to learn everything about
anything.

—*Nathaniel Emmons*

CHAPTER 11

# Tropism

In the literature on the subject of normal facings of the lumbar articular facets,
there is a variance of opinion. Some investigators believe that sagittal facings are
normal, whereas others believe that coronal facings are normal. In our clinical
study (1) of patients with vertebral disc
lesions, we recorded which facet findings
were involved at all lumbar levels. We
believe that this is the first controlled
study documented in the chiropractic
and, perhaps, the medical literature concerning which facet facings are involved
in lumbar disc lesions. It must be stressed
that these findings are based on x-rays of
patients with disc protrusion or prolapse.

Tropism (from the Greek word *trope*, a
turning) refers to an anomaly of articular
formation in which the two articular facings are not the same; i.e., instead of both
being sagittal or both coronal, each side
assumes a different facing, as shown in
Figure 11.1.

From Tables 11.1 and 11.2, it can be
inferred that sagittal facet facings are typical in the upper lumbar spine, whereas
coronal facet findings are typical in the
lower lumbar spine. In 18 of 56 cases of
disc lesion (32%), anomalies of articular
tropism were present. The most difficult
cases to treat were those involving the
sagittal facet facings at the level of discal
protrusion or prolapse, especially when a
medial disc was involved.

The directional plane of articulation of
the facets allows for specific movement.
Sagittal facets flex and extend while coronal facets bend laterally. The combining
of these two directional opposing forces
places excessive stress on the annular fibers of the intervertebral disc (IVD),
which tear in nuclear protrusion. The axis
of rotation of a lumbar vertebral unit is
between the articular facets, with the
body rotating forward of this axis (1a).
Therefore, the altered motoricity of a sagittal and coronal combination creates
stress on both the disc and articular facets
in all motions of the lumbar spine.

Facet tropism, therefore, creates stress
on the lumbar spine during motion. In
this situation, rotation takes on added importance, since it places maximum stress
on the annular fibers which must tear in
order for the nucleus pulposus to protrude, creating the typical disc syndrome
with sciatica.

According to Farfan et al. (2), the IVD is
capable of great compressive loads. They
also believe that Schmorl and Beadle
were inaccurate when they stated that the
compressive load was the mechanical
basis of disc degeneration.

By application of torsional loading to 90
IVD joints (proven normal by discogram)
from 66 necropsy specimens, the amount
of rotation needed to cause failure of the
normal disc was determined to be 22.6°;
in cases of degenerated disc, the angle of
failure was 14.3°. Degenerated discs show
a consistently smaller torsional angle of
failure. Farfan et al. concluded that the
IVD is injured by rotation within a small
normal range of movement and that disc
protrusion is a manifestation of annular
tearing by torsional injury.

According to Cailliet (3), 75% of lumbar
flexion occurs at the lumbosacral articulation. He further states that the shearing
stress of the 5th lumbar vertebra on the
sacrum increases proportionately to the
anterior angulation of the sacrum. We

275

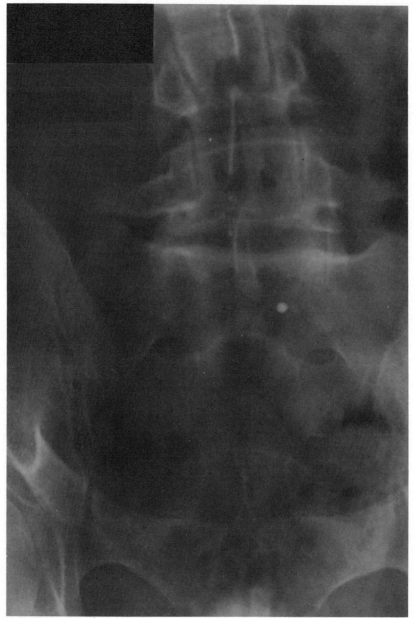

**Figure 11.1.** X-ray study reveals tropism of the articular facets, with the right L5-S1 facet facings being sagittal and the left being coronal. Note that the facet facings at L4-L5 are bilaterally sagittal.

**Table 11.1.**
**Percentage of Facet Facings in 56 Cases of Lumbar Disc Lesion, by Location and Position**

|  | L1-L2 | | L2-L3 | | L3-L4 | | L4-L5 | | L5-S1 | |
|---|---|---|---|---|---|---|---|---|---|---|
|  | Right | Left | Right | Left | Right | Left | Right | Left | Right | Left |
| Sagittal | 74 | 72 | 55 | 64 | 47 | 43 | 29 | 29 | 7 | 5 |
| Coronal | 23 | 26 | 40 | 34 | 41 | 53 | 64 | 65 | 91 | 95 |
| Semisagittal | 3 | 2 | 5 | 2 | 12 | 4 | 7 | 6 | 2 | |

**Table 11.2.**
**Average Percentage of Facet Facings at Each Level in 56 Cases of Lumbar Disc Lesion**

|              | L1-L2 | L2-L3 | L3-L4 | L4-L5 | L5-S1 |
|--------------|-------|-------|-------|-------|-------|
| Sagittal     | 73    | 59.5  | 45    | 29    | 6     |
| Coronal      | 24.5  | 37    | 47    | 64.5  | 93    |
| Semisagittal | 2.5   | 3.5   | 8     | 6.5   | 1     |

have applied these ideas on stress to our knowledge of the facet articular plane and believe that the coronal facet facing at L5-S1 allows greater stability than does the sagittal facet facing at L5-S1.

We believe, therefore, that the following conclusions are justified.

1. Sagittal facet articulation facings are normal for the upper lumbar spine, and coronal facet articulation facings are normal for the lower lumbar spine.

2. Even with the lesser number of sagittal facings in the lower lumbar spine, tropism at the level of disc lesion occurred in 32% of the cases; therefore, there is a prominence of disc lesions in cases of sagittal facings and of tropism.

3. Rotation is the most damaging motion of the low back, resulting in tearing of the lumbar disc annular fibers which allows for nuclear protrusion.

4. Sagittal facets or anomalies of tropism create additional stress on the spine during rotation. Rotation in this situation may be much less than normal before annular disc fibers tear.

5. Patients with anomalous facet facings are at high risk for developing a disc lesion on rotation.

6. In 1 of every 5 patients, there is an asymmetrical orientation of the articular facets of the spine at a single level and abnormal spinal motion; these patients, therefore, are predisposed to develop low back and sciatic pain syndromes (4).

7. In patients with articular tropism, the joints rotate toward the side of the more oblique facet (5). Figures 11.4 and 11.5 reveal how tropism changes the force distribution and applies additional torsion to the disc. Furthermore, tropism may predispose to degenerative arthrosis at these facets.

Finally, articular tropism or asymmetry

of the articular facets can lead to the manifestation of lumbar instability as joint rotation. This rotation occurs toward the side of the more oblique facet and can place additional stress on the annulus fibrosus of the intervertebral disc and capsular ligaments of the apophyseal joints.

Because the posterior elements maintain stability of the spine, they play an important role in the triple joint complex of the facets and disc. Tropism occurs most commonly in the two lowest lumbar levels (6–9). Keep in mind that these are synovial joints and shearing forces place compression on facet surfaces. This compression is greater in less obliquely facing facets. Less oblique facets have greater interfacet forces, predisposing them to degenerative forces.

Arthrosis of the facets is rare in patients under 30 and is found progressively more frequently and is more severe as these patients age (10). Also, intervertebral arthritis is more common at L3-L4 and L4-L5 than at L5-S1 where the facets are less obliquely faced. Badgley (6) reports that arthritis of the facets is more common in cases of tropism and lesions of articular capsules, granular ossification, calcification, and adhesions of the meningeal covering of the nerve root adjacent to it.

The normal plane of articulation of the lower lumbar facets (Fig. 11.2) is 45° to the body sagittal or coronal planes (11). The inferior facets are convex, whereas the superior facets are concave.

Figure 11.3 shows the normal 45° angle of inclination (5). Figure 11.4 shows that the vector forces are equally balanced on the two facets in the case of a symmetrically oriented articular facet, whereas Figure 11.5 shows that the forces shift to the side of the more obliquely faced facet in the case of tropism. It is on the side of the more obliquely faced facet that the posterolateral annular fibers tear.

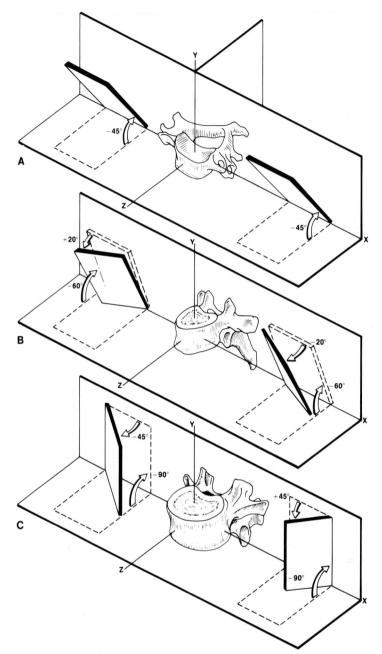

**Figure 11.2.** Orientation of the facet joints. A graphical representation of the facet joint inclinations in various regions of the spine is obtained by rotating two cards lying in the horizontal plane through two consecutive angles, i.e., x-axis rotation followed by y-axis rotation. Typical values for the two angles for the three regions of the spine follow. A. Cervical spine: −45° followed by 0°. B. Thoracic spine: −60° followed by +20° for right facet rotation, or −20° for left facet rotation. C. Lumbar spine: −90° and −45° for right facet rotation or +45° for the left facet rotation. (These are only rough estimates.) There are variations within the regions of the spine and between different individuals. (Reproduced with permission from A. A. White and M. M. Panjabi: *Clinical Biomechanics of the Spine.* Philadelphia, J. B. Lippincott, 1978, p. 22.)

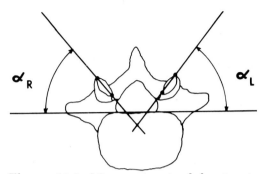

**Figure 11.3.** Measurement of facet orientation. (Reproduced with permission from B. M. Cyron and W. C. Hutton: Articular Tropism. *Spine* 5(2):170, 1980.)

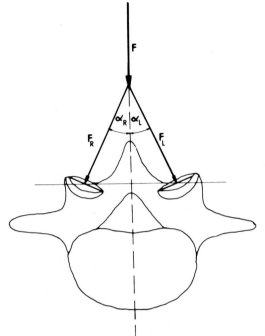

**Figure 11.4.** Forces (*F*) acting on symmetrically oriented superior articular facets. (Reproduced with permission from B. M. Cyron and W. C. Hutton: Articular Tropism. *Spine* 5(2):170, 1980.)

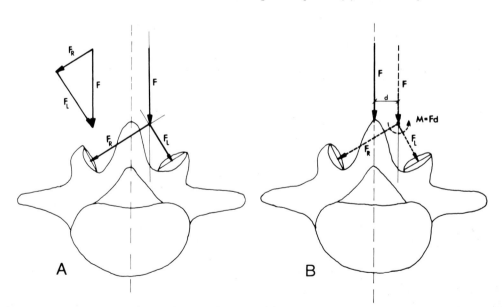

**Figure 11.5.** Forces (*F*) acting on asymmetrically oriented superior articular facets. A. The force *F* acts at the point of concurrency and is distributed unevenly to the articular facets. B. The force is offset from the point of concurrency, and additional torsion is applied to the joint. (Reproduced with permission from B. M. Cyron and W. C. Hutton: Articular Tropism. *Spine* 5(2):171, 1980.)

# References

1. Cox JM: Statistical data on facet facings of the lumbar spine and tropism. *ACA J Chiropractic* 14(4):S-39, 1977.

1a. Finneson BE: *Low Back Pain.* Philadelphia, JB Lippincott, 1973, p 25.

2. Farfan HF, Cossette JW, Robertson GH, Wells RV, Kraus H: The effects of torsion on the lumbar intervertebral joints: the role of torsion in the production of disc degeneration. *J Bone Joint Surg* 52A(3):468 and 494–496, 1970.

3. Cailliet R: *Low Back Pain Syndrome.* Philadelphia, FH Davis, 1962, pp 20 and 33.

4. Ehni G, Weinstein PR, Wilson CB: *Lumbar Spondylosis: Diagnosis, Management and Surgical Treatment.* Chicago, Year Book Medical Publishers, 1977, p 19.

5. Cyron BM, Hutton WC: Articular tropism and stability of the lumbar spine. *Spine* 5(2):168–172, 1980.

6. Badgley CE: The articular facets in relation to low-back pain and sciatic radiation. *J Bone Joint Surg* 23:481–496, 1941.

7. Brailsford JF: Deformities of the lumbosacral region of the spine. *Br J Surg* 16:562–568, 1928–1929.

8. Farfan HF, Sullivan JD: The relation of facet orientation to intervertebral disc failure. *Can J Surg* 10:179–185, 1967.

9. Willis TA; Lumbosacral anomalies. *J Bone Joint Surg* 41A:935–938, 1959.

10. Putti V, Logroscino D: Anatomia dell'artritismo vertebrale apofisario. *Chir Organi Mov* 23:317–321, 1937–1938.

11. White AA, Panjabi MM: *Clinical Biomechanics of the Spine.* Philadelphia, JB Lippincott, 1978, p 22.

CHAPTER **12**

# Spondylolisthesis

Herbinaux (1) in 1782 was the first to recognize spondylolisthesis as a cause of obstruction in his obstetric cases, but Kilian (1a) was the first to describe and name it, calling it a slow subluxation of the posterior facets. Robert (1b) believed that some defect in the neural arch must be present, and Neugebauer (1c) recognized that the slip could occur with or without a neural defect.

Figure 12.1 is an illustration of the normal L5-S1 locking mechanism of the intact intervertebral disc stabilizing the L5 vertebral body to the sacrum, of the neural arch solid bone stabilizing the anterior body to the arch, and of the articular facets locking the entire functional splint units of L5 and the sacrum. Figure 12.2 is an illustration of the progressive slippage that occurs in a person from birth through development.

## CLASSIFICATION (2)

In 1963, Newman (3) classified spondylolisthesis into 5 types. His classification, which follows, is still valid and useful today.

I. Dysplastic (congenital). Congenital abnormalities of the upper sacrum or the arch of L5 permit the "olisthesis" to occur.
II. Isthmic, in which the lesion is in the pars interarticularis. Three kinds can be delineated:

    a. Lytic, which is a fatigue fracture of the pars.
    b. Elongated but intact pars.
    c. Acute fracture of the pars (not to be confused with "traumatic," see IV).

III. Degenerative, due to a long-standing intersegmental instability.

IV. Posttraumatic, due to fractures in areas of the bony hook other than the pars.
V. Pathologic, i.e., generalized or localized bone disease.

## Dysplastic Spondylolisthesis

Congenital or dysplastic spondylolisthesis ocurs at L5-S1, with defects of fusion of the neural arch occurring in the upper sacral vertebrae as well as at L5. There is hypoplastic facet development of the sacrum which fails to provide sufficient resistance to the forward shear force of L5 on S1 (4). The L5 arch may reveal spina bifida which occurs in girls twice as frequently as it occurs in boys. During the growth spurt between ages 12 and 16, the condition commonly manifests itself probably due to increased weight bearing and stress. The pars interarticularis either elongates or separates (2). The dysplastic type of spondylolisthesis can be difficult to differentiate from the isthmic type on radiography. There is a strong genetic association in dysplastic spondylolisthesis (5), and a study by Wynne-Davies and Scott (6) showed that 1 in 3 (33%) relatives of patients with dysplastic spondylolisthesis will be affected.

## Isthmic Spondylolisthesis

Isthmic spondylolisthesis is the most common type of spondylolisthesis and is due to a defect in the ossification of the pars interarticularis. Three subdivisions of isthmic spondylolisthesis have been delineated: the lytic (Subtype A), an elongated pars without separation (Subtype B), and an acute pars fracture (Subtype C). Subtype A can be seen in Figures 12.3

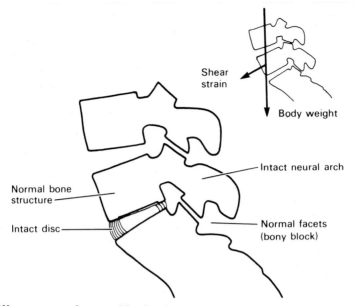

**Figure 12.1.** Illustration of normal locking mechanisms resisting forward displacement of the 5th lumbar vertebral body. (Reproduced with permission from I. Macnab: *Backache*. Baltimore, Williams & Wilkins, 1977, p. 45.)

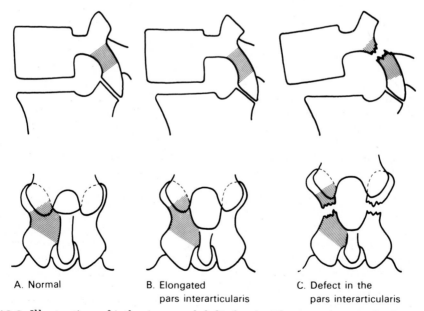

**Figure 12.2.** Illustration of isthmic spondylolisthesis. The pars interarticularis, which was normal at birth (A), becomes attenuated and elongated, allowing the vertebral body to slip forward in relation to the vertebral body below (B). Eventually, the elongated pars interarticularis may break (C). This defect in the pars interarticularis is, however, secondary to the slip and is not the cause of the forward displacement of the vertebral body. (Reproduced with permission from I. Macnab: *Backache*. Baltimore, Williams & Wilkins, 1977, p. 46.)

through 12.6. Note that although there are defects of the pars (spondylolysis) at L2 and L3, there is no forward slippage of the superior body on the one below. In this instance, the intervertebral disc is resisting the forward slippage of the vertebral body, although there may be some fibrous union of the pars interarticularis.

Spondylolysis is a term applied to the mechanical failure of an apparently normal isthmus. This occurs most frequently at the L5 level, less frequently at the L4 level, and rarely at levels above L4. It is no longer questioned that spondylolysis is a fracture that may or may not heal. These fractures are postulated to occur due to the assumption of the upright posture by the infant, allowing a fatigue type of fracture to occur when stress beyond the strength of bone occurs. Rosenberg (7) obtained radiographs of the lumbosacral spines of 143 patients who had never walked. The frequency of spondylolysis and spondylolisthesis as well as of other spinal abnormalities was determined. The average age of the patients was 27 years, with an age range from 11 to 93 years. The underlying diagnosis responsible for the nonambulatory status varied, but cerebral palsy predominated. No case of spondylolysis or spondylolisthesis was detected, and this is significant when it is compared with the 5.8% incidence in the general population. The incidences of spina bifida (8.4%) and of transitional vertebra (10.9%) were similar to those found in the general population. Scoliosis was found in 49%, and vertebral body height was increased in 33%. Degenerative changes occurred in only 2.8%. These results support the theory that spondylolysis and isthmic spondylolisthesis represent fatigue fractures resulting from activities associated with ambulation.

According to Scoville and Corkill (8), King studied 500 normal school children whom he x-rayed at the ages 6, 12, and 18. He also x-rayed 25 children with back problems. He found almost no progression or development of spondylolisthesis after the age of 6 years in any of these children. True spondylolisthesis rarely if ever progressed after the patient reached maturity. Pfeil (9) showed that the infant spine is susceptible to fatigue fracture in the isthmus.

The isthmus can be seen in Figure 12.7. There are two layers of cortical bone, the anterolateral and the posteromedial, which are joined by parallel thick trabeculae directed inferolaterally and anteriorly from the base of the superior articular process (10). The anterolateral layer is the thicker of the two and appears to be capable of resisting forces that tend to bend the inferior articular processes posteriorly or posteromedially, are induced whenever the effect of gravity is transmitted to a vertebra inclined below the horizontal anteriorly, and are induced when the vertebra is exposed to axial torque. Sullivan and Farfan (11) have studied the effect of axial torque which tends to disrupt the inferior articular processes; they believe that such damage predisposes to spondylolysis.

## Degenerative Spondylolisthesis

In degenerative spondylolisthesis, the pars interarticularis is intact but the degenerated disc allows subluxation of the inferior facet of the superior vertebra on the superior facet below.

In Figures 12.8 to 12.10, degenerative spondylolisthesis of L4 on L5 can be seen. On the oblique views (Figs. 12.9 and 12.10), the pars interarticularis is shown to be intact, but there is slippage due to degeneration of the L4-L5 disc resulting in intersegmental instability. Farfan (12, 13) believes that there are multiple small compression fractures of the inferior articular facets of the vertebra that slips forward. This causes the articular processes of the bone to grossly resemble Paget's disease in appearance. As the slip progresses, the articular processes change direction and become more horizontal. One side slips forward more than the other, allowing rotosubluxation of L4 on L5. Interestingly, Farfan (13) found that 43% of 19 patients with degenerative spondylolisthesis were diabetic.

Degenerative spondylolisthesis occurs 6 times more frequently in females than in males, 6 to 9 times more frequently at the L4 interspace than at the adjoining levels,

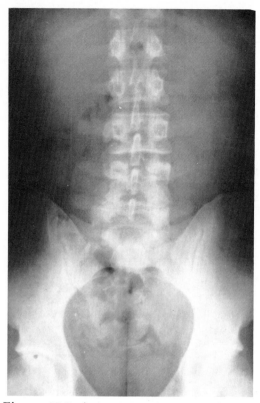

**Figure 12.3.** Anteroposterior view showing defects of the pars interarticularis.

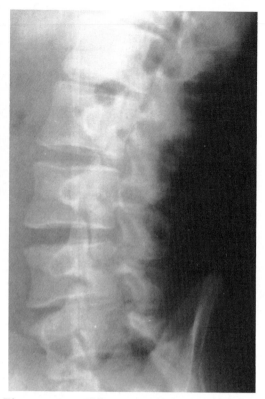

**Figure 12.5.** Oblique view revealing defects of the pars at L2, L3, L4, and L5.

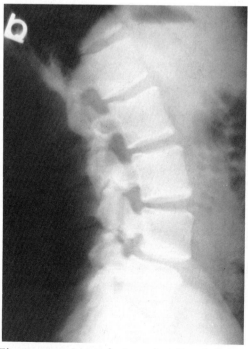

**Figure 12.4.** Lateral view showing defects of the pars at L2, L3, L4, and L5, with a 10% slippage of L4 on L5 but with no slippage of L2 on L3 or L3 on L4.

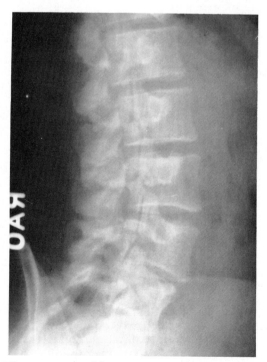

**Figure 12.6.** Oblique view revealing defects of the pars at L2, L3, L4, and L5.

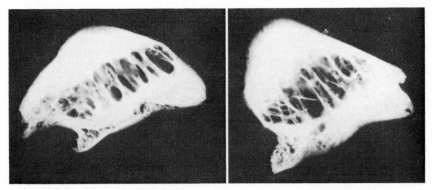

**Figure 12.7.** Photograph of two slices through the isthmus from the 5th lumbar vertebra of a 66-year-old man, which were cut parallel to the plane of the narrowest perimeter of the isthmus (i.e., the plane of a spondylolytic defect). This is typical of the normal appearance of the isthmus. The anterolateral layer of cortical bone can be seen in the *upper left region* of the slices. (Reproduced with permission from J. Krenz and J. D. G. Troup: The Structure of the Pars Interarticularis of the Lower Lumbar Vertebrae and Its Relation to the Etiology of Spondylolysis. *Journal of Bone and Joint Surgery* 55B:735, 1973.)

and 4 times more frequently when L5 is sacralized than when it is not (14). It is believed that the predisposing factor is a straight, stable lumbosacral joint which sits high between the ilia. This arrangement puts increased stress on the joint between L4 and L5, leading to decompensation of the ligaments, hypermobility and degeneration at the articular processes, and multiple microfractures of the inferior articular processes of L4, allowing forward slippage (13).

### Traumatic Spondylolisthesis

Traumatic spondylolisthesis is a fracture of any part of the vertebral arch other than the pars, which allows forward displacement to occur. This type of spondylolisthesis is rare.

### Pathological Spondylolisthesis

If the bony hook mechanism (articular facet, pedicle, pars) fails to hold the body of the articulation in place because of local or generalized bone disease, pathological spondylolisthesis can occur. Since pathological spondylolisthesis is rare, only one variant, spondylolisthesis adquisita, is mentioned here. In this type, there is a fatigue fracture of the pars at the upper end of a lumbar surgical fusion that allows forward slipping.

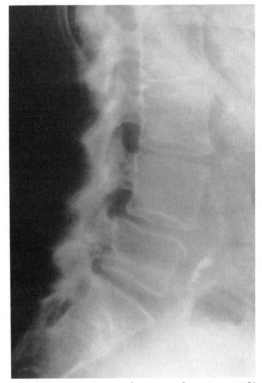

**Figure 12.8.** Lateral view showing 10% forward slippage of L4 on L5.

### CAUSES OF SPONDYLOLISTHESIS

Figure 12.11 reveals a 60% forward slippage of the lumbar vertebral body on the

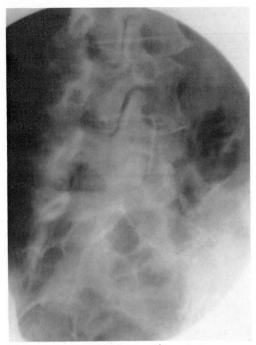

**Figure 12.9.** Oblique view of the same patient as in Figure 12.8 reveals no evidence of a pars interarticularis defect of ossification.

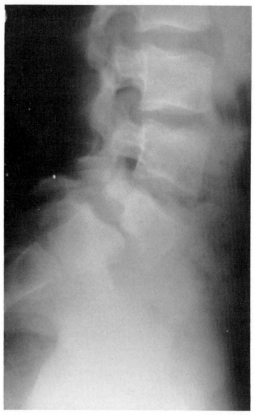

**Figure 12.11.** X-ray showing a 60% spondylolisthesis of L5 on the sacrum. Note the facet syndrome at L4-L5.

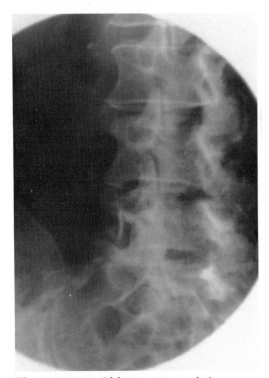

**Figure 12.10.** Oblique view of the same patient as in Figure 12.8 reveals no evidence of a pars interarticularis defect of ossification.

sacrum with a massive defect within the pars interarticularis. The only structure which could have kept this vertebral body from slipping forward was the intervertebral disc, which had to have been totally torn to allow this forward slippage. The inferior facets of L5 have glided over the rudimentary superior articular facets of the sacrum. The spinous processes of L5 rest upon the dorsal aspect of the 1st sacral arch. Here the pars interarticularis is not only fractured, but it is also greatly elongated, as this degree of slippage would not have been possible otherwise. Also note that the superior facet of L5 has entered the upper third of the intervertebral foramen between L4 and L5, thus producing a facet syndrome at this level and potential compression of the 4th lumbar nerve root existing here.

A pars defect is visible on the x-ray and of a cadaver specimen (Fig. 12.12), and the actual specimen dissected out at necropsy can be seen on Figure 12.13. A discogram (Fig. 12.14) of the same specimen reveals degenerative spondylolisthesis.

The 32-year-old woman in Figures 12.15 to 12.17 had never had low back pain until her pregnancy; she later delivered triplets. There is a 25% isthmic spondylolisthesis shown in Figure 12.15. The patient also had a 20-mm left short leg (Fig. 12.16); its correction is shown in Figure 12.17. Flexion distraction and flexion exercises produced complete relief of this patient's symptomatology. The appearance of a vertebra like the one in this patient is demonstrated in a dry specimen (Fig. 12.13) well defining the interruption of the pars interarticularis.

## INCIDENCE OF SPONDYLOLYSIS AND SPONDYLOLISTHESIS

In a study (15) reported by Wiltse, it was stated that if 100 children aged 5 were to be studied roentgenographically, there probably would not be one with a defect of the pars. If the same children were examined toward the end of the first grade (age 7), however, the incidence would be around 4.4%, which is just slightly below the national average. Baker (as reported in Finneson (16)) found that

as those children reached 18, only 1.4% more showed spondylolisthesis, with most of the increase occurring between ages 11 and 16, the time of greatest strenuous athletics which produce fatigue fractures.

One reason that forward slippage occurs most often in children 5 to 7 years old may be due to the increased activity or to the increased sitting in the lordotic posture done by children. It is known that fracture never occurs in animals other than humans, and only humans have lordosis (5, 12, 17, 18).

The average age of onset of symptoms of spondylolisthesis is 14 in girls and 16 in boys (19). A sudden onset is termed the "listhetic crisis." The pelvis is rotated anteriorly, the sacrum is flat, and the hamstring is found to be in spasm, frequently making the patient walk with bent knees. The patient with an isthmic spondylolisthesis producing severe symptoms before age 21, with or without past symptoms, probably will not recover completely without surgery.

The severity of symptoms and the treatment of spondylolisthesis in the child vary greatly from that in the adult. Surgery may be more imperative in the child than in the adult because further slippage occurs more often in the child than in the adult. Furthermore, the outcome of fusion is better in the child than in the adult, with the adult being more willing to curtail activities, so as to prevent further aggravation of the condition, than would be the child. It is also known that, following surgery, there is a greater relief from pain for the child than there is for the adult. For the adult, the prime reason for surgical treatment is to relieve pain, not to prevent progression of slippage. Slippage rarely increases in the adult (20).

Semon (21) found that in a large group of college football players, spondylolysis was not a predisposing factor to low back pain. Furthermore, the mere indication of spondylolysis or spondylolisthesis on x-ray did not mean that spondylolysis or spondylolisthesis was the cause of the person's low back pain. Newman (22) observed that despite the obvious displacement at the L5-S1 intervertebral joint, the symptomatology seems to derive from the

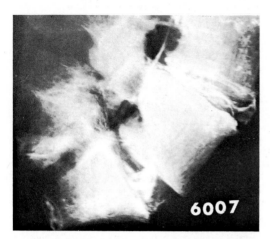

6007

**Figure 12.12.** X-ray showing spondylolysis in a cadaver specimen. A defect of the inferior articular process is clearly visible. The lumbosacral disc shows degeneration, but this does not appear to be as advanced as that at the L4-L5 level. (Reproduced with permission from H. F. Farfan: *Mechanical Disorders of the Low Back*. Philadelphia, Lea & Febiger, 1973, chap. 7, p. 164.)

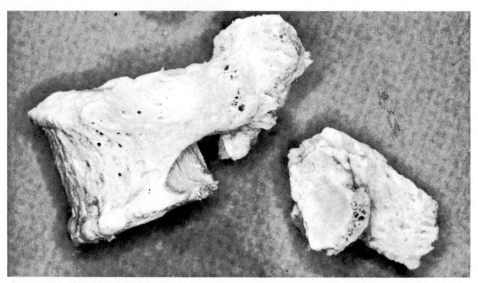

**Figure 12.13.** Photograph of L5 isolated from the same specimen as in Figure 12.12. (Reproduced with permission from H. F. Farfan: *Mechanical Disorders of the Low Back*. Philadelphia, Lea & Febiger, 1973, chap. 7, p. 165.)

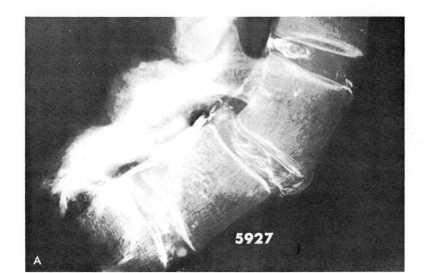

**Figure 12.14.** A, Discogram showing spondylolisthesis of L4 on L5 in a cadaver specimen. There is no defect in the pars interarticularis; however, there appears to be a prolonged inferior articular process. The disc is degenerated. *B*, Skeletal arrangement. The specimen does not show a true elongation. The apparent elongation is due to superimposition of subluxated superior and inferior articular facets and to the widening of the angle between the lamina and pedicle (*C*). (Reproduced with permission from H. F. Farfan: *Mechanical Disorders of the Low Back.* Philadelphia, Lea & Febiger, 1973, p. 167.)

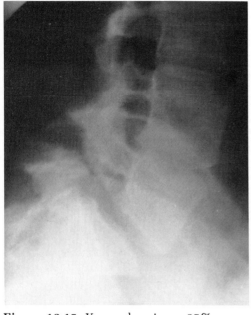

**Figure 12.15.** X-ray showing a 25% spondylolisthesis of L5 on the sacrum, with an isthmic defect present.

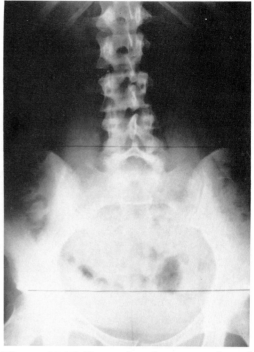

**Figure 12.17.** X-ray showing correction of the left short leg of the same patient as in Figure 12.16. The correction was accomplished with a 9-mm lift.

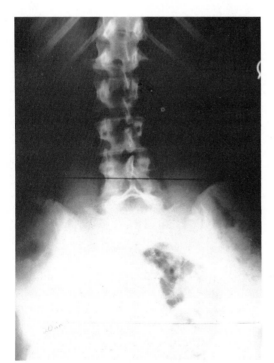

**Figure 12.16.** Posteroanterior view of the same patient as in Figure 12.15 reveals a 20-mm left short femoral head.

L4-L5 joint. This would be logical, since the forward slippage of L5 does allow the superior facet of L5 to enter the intervertebral foramen in a telescoping effect at the L4-L5 level. Furthermore, at the time of the slippage, either or both discs, i.e., either the L4-L5 of L5-S1 discs, must break down, allowing annular stretching and tearing. Without this phenomenon, there could be no forward slippage of the vertebra. This would be true even if there were growth defects within the arch, namely, pars interarticularis fracture. The disc, being a very pain-sensitive structure, certainly creates symptomatology as the slippage occurs. Perhaps it is understandable why in the adult, after this slippage occurs and there is a healing of the annular fibers, the pain lessens or disappears. In Figure 12.14, a discogram of the L4-L5 level, there certainly is disruption of the annular fibers, allowing escape of the dye from the nucleus into the perimeter of the disc. This certainly

demonstrates the tearing that would occur in the annulus at the time of slippage.

In a study of facet joints with the use of
arthrography, an abnormal communication between the two facet joints border-
ing the separated pars interarticularis was
observed in 9 of 11 patients. This communication occurred in the area of the
defect. In one patient with bilateral spondylolysis of the L5 vertebra, both left adjacent apophyseal joints were observed to
communicate not only with one another
but also with the contralateral facet joints
through a transverse channel joining the
isthmic areas of L5 (23). Furthermore, it
was found that spondylolysis considerably altered the soft tissues of the adjacent
facet joints. Irritation of these structures
might explain certain complaints such as
low back and scleratogenous pain in patients with spondylolysis.

Among the causes of spondylolisthesis,
the 5th lumbar vertebra, placed at the
apex of the lumbar curve, is probably the
recipient of the highest stress on flexion
and rotation movement. If L5 is well an-
chored to the pelvis by enlarged transverse processes, the same findings may
well be seen at the L4 level. According to
Farfan (24), during forced rotation the
neural arch is placed under such stress
that a permanent sprain of the neural arch
can occur. This sprain could take two
forms:

1. The interarticular distance between
the inferior facet articulations is reduced.
This may allow the sprained neural arch
to slip through the other.

2. The angle of these processes to the
axis of the pedicle would be increased
from a normal angle of about 90° to an
abnormal angle of about 130°

This produces an apparent lengthening of
the pedicles, which in turn could allow
the forward slip of the affected vertebra.
Farfan further believes that the defect in
the lamina is probably a fracture at the
junction between the laminae and the
pedicle, as the angle between these structures is opened up. Furthermore, the injury at the disc is an epiphyseal separation
of the upper epiphysis of the sacrum.

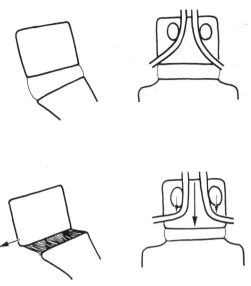

**Figure 12.18.** Illustration of kinking of the
nerve roots by the pedicles as the body of
L5 slips downward and forward. (Reproduced with permission from I. Macnab:
*Backache.* Baltimore, Williams & Wilkins,
1977, p. 54.)

## CAUSES OF PAIN IN SPONDYLOLISTHESIS

Spondylolytic spondylolisthesis, i.e., a
defect in the pars interarticularis allowing
forward slippage, can and does occur
without symptoms. It is known that Es-
kimos have a 40% to 50% occurrence of
spondylolisthesis but not that high an incidence of pain with it. Forward slippage
of the body will not occur without degenerative changes occurring in the underlying disc; i.e., forward slippage is not
possible without annular tearing or breakdown. The disc is not capable of with-
standing the shearing stresses of the body
above on the one below.

In a study comparing the incidence of
pain in patients with spondylolisthesis by
age, Macnab (19) divided patients into
three age groups (under 26, 26 to 39, and
40 and older). In the 40 and older group,
the incidence of spondylolisthesis in patients with back pain was about the same
as it was in the general population,
whereas in the under-26 group, the incidence was nearly 19% of back pain pa-

tients exhibiting spondylolisthesis. Thus, if spondylotic spondylolisthesis is found in a patient under 26 years of age who does have back pain, it probably is the cause of the symptoms; if it is found in patients 26 to 39 years of age, it is a possible cause; and if it is found in patients 40 years of age or older, it rarely, if ever, is the sole cause of symptoms.

Figure 12.18 shows how L5 spondylolisthesis kinks the L5 nerve root passing under the L5 pedicles. This can be confused with root symptoms, due to L4-L5 disc protrusion. In a patient with L5 nerve root symptoms, however, a negative myelogram at L4-L5 would lead to the suspicion that the L5 spondylolisthesis is kinking the L5 nerve root. An L4 spondylolisthesis could kink the L4 nerve root and cause femoral nerve paresthesia.

In summary, pars interarticularis defects are not the cause of spondylolisthesis. Spondylolisthesis can occur without pars interarticular defects, but the presence of a defect can allow greater slippage. Spondylolisthesis is due to instability of the lumbar spine in one of or a combination of the following: intervertebral disc, pars interarticularis, or articular facets.

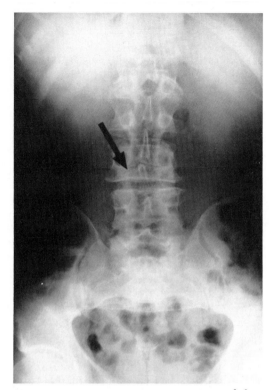

**Figure 12.19.** Anteroposterior view of the isthmic spondylolisthesis of L3 on L4. Note the break within the pars interarticularis (*arrow*).

## TREATMENT OF SPONDYLOLISTHESIS

Figures 12.19 through 12.22 reveal a pars interarticularis break in continuity, with an approximately 10% slippage of the 3rd lumbar vertebral body occurring between the 2nd and 4th vertebral bodies. There is also thinning of the L3-L4 disc with anterolateral lipping and spurring and a left posterior rotation of the vertebral body and of those segments cephalad from it. The articular facets are fairly well maintained in their joint spaces, although there is a decrease in both the sagittal and the vertical height of the intervertebral foramen at this level.

In the treatment of both true and false spondylolisthesis, the basic Cox flexion distraction manipulations are applied (Figs. 12.23 to 12.26). A Dutchman roll is placed under the spondylolisthetic segment. In the absence of sciatica, which is quite unusual due to spondylolisthesis, the full range of motion of the articular facets is utilized, but flexion distraction as demonstrated in Figure 12.23 is the first movement.

The contact hand for flexion distraction will be on the spinous process directly above the forward slippage, in this case at the L2 level. With the fulcrum effect of the Dutchman roll, the leverage needed to distract these segments is minimal. This author suggests that no more that 1 inch to 2 inches of downward caudal distraction of the table be utilized in this treatment. Following flexion distraction, lateral bending of the articular facets is applied at each segment (Fig. 12.24). The foramen magnum "pump" or, in this case, full spinal distraction as demonstrated in Figure 12.25 was utilized. Again note the fulcrum effect of the Dutchman roll under the forward slipped segment. Lastly, flexion distraction as demonstrated in Figure 12.26 is applied to each segment cephalad from the L3 level.

The desired effect of this treatment is to create minimal flexion of the segments,

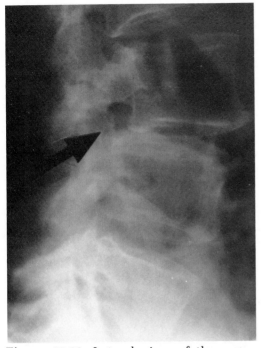

**Figure 12.20.** Lateral view of the same patient as in Figure 12.19, showing a 10% anterior body slippage of L3 on L4.

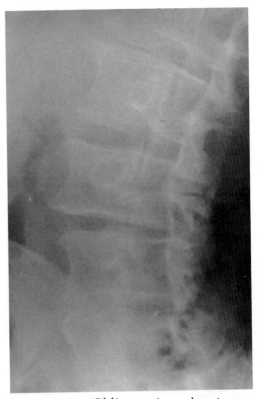

**Figure 12.22.** Oblique view showing a pars interarticularis defect at L3.

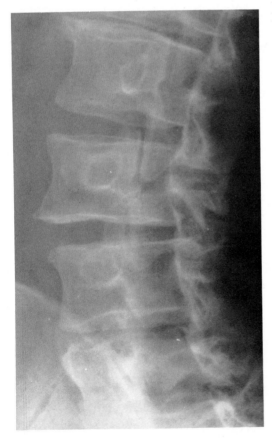

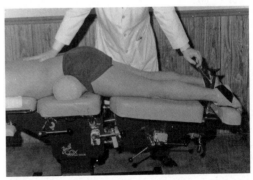

**Figure 12.23.** Flexion distraction of a patient with spondylolisthesis; a Dutchman roll can be seen in place.

with the Dutchman roll acting as a reduction force on the forward slippage.

The frequency of distraction at each session is as follows: The distraction is applied on an average of three 20-second

**Figure 12.21.** Oblique view showing a pars interarticularis defect at L3.

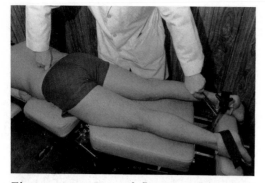

**Figure 12.24.** Lateral flexion is being applied.

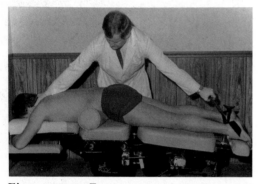

**Figure 12.25.** Foramen magnum "pump."

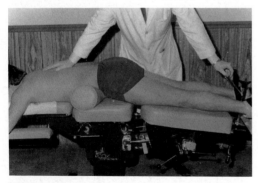

**Figure 12.26.** Flexion distraction is being applied to segments cephalad to the L3 level.

periods while the contact hand is on the spinous process directly above the forward slipped segment. During this 20-second distraction, a "milking" action is applied to the segment by maintaining a firm

spinous contact while slowly moving the caudal section of the table up and down, thus achieving a push-pull pumping effect on the posterior elements and intervertebral disc space. This can be sensed under the treating hand, and the relaxation of the patient during this application can be felt. It is important not to fight any resistance of the paravertebral muscles or the voluntary or involuntary contraction of these muscles by the patient. At the outset of care, it is important to gain the patient's confidence so that the patient can relax to allow this manipulation.

Note: A 1- to 2-inch downward movement on the caudal section of the table is maximum in the treatment of spondylolisthesis. This is not the time to be a "macho" clinician. It is recommended that the pressure of 1 finger on the caudal section is adequate. The Dutchman roll acts as a fulcrum that reduces the need for strong distractive force.

Lateral flexion is applied to check for hypomobility of the articular facets; if hypomobility is found, the facets are put through their full range of motion so as to bring them back to their physiological mobility.

The paravertebral muscles can then be treated with physical modalities if needed. These modalities might well include positive galvanism to reduce inflammation and sedate irritated tissues or sinusoidal currents to return normal tone to the musculature.

A belt support may be worn if the patient is in acute pain, but this is only a temporary measure. Exercises for the spondylolisthesis patient are extremely important. We most often use the first three Cox exercises in the treatment of spondylolisthesis.

In a study of 47 patients with symptomatic back pain secondary to spondylolisthesis who were treated with flexion and extension exercises of the lumbar spine, it was found that patients treated with flexion type exercises were less likely to require back supports, require modification of their jobs, or limit their activities because of pain (25). In this study, 19 patients were treated with extension type exercises in addition to flexion exercises, and 28 patients were treated with only flexion exercises of the lumbar spine. At follow-up evaluation, treatment results from the two groups were compared. Eighty-two percent of those who underwent flexion exercises stated that they had less pain, whereas 37% of those who did only extension exercises stated that they had less pain. The flexion group was found to have less pain, less need to modify their work, less need for continued use of bracing, and a greater chance of recovery. The type of spondylolisthesis had no effect on the response to flexion exercises.

Figures 12.27 and 12.28 reveal the effects of flexion exercises on the lumbar spine in a patient performing abdominal

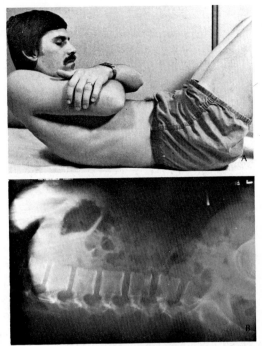

**Figure 12.28.** A, Photograph of the subject performing abdominal strengthening exercise. B, Roentgenogram of spinal column while the subject performs abdominal strengthening exercise. (Reproduced with permission from R. R. Gramse, M. Sinaki, and D. M. Ilstrup: Lumbar Spondylolisthesis—A Rational Approach to Conservative Treatment. *Mayo Clinic Proceedings* 55:681–686, 1980.)

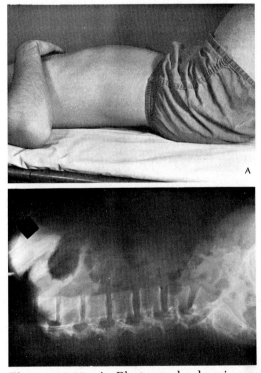

**Figure 12.27.** A, Photograph showing a decrease in lumbar lordosis while the subject is lying supine with the knees bent. B, Roentgenogram of spinal column while the subject is lying supine with the knees bent and is performing the pelvic-tilting exercise. (Reproduced with permission from R. R. Gramse, M. Sinaki, and D. M. Ilstrup: Lumbar Spondylolisthesis—A Rational Approach to Conservative Treatment. *Mayo Clinic Proceedings* 55:681–686, 1980.)

strengthening exercises. Please note that extension exercises are to be avoided in spondylolysis and spondylolisthesis, as they have been shown to increase the pain not only in gymnasts but also in the general public (26).

## ANALYSIS OF THE RESULTS OF CHIROPRACTIC TREATMENT OF SPONDYLOLISTHESIS

In 1981, Lenz (27) reported on the results of chiropractic treatment of spondylolisthesis. The following notes are given from his report.

Using the "time-honored" specific side posture technics, we treated 10 cases of "olisthesis" (3 males, 7 females) and achieved the following results: 4 of the 10 (40%) showed excellent, good, or fair results and 6 of the 10 (60%) either showed no change or, unfortunately, were made worse.

Since learning the lumbar flexion distraction technic as taught by J. M. Cox, D.C., Fort Wayne, Indiana, we can now report a more favorable outcome in 15 cases of olisthesis and 1 case of "oloptosis": 86.6% showed a favorable outcome (excellent, good, or fair results) and only 13.4% showed poor outcome.

The age of these patients ranged from 20 years (8 years since onset of symptoms) to 62 years (30 years since onset of symptoms). Of these 15, 4 were men and 11 were women. The sex or age of the patient did not affect the results.

In only 2 cases could we detect any measurable difference in the olisthetic movement following treatment and that was only a 3% and a 5% improvement in position. In all of the other cases, there was no measurable difference. In the 1 case of oloptosis, there was also no detectable change of position.

The procedure used was mild lumbar flexion distraction with the use of a Dutchman roll under the abdomen. After distraction, any severe lateral misalignment of adjacent bony structures was specifically corrected (as much as possible) by a mild side posture technique. The patient was then instructed in a simple exercise to do at home to loosen the hamstring muscles.

The patient was then placed in a supine position with both the hips and the knees flexed at 90°, with the calf of the leg supported in that position. While in this position the patient was given a 20- to 30-minute period of very mild short-wave diathermy, with one pad under the cervical area and the other under the lumbar area. Only one patient required the use of an orthopedic lumbar restraint, and that was used more for abdominal support than for lumbar support.

When looking back over the 34 years of chiropractic practice, "I must confess to many years of trepidation" in treating patients with extremely acute low back problems. Since learning Dr. Cox's distraction methods, however, "I have to admit that I am finally enjoying all of my work with patients."

## References

1. Newman PH: Spondylolisthesis: its cause and effect. *Ann Coll Surg Engl* 16:305, 1955.
1a. Kilian HF: Schilderungen neuer Beckenformen and ihres Verhalten im leben Bassermann und Mathy. Mannheim, 1854 (cit da Brocher).
1b. Robert (zu Koblenz): Eine eigentumliche angeborene Lordose, wahrseheinlich bedingt eine Verschiebung des Korpers des letzten Lindenwirbels auf die vordere Flache des ersten Kreuzheinwirbels (Spondylolisthesis Kilian), nebst Bermerlsungen über die Mechanik dieser Beckenformation. *Monatsschr Geburtskunde Frauenkrank* 5:81–94, 1855.
1c. Neugebauer F: Die Entschung der Spondylolisthesis. *Zentrable Gynaekol* 5:260–261, 1881.
2. Wiltse L, Newman PH, Macnab I: Classification of spondylosis and spondylolisthesis. *Clin Orthop* 117:23–29, 1976.
3. Newman PH: The aetiology in spondylolisthesis. *J Bone Joint Surg* 45B:39–59, 1963.
4. Newman PH: Spondylolisthesis. *Physiology* 60:14, 1974.
5. Wiltse LL: Spondylolisthesis and its treatment. In Finneson BE: *Low Back Pain*. Philadelphia, JB Lippincott, 1980.
6. Wynne-Davies R, Scott JHS: Inheritance and spondylolisthesis; a radiographic family survey. *J Bone Joint Surg [Br]* 61B:301–305, 1979.
7. Rosenberg NJ, Bargar WL, Friedman B: The incidence of spondylolysis and spondylolisthesis in non-ambulatory patients. *Spine* 6(1):35–38, 1981.
8. Scoville WB, Corkill G: Lumbar spondylolisthesis with ruptured disc. *J Neurosurg* 40:529–534, 1974.
9. Pfeil E: Experimentelle Untersuchunngen zur Frage der Entstehung der Spondylolyse. *Z Orthop* 109:231, 1971.
10. Krenz J, Troup JDG: The structure of the pars interarticularis of the lower lumbar vertebrae and its relation to the etiology of spondylolysis: with a report of a healing fracture in the neural arch of a fourth lumbar vertebra. *J Bone Joint Surg* 55B:735, 1973.
11. Sullivan JD, Farfan HF: The crumpled neural arch. *Orthop Clin North Am* 6:199, 1975.
12. Farfan HF: *Mechnical Disorders of the Low Back.* Philadelphia, Lea & Febiger, 1973, chap 7, pp 164–165.
13. Farfan HF: The pathological anatomy of degenerative spondylolisthesis. *Spine* 5(5):412–418, 1980.
14. Rosenberg NJ: Degenerative spondylolisthesis, predisposing factors. *J Bone Joint Surg* 57A:467, 1978.
15. Rowe GG, Roche MB: The etiology of separate neural arch. *J Bone Joint Surg* 35A:102, 1953.
16. Finneson BE: *Low Back Pain*, ed 2. Philadelphia, JB Lippincott, 1980, p 453.
17. Troup D: Paper read at the meeting of the International Society for the Study of the Lumbar Spine, London, 1975.
18. Hutton WC, Cyron BM: Spondylolysis: the role of the posterior elements in resisting the intervertebral force. *Acta Orthop Scand* 49:604–609, 1978.

19. Macnab I: *Backache.* Baltimore, Williams & Wilkins, 1977, p 47–52.
20. Finneson BE: *Low Back Pain*, ed 2. Philadelphia, JB Lippincott, 1980, chap 15, pp 457–476.
21. Semon RL, Spengler D: Significance of lumbar spondylolysis in college football players. *Spine* 6(2):172–174, 1981.
22. Newman PH: Spondylolisthesis: its cause and effect. *R Coll Surg Engl* 16:305, 1955.
23. Maldague B, Mathruin P, Malghem J: Facet joint arthrography in lumbar spondylosis. *Diag Radiol* 140:29–36, 1981.
24. Farfan HF: *Mechanical Disorders of the Low Back.* Philadelphia, Lea & Febiger, 1973, chap 7, p 164.
25. Granse RR, Mehrsheed S, Ilstrup DM: Lumbar spondylolisthesis: a rational approach to conservative treatment. *Mayo Clin Proc* 55:681–686, 1980.
26. Jackson DW, Wiltse LL, Cerincione RJ: Spondylolysis in the female gymnast. *Clin Orthop* 117:68–73, 1976.
27. Lenz W: Spondylolisthesis and spondyloptosis of the lower lumbar spine: a microstudy. *ACA J Chiropractic* 15:S107–S110, 1981.

*Have the courage to be ignorant of a great many things, in order to avoid the calamity of being ignorant of everything.*

*—Sidney Smith*

CHAPTER **13**

# Specific Low Back Conditions: Discogenic Spondyloarthrosis, Failed Back Surgery Syndrome, Compression Fracture, and Sacroiliac Joint Positioning

## DISCOGENIC SPONDYLOARTHROSIS

Discogenic spondyloarthrosis may be the most common condition seen in clinical practice. Middle-aged to elderly people are extremely prone to degenerative disc disease; as the nucleus pulposus dehydrates, the opposing vertebral body plates approximate one another, resulting in loss of disc space height and subchondral sclerosis. The person thus becomes shorter and may become stooped. Patients with this condition often state that it would feel good to be "pulled apart" or tractioned. This condition can be effectively treated by flexion distraction manipulation.

*Every vertebra and its articulations are capable of performing certain movements, namely, flexion, extension, lateral bending, rotation, and circumduction.* A vertebra capable of its normal motions is one less encumbered with subluxation and with the resulting nerve root irritations accompanying it.

By working within patient tolerance from the outset of Cox traction manipulation, the doctor can shortly increase the range of motion of a previously considered degenerated joint until the patient not only is pain-free or close to it but also realizes a range of motion which he had not enjoyed for months or years. With use of the Zenith-Cox table, it takes a minimum of traction to elicit these various motions and to achieve a relaxation and control of the patient that is desired. The Zenith-Cox table is capable of affording the doctor these passive motions without the necessity of thrust adjusting.

Figures 13.1, *A* and *B*, and 13.2, *A* and *B*, reveal marked degenerative spondylolarthrosis of the lumbar spine.

**Case 1** is of a 50-year-old white woman who developed low back pain after shoveling snow 1 month previously. Her family doctor had given her pain pills and, when no relief was obtained, ordered a bone scan and x-rays of the low back. An orthopedic surgeon had recommended heat and exercises following a myelogram, CT scan, and EMG which were all negative. She had been hospitalized for 5 days of traction. She had made an appointment to visit a neurosurgeon but, in the meantime, had decided to visit a chiropractor. She had had a malignant breast removed in 1973.

On examination, range of motion is 30° on flexion, 10° on extension, 10° on right lateral flexion, 10° on left lateral flexion, 30° on right rotation, and 30° on left rotation. Déjérine's triad is negative. The straight leg raise is negative bilaterally. Motor and sensory findings of the lower extremities are normal. Vital signs are normal.

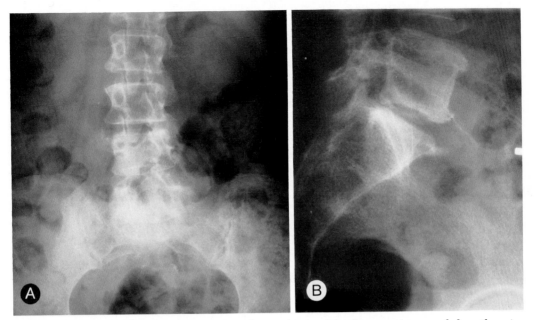

**Figure 13.1.** *A,* Anteroposterior view of a patient with discogenic spondyloarthrosis. *B,* Lateral view. Traction spurs and narrowing of the disc space are noted at the anterolateral body margins. Vertebral body plate sclerosis of L5 and the sacrum is present especially posteriorly.

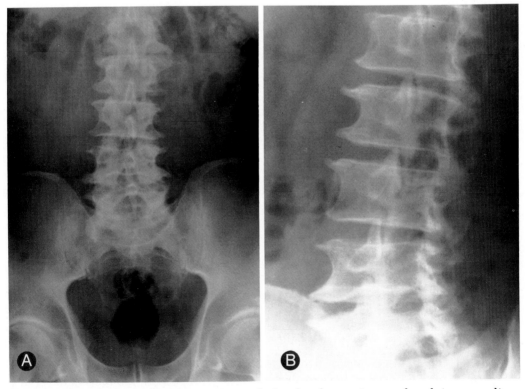

**Figure 13.2.** *A,* Anteroposterior view of the lumbar spine and pelvis, revealing extensive anterolateral hypertrophic osteophytes of the body margins. *B,* Oblique view showing how extensive the projection of these traction spurs can become.

X-rays reveal:

1. Left lateral flexion subluxation of L4 on L5 (Fig. 13.3), with left lateral bending (Fig. 13.4) revealing failure of the spinous process of the lumbar vertebra to rotate left into the concavity and of the bodies to rotate right to the convexity. Figure 13.5 shows good Lovett posture and normal right lateral bending.

2. Thinning of the L3-L4, L4-L5, and L5-S1 disc spaces (Fig. 13.6).

3. Arthrotic facet changes, namely, loss of joint space and subchondral sclerosis (Fig. 13.7).

This patient has degenerative disc disease at L3-L4, L4-L5, and L5-S1 with arthrosis of the articular facets and aberrant lateral bending.

Treatment consisted of:

1. Cox flexion distraction manipulation (Figs. 13.11 to 13.17).

2. Exercises 1 to 5 (see Chapter 8).

3. Goading of acupressure points B24 to B54 (Figs. 13.18 to 13.21).

4. Hydrocollation with positive galvanic current to the L5-S1 disc.

5. Discat including 800 mg of $MnSO_4$ daily.

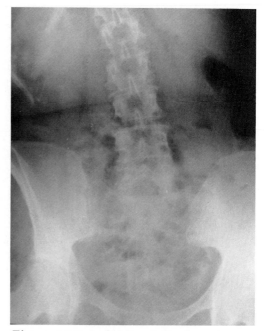

**Figure 13.4.** Left lateral flexion view revealing minimal L4 spinous process left rotation.

**Case 2** is of an 86-year-old woman who has had low back and bilateral leg pain for several

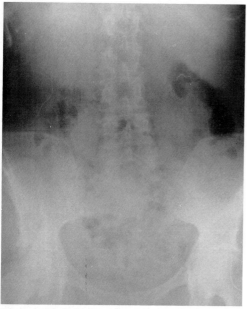

**Figure 13.3.** Neutral posteroanterior view revealing L4 left lateral flexion subluxation on L5.

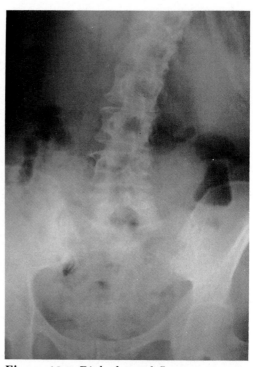

**Figure 13.5.** Right lateral flexion view revealing strong rotation of the lumbar segments.

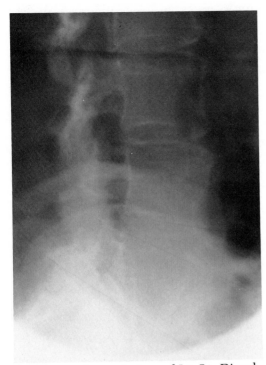

**Figure 13.6.** Lateral view of L5-S1. Discal thinning is noted.

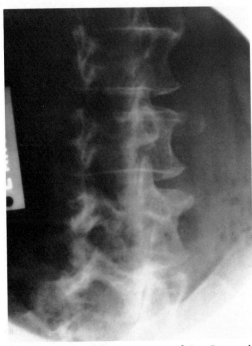

**Figure 13.7.** Oblique view of L5-S1 and L4-L5 facet arthrosis. Note the loss of joint space and sclerosis of the facet facings.

weeks. She has not been able to sleep because of leg ache.

On examination, dextroscoliosis of the thoracolumbar spine is noted. Range of motion is 30° on flexion, 5° on right lateral bending, 10° on left lateral bending, 10° on right rotation, and 10° on left rotation. Palpation reveals adequate posterior tibialis and dorsalis pedis pulses. Vital signs are within normal limits.

X-rays reveal:

1. Dextroscoliosis of the thoracolumbar spine with advanced degenerative disc disease and L3 right lateral listhesis subluxation (Figs. 13.8 and 13.9).

2. Atherosclerosis of the abdominal aorta.

Treatment consisted of the following:

1. Gentle Cox distraction manipulation of the thoracolumbar spine (Figs. 13.11 to 13.17).
2. Goading of acupressure points B24 to B49 (Figs. 13.18 to 13.21).
3. Application of sinusoidal currents to the paravertebral muscles in the lumbar area (Fig. 13.42).
4. Hydrocollator packs (Fig. 13.43).
5. Mild exercises 1 to 3 (see Chapter 8).

The patient was seen twice weekly for 1 month. She obtained a 75% subjective relief from pain, which was the goal of therapy. She continues weekly visits for distraction and therapy to maintain relief.

Figure 13.10 reveals the vacuum phenomenon of gas formation which occurs during the degenerative process of the nucleus pulposus.

## Treatment of Discogenic Spondyloarthrosis

In Figure 13.11, flexion is being applied to each lumbar disc space and facet facing. By maintenance of hand contact with the spinous process of each lumbar and thoracic vertebra, the downward pressure on the caudal section of the table allows stretching and spreading apart of each functional spinal unit.

Testing for patient tolerance of traction, as demonstrated in Figure 13.12, is performed before the cuffs are applied. This is done by grasping the ankle and applying traction while asking whether the patient feels any pain in the low back. Muscle resistance can be felt in patients who cannot tolerate traction. If there is no pain,

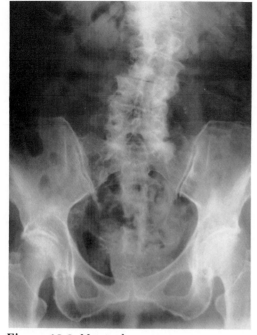

**Figure 13.8.** Neutral posteroanterior view showing advanced discogenic spondyloarthrosis of the lumbar spine with dextroscoliosis.

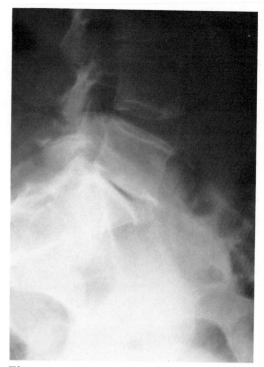

**Figure 13.10.** X-ray showing vacuum phenomenon.

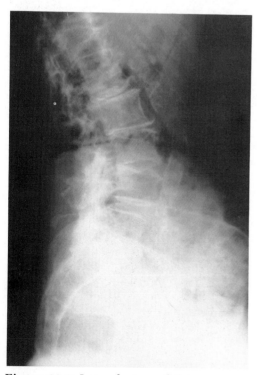

**Figure 13.9.** Lateral view of the same patient as in Figure 13.8.

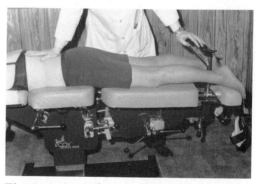

**Figure 13.11.** Flexion distraction manipulation.

the cuffs are attached and flexion, as demonstrated in Figure 13.11, is carried out.

Lateral flexion is demonstrated in Figure 13.13 and is performed by grasping the spinous process of each lumbar segment individually between the thumb and index finger (Fig. 13.14). Motion palpation is elicited by testing the ability of the articular facets to lateral bend during movement of the caudal section of the table in lateral flexion. Hypomobility is

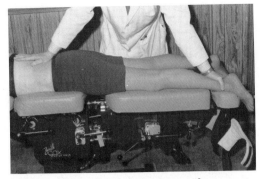

**Figure 13.12.** Testing patient tolerance to distraction before applying distraction cuffs.

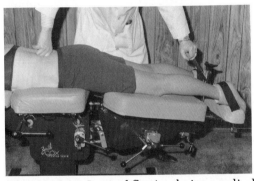

**Figure 13.13.** Lateral flexion being applied to the articular facets.

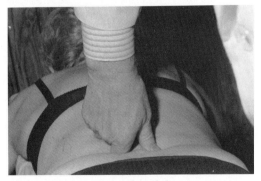

**Figure 13.14.** Grasping of the spinous process above the facets to be motion-palpated and manipulated.

evidenced by resistance to movement laterally, pain to the patient, or both.

Circumduction which is a combination of lateral flexion and plain flexion is demonstrated in Figure 13.15. This coupled movement of the table allows full range of motion of the facet and is very effective in restoring mobility to the facet.

Rotation, as demonstrated in Figure 13.16, is applied by rotating the caudal section of the table while the vertebral segment is held in resistance. Traction can be applied prior to this movement and maintained during rotation by leaving the ankle cuffs on the patient and opening the caudal section of the table. Keep in mind that L4-L5 and L5-S1 have very restricted ranges of motion in rotation and should not be forced into rotation. The upper lumbar and thoracic segments are capable of rotation.

Rotation and flexion as applied simultaneously to the upper lumbar and thoracic segments are demonstrated in Figure 13.17. This coupled mobilization is powerful and must be done to patient tolerance.

Goading of acupressure bladder meridian points B24 and B35, as demonstrated

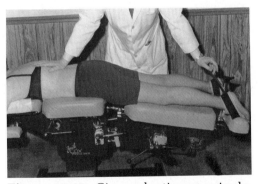

**Figure 13.15.** Circumduction manipulation.

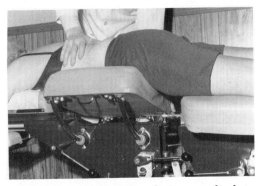

**Figure 13.16.** Rotation being applied to the thoracolumbar spine.

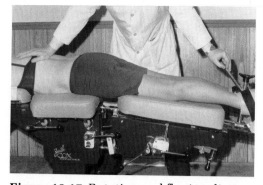

**Figure 13.17.** Rotation and flexion distraction being applied simultaneously.

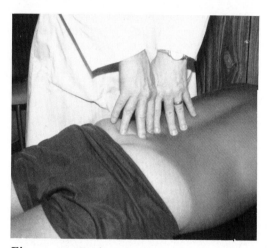

**Figure 13.18.** Acupressure points B24 to B35 being goaded.

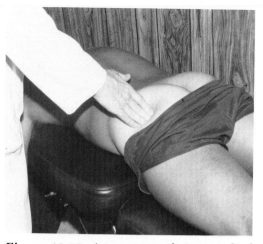

**Figure 13.19.** Acupressure being applied to the gluteus maximus and bladder meridian point B49.

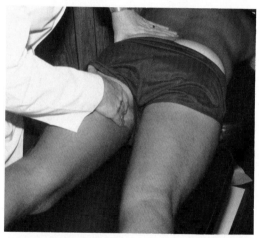

**Figure 13.20.** Goading of the adductor and gracilis tendons at their origins.

in Figure 13.18, is performed prior to and after distraction.

Deep pressure into the belly of the gluteus maximus muscle and bladder meridian point B49, as demonstrated in Figure 13.19, is used to relieve the pain of sciatica.

Pressure being applied to the adductor and gracilis tendons at their origins is demonstrated in Figure 13.20; pressure being applied to the their insertions on the medial femur and medial condyle of the tibia is demonstrated in Figure 13.21.

Application of the "foramen magnum pump" is demonstrated in Figure 13.22 and is performed by grasping the occiput while applying traction to the full spine with caudal distraction.

The application of heat and sinusoidal muscle stimulation or ultrasound with sinusoidal currents, either before or after

manipulation, also provides relief from pain for patients with discogenic spondyloarthrosis.

Other considerations in the treatment of patients with the degenerative low back are important.

1. Nutrition. Osteoporosis is a common accompanying factor with the older spine. Therefore, amino acids to build osteoid tissue and calcium to aid in bone ossification are recommended and prescribed. Manganese (500 to 800 mg/day) which is an ingredient of Discat, a nutritional supplement, is also prescribed. Niacin (200

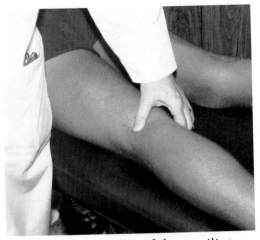

**Figure 13.21.** Insertion of the gracilis tendon being goaded at the medial tibal condyle.

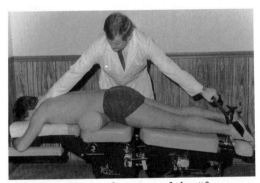

**Figure 13.22.** Application of the "foramen magnum pump" in full-spine occipital distraction.

mg/day) and vitamin B₆ (150 mg/day) are also recommended. The alkalinity of the bowel depresses the absorption of calcium. This is due to the low output of HCl and enzymes in the elderly and may account for the etiology of osteoporosis along with endocrine hyposecretion. Thus, digestive enzymes are also prescribed.

2. Exercise. Walking improves the circulation and increases the muscular activity of the paravertebral musculature, thereby enhancing the flow of nutrients to the bone tissue as well as the removal of waste materials. Thus, it is recommended for patients with discogenic spondyloarthrosis.

3. Check and strengthen the gracilis tendon to enhance the adrenal output and, thereby, the general well being of the patient. This is shown later in this chapter.

## FAILED BACK SURGERY SYNDROME

As cited in Chapter 1, up to 50% of the patients who have had surgery to relieve low back pain have recurrence of symptoms. To these patients who want to avoid further surgery, if possible, conservative care is most appealing. They, consequently, are most cooperative and follow instructions better than patients who have not had surgery. As "good patients," they are, of course, a pleasure to treat.

**Case 3** is of a 61-year-old white man who has low back and left S1 dermatome pain. Two laminectomies for removal of the L4-L5 disc had been performed 4 and 7 years previously. The neurosurgeon does not wish to operate again if conservative care is successful.

On examination, range of motion is 90° on flexion, 5° on extension, 10° on right lateral bending, 20° on left lateral bending, 10° on right rotation, and 10° on left rotation. The straight leg raise is 90° on the right and 45° on the left; it causes left leg pain. There is marked shortness of the hamstring muscles. Muscle strength is equal and good during dorsiflexion and plantar flexion of the feet and great toes. There is gluteus maximus muscle weakness with a gluteal skyline sign on the left. Deep reflexes are active and ++ for the ankle and knee. Déjérine's triad is negative. Kemp's sign is bilaterally positive.

X-rays reveal that right lateral bending (Fig. 13.25) compared with the left lateral bending (Fig. 13.24) is restricted. In Figure 13.23, L4 can be seen in left lateral flexion subluxation on L5, and L3 can be seen in right lateral flexion subluxation on L4. There is also marked loss of L4-L5 and L1-L2 disc spaces (Figs. 13.26 and 13.27) and arteriosclerosis of the abdominal aorta and iliac vessels. A defect in the anterior subarachnoid space at L4-L5 indicates nuclear protrusion at that level (Figs. 13.28 and 13.29).

This patient has L4-L5 nuclear protrusion and perhaps development of an old adhesion.

Treatment consisted of flexion distraction manipulation at the L4-L5 level following goading of acupressure points B24 to B35, B49, and B54, and kinesiology of the adductors, gluteus maximus, abductors, and hamstring group. Physical therapy was applied in the

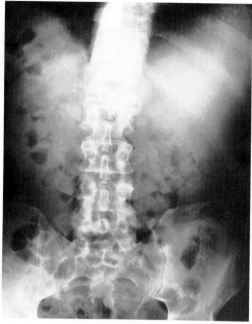

**Figure 13.23.** Neutral posteroanterior view of the lumbar spine and pelvis reveals that L4 is in left lateral flexion on L5 and L3 is in right lateral flexion on L4.

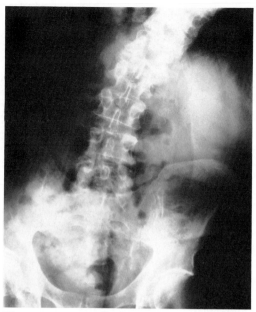

**Figure 13.25.** Right lateral flexion view of the same patient as in Figure 13.23. Hypomobility is present at the L4-L5 level.

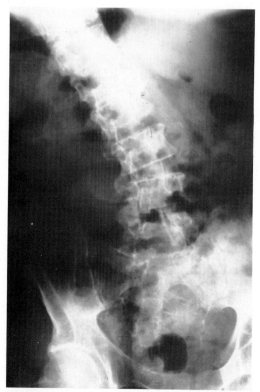

**Figure 13.24.** Left lateral flexion view of the same patient as in Figure 13.23. Marked mobility is noted.

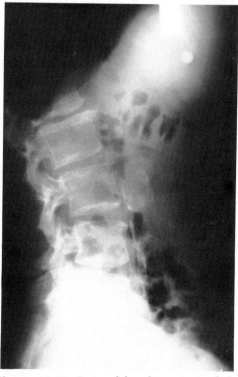

**Figure 13.26.** Lateral lumbar view of the same patient as in Figure 13.23. L1-L2 and L4-L5 disc degeneration is noted.

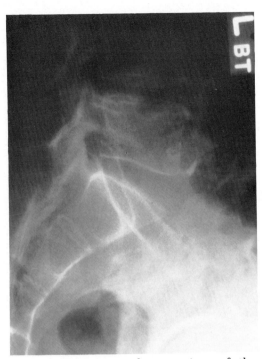

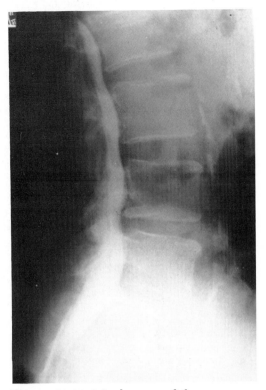

**Figure 13.27.** Lateral spot view of the same patient as in Figure 13.23.

**Figure 13.28.** Myelogram of the same patient as in Figure 13.23 shows an L4-L5 defect in the dye-filled subarachnoid space.

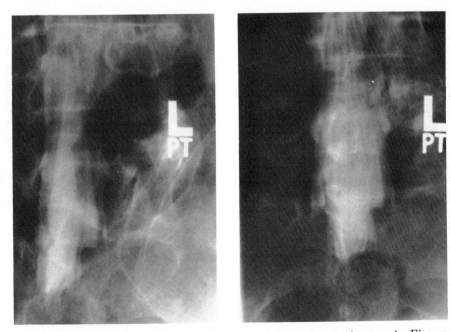

**Figure 13.29.** Oblique view of the myelogram of the same patient as in Figure 13.23 fails to reveal a marked defect.

form of positive galvanism to L4-L5 and hot and cold alternating packs. Treatment was given 3 times a week for 4 weeks.

The patient received distraction treatments which resulted in a more than 50% relief from low back and leg pain. The patient was originally told that 50% relief from pain would be an excellent response in 3 months of care; he exceeded that in 2 weeks.

**Case 4** is of a 53-year-old man who 12 years ago had had a fusion for spondylolisthesis because of prolonged low back pain. Now he has low back pain and anterior and lateral right thigh numbness paresthesias.

On examination, range of motion is 90° on flexion, 10° on extension, 10° on right lateral bending, and 10° on rotation bilaterally. All motion takes place at the femoral heads and upper lumbar spine. There is an incision over the S2 and S1 spinous process with a right ilial incision where iliac bone was removed for fusion. Deep reflexes and muscle strengths of the lower extremities are active and equal. Hypoesthesia of the right anterolateral thigh in L3 and L4 dermatomes is noted. The hamstring muscles are very shortened. The straight leg raise is negative otherwise. Kemp's sign is negative. Déjérine's triad is negative.

X-rays (Figs. 13.30 to 13.33) reveal that there is a surgical intertransverse bone fusion and interspinous wiring of L4-L5 and L5-S1. Lateral bending reveals motion of L3 and L4 on the segments cephalad. There is posterior disc thinning of the L3-L4 disc space, with a retrolisthesis subluxation of L3 on L4 indicative of instability at this level, especially when this finding is combined with the traction spurs at the L3-L4 anterolateral body plates. The body of L5 is displaced 10% anteriorly on the sacrum. Also, there is a facet syndrome at the L3-L4 level.

The fusion of L4-L5-S1 has placed all lumbar mobility at the L3-L4 level which is now unstable, as noted in the x-ray findings. There is a 10% spondylolisthesis (either true or degenerative or a combination) of L5. The femoral nerve is involved as indicated by the numbness of the anterolateral thigh, perhaps by the facet syndrome at the L3-L4 level or a discal protrusion at L3-L4.

Treatment consisted of motion palpation of L3-L4 performed on the Cox table. Distraction was then applied at the L3-L4 segment while the facets at L3-L4 and L2-L3 were placed through physiological motion. Acupressure points B24 to B35 and B49 were goaded. Blocking of the pelvis for a left posterior ilium and a right anterior ilium was given. Stretching of hamstring muscles and the performance of

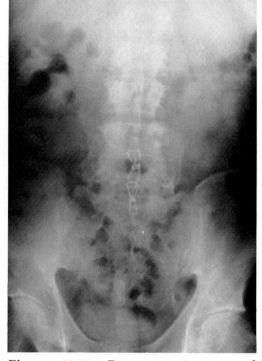

**Figure 13.30.** Posteroanterior neutral view revealing intertransverse fusion and interspinous wiring.

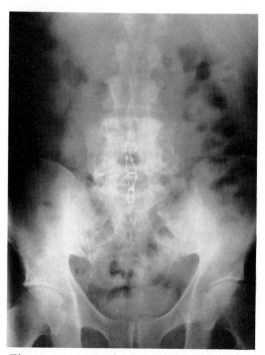

**Figure 13.31.** Right lateral bending view revealing mobility above the fusion.

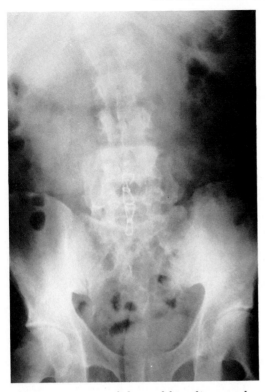

**Figure 13.32.** Left lateral bending study.

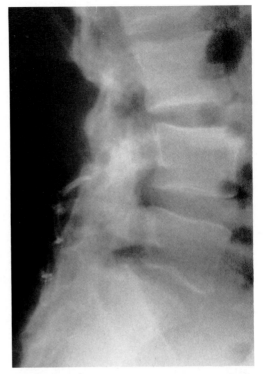

**Figure 13.33.** Lateral projection of the same patient as in Figure 13.30. Note L3-L4 disc thinning and retrolisthesis of L3 on L4. L5 is displaced 10% anteriorly on the sacrum (spondylolisthesis).

other exercises were started. Physical therapy consisting of positive galvanism at the L3-L4 level was given.

This patient was seen 3 times a week for 3 weeks. At the end of 3 weeks treatment, he had no right thigh paresthesias. He felt such relief from low back pain that he was able to golf 3 times weekly and stated that he felt better than he had in many years.

**Case 5** is of a 67-year-old white woman who had had low back and left leg pain for 3 years. In 1969, a laminectomy and fusion had been performed with removal of L4-L5 and L5-S1 discs. She had consulted two chiropractors who would not treat her due to the fusion. She has recently experienced numbness of her left great toe. Neurosurgical consultation yielded the diagnosis of back strain.

On examination, range of motion is 20° on flexion, 10° on extension, 20° on right lateral flexion, 5° on left lateral flexion, 20° on right rotation, and 20° on left rotation. Straight leg raise is positive for low back pain on the right at 45° and on the left at 25°. Déjérine's triad is positive. Walking increased low back and left leg pain. Deep reflexes are ++ bilaterally. Sensory examination reveals hypoesthesia of

the left L4-L5 dermatomes. Kemp's sign is positive on the left.

X-rays reveal:

1. Dextroscoliosis of the lumbar spine (Fig. 13.34). (Figure 13.38, an overlay of the original scoliosis to the correction at the end of 6 weeks care, i.e., from 9/28/82 to 11/9/82, shows reduction of the dextrorotation.)

2. A 24-mm shortness of the left femoral head and hemipelvis (Fig. 13.35). (Correction of this shortness with a 12.5-mm lift can be seen in Figure 13.36. Note it took one-half the shortness to correct the deficiency; this measurement is best found by x-ray with heel and sole lifts in place. Afterwards, the patient is sent for the buildup.)

3. Intertransverse fusion of L4-L5 and the sacrum, which has placed all motion at the L3-L4 level and above. These levels are normally not asked to flex and extend, and when this type of movement is placed on them, a resultant degenerative disc disease sets in. Note the right lateral flexion subluxation of L3 on L4 and the right rotosubluxation of L2 on L3.

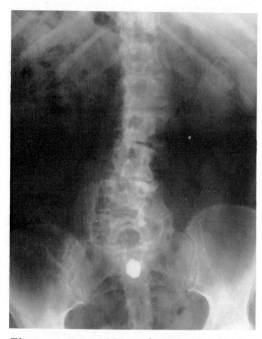

**Figure 13.34.** Neutral posteroanterior view of the lumbar spine and pelvis. Dextroscoliosis and intertransverse fusion of L4 through the sacrum are noted. L2 is in right rotation, and there is right lateral listhesis subluxation on L3.

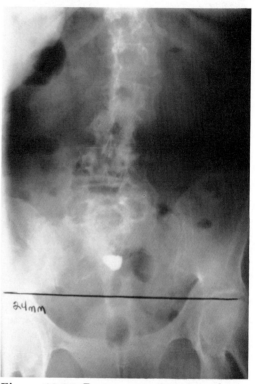

**Figure 13.35.** Posteroanterior view showing a 24-mm shortness of the left femoral head and hemipelvis.

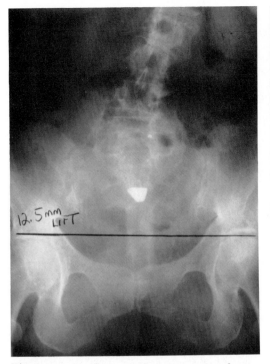

**Figure 13.36.** Posteroanterior view showing that a 12.5-mm lift placed under the left shoe has corrected the shortness.

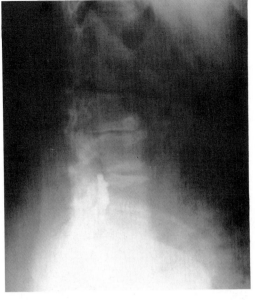

**Figure 13.37.** Lateral view of the same patient as in Figure 13.34.

4. L2-L3 and L3-L4 disc degeneration and rotation deformities of L2 on L3 (Fig. 13.37).

Treatment consisted of Cox distraction without the ankle cuffs. Rotation and lateral bending to the right were used with gentle caudal traction. Sinusoidal current was applied to the right thoracolumbar spine.

In 3 months, the patient obtained much more than 50% relief from low back and leg pain. Originally, she had been told not to expect 100% relief and that 50% relief could be considered an excellent response. After the first 3 months of care, she received treatment once every 2 weeks.

## Treatment of Failed Back Surgery Syndrome

Spinal manipulative therapy for the patient with the failed back surgery syndrome is applied under strict parameters:

1. Never is the caudal section of the table lowered over 2 inches.
2. Rotation is never applied to the lower lumbar spine.

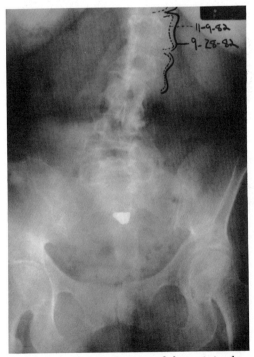

**Figure 13.38.** Overlaying of the original x-ray (Fig. 13.34) with this x-ray reveals some reduction of the rotational subluxation after 6 weeks of treatment.

3. No electrical intermittent traction is used—only hand-controlled manual manipulation.

4. Any lateral flexion is restricted to facet capability; lateral bending should never be forced.

5. The primary motion used is flexion.

6. Traction is applied above the fused segments.

Figure 13.39 is a photograph of the back of the patient discussed in Case 5 who had had surgery. Flexion to the spinous process is applied above the fusion, as is demonstrated in Figure 13.40. The rules for application of traction, which were given previously, are followed. In Figure 13.41, lateral flexion of the segments is demonstrated.

Sinusoidal currents are applied to the paravertebral muscles as demonstrated in Figure 13.42. Hydrocollator packs are applied over the sinusoidal current pads for 10 minutes (Fig. 13.43). Cold packs are then applied for 5 minutes (Fig. 13.44). Hot and cold packs, beginning and ending with heat, are applied alternately.

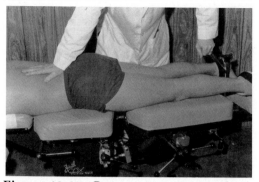

**Figure 13.40.** Contact is maintained on the spinous process above the surgical fusion shown in Figure 13.39.

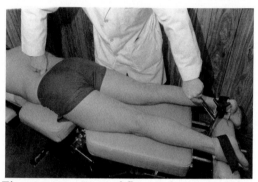

**Figure 13.41.** Lateral flexion being applied to the same patient as in Figure 13.39.

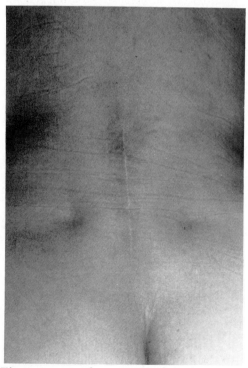

**Figure 13.39.** Photograph of the back of a patient with failed back surgery syndrome.

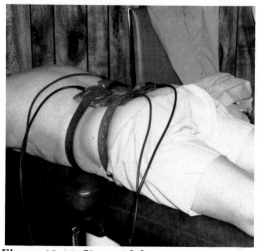

**Figure 13.42.** Sinusoidal current being applied to the same patient as in Figure 13.39.

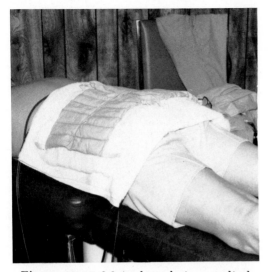

**Figure 13.43.** Moist heat being applied.

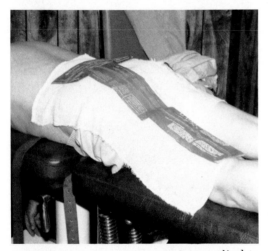

**Figure 13.44.** Cold packs being applied to the low back and sciatic distribution.

In Figure 13.45, unilateral traction being applied without the ankle cuffs is shown; the ankle is held while distraction is being applied. By the holding of each lower extremity, the facets can be more strongly tractioned unilaterally.

Figures 13.46 and 13.47 are x-rays of a patient with hip arthroplasty. Commonly, these patients also have degenerative disc disease and are best treated unilaterally, as shown in Figure 13.45, in order to control traction on the involved replaced hip socket.

Patients with the failed back surgery syndrome are treated by goading of acupressure kinesiology points, as shown in

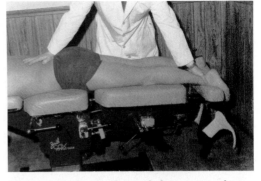

**Figure 13.45.** Unilateral distraction being applied.

Figures 13.18 to 13.21. Treatments are given daily until the pain subsides in the lower extremities; then they are reduced to 3 visits daily until 50% relief is obtained. We tell these patients that 50% relief is an excellent clinical response.

## COMPRESSION FRACTURE

**Case 6** is of a 76-year-old white woman who had developed thoracolumbar spine pain following a fall down her basement steps. She had had 13 chiropractic adjustments and found that they hurt her, causing her to seek a second opinion. No x-rays had been taken prior to treatment.

X-rays reveal about a one-third loss of height with central and left body compression deformity at the T12 vertebral body. Generalized osteoporosis is also present (Figs. 13.48 and 13.49).

This patient has a compression fracture of the T12 vertebral body (35%).

Treatment consisted of extension manipulation on the Cox table (see Figs. 13.50 and 13.51) and home hyperextension exercises. Also, nonphosphorous calcium (1000 mg daily) and amino acids were prescribed.

The patient obtained complete relief from pain in 2 months. She was advised to avoid carrying heavy packages or hyperflexing at the waist.

## SACROILIAC JOINT POSITIONING

### Evaluation and Treatment of the Innominates

ANTERIOR INNOMINATE

When the innominate ilium portion is anterior and the ischium is posterior, the following findings will be noted:

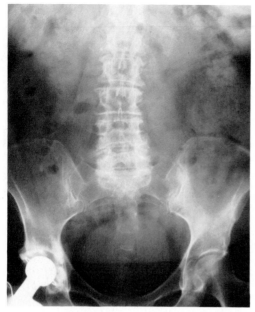

**Figure 13.46.** Anteroposterior view of the lumbar spine and pelvis of a patient with hip arthroplasty.

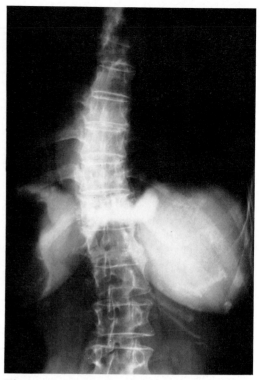

**Figure 13.48.** Anteroposterior view showing compression fracture at T12.

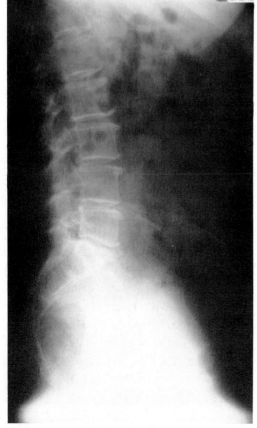

**Figure 13.47.** Lateral view of the same patient as in Figure 13.46.

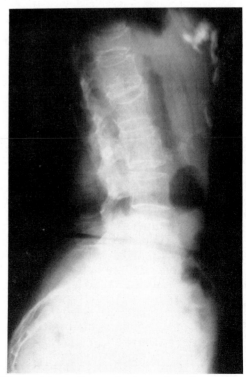

**Figure 13.49.** Lateral view showing compression fracture at T12 of the same patient as in Figure 13.48.

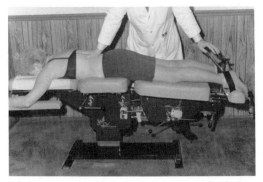

**Figure 13.50.** Mild flexion distraction being applied.

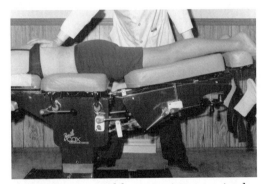

**Figure 13.51.** Mild extension manipulation being applied.

1. Long leg on mensuration.

2. A low ilium and an anterior ilium on visual examination.

3. Spasm of the gluteus medius and minimus muscles and the quadriceps muscles and weakness of the gluteus maximus muscle, the hamstring muscles, and the gracilis muscle on testing are probable.

4. Spasm of the gluteus medius and minimus muscles and/or weakness of the gluteus maximus muscle and piriformis muscle can result in internal rotation of the foot.

5. Spasm of the gluteus maximus muscle and piriformis muscle and/or weakness of the gluteus medius and minimus muscles can result in external rotation of the foot.

6. Bilateral anterior iliae of the anterior pelvis on x-rays (see Fig. 13.52, A and B). The pelvic outlet is vertically increased in height, and the obturator foramina are smaller.

Treatment of the anterior innominate is accomplished in the following way:

1. Balance the gluteal muscles by strengthening the gluteus maximus muscle and relaxing the gluteus medius and

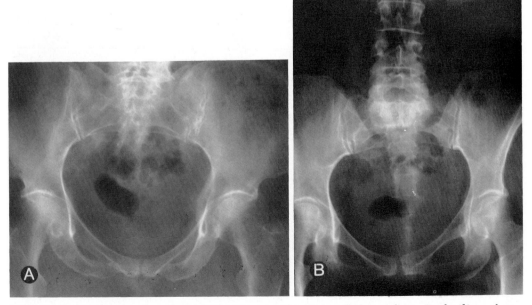

**Figure 13.52.** X-ray showing bilateral anterior iliae of the pelvis. Both iliae show anterior motion in two different cases.

minimus muscles as described later in this chapter.

2. Strengthen the hamstring muscles and relax the quadriceps muscles as described later in this chapter.

3. Balance the piriformis muscle as described later in this chapter.

4. Place a block under the anterior superior iliac spine (ASIS) and traction the innominate as shown in Figure 13.53. This can be done while a disc lesion, facet syndrome, or other low back condition is being reduced. If both innominates are anterior (anterior pelvis), a Dutchman roll can be placed under the iliae and both iliae can be distracted simultaneously (Fig. 13.54).

5. Maintain hand contact on the L5 spinous process with cephalad pressure for 20 seconds while pumping the caudal section of the table up and down 2 inches. This 20-second distraction is repeated 3 times.

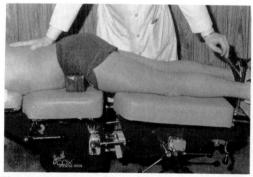

Figure 13.53. Unilateral correction being applied to the anterior ilium.

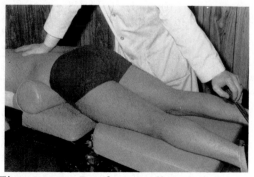

Figure 13.54. Dutchman roll is placed under the iliae for correction of a bilateral anterior pelvis.

## POSTERIOR INNOMINATE

When the innominate ilium portion is posterior and the ischium is anterior, the following findings will be noted:

1. Short leg mensuration.

2. A high and posterior ilium on visual examination.

3. Spasm of the gluteus maximus muscle, weakness of the gluteus medius and minimus muscles, the gracilis muscle, and possibly the quadriceps muscles, tenderness of the gracilis muscle over the medial tibial insertion, and strength in the hamstring muscles on testing are probable.

4. The feet will rotate inward or outward according to the muscle changes described under #4 of the anterior innominate.

5. Enlargement of the obturator foramen and lessening of the pelvic outlet vertical height on x-rays (Figs. 13.55, 13.56, and 13.57).

Treatment of the posterior innominate is accomplished in the following way:

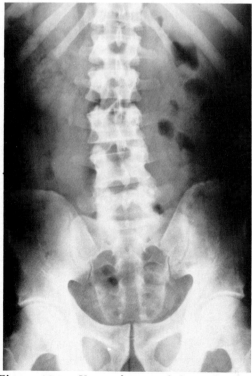

Figure 13.55. X-ray showing bilateral posterior iliae.

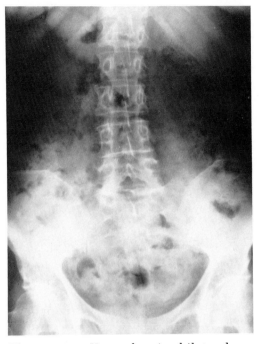

**Figure 13.56.** X-ray showing bilateral posterior iliae.

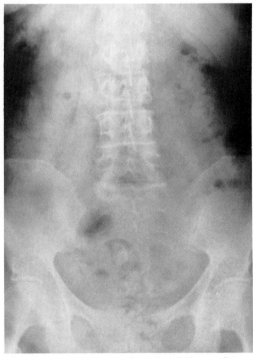

**Figure 13.57.** X-ray showing bilateral posterior iliae.

1. Balance the gluteal muscle by relaxing the gluteus maximus muscle and strengthening the gluteus medius and minimus muscles as described later in this chapter.

2. Relax the hamstring muscles and strengthen the quadriceps muscles as described later in this chapter.

3. Balance the piriformis muscle, after foot rotation and testing, as described later in this chapter.

4. Place a block under the acetabulum and traction the innominate (Fig. 13.58). This can be done while a disc lesion, facet syndrome, or other low back condition is being treated.

5. Maintain hand contact on the L5 spinous process with cephalad pressure for 20 seconds while pumping the caudal section of the table up and down 2 inches. This 20-second distraction is repeated 3 times.

## RETROLISTHESIS

Retrolisthesis can be caused by three primary factors:

1. Congenital underdevelopment of the pedicles of the lumbar vertebrae, the so-called pedicogenic spondylosis, may result. This underdevelopment certainly creates alteration of motion function and can be relieved only by the best of treatment.

2. Multifidus and rotatores muscle spasm.

3. Subluxation of a primary traumatic etiology, such as hyperflexion.

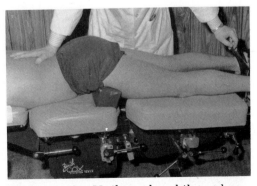

**Figure 13.58.** Unilateral or bilateral correction of the posterior ilium being applied.

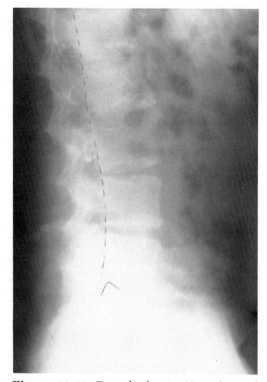

**Figure 13.59.** Retrolisthesis. Note loss of lumbar lordosis as revealed by George's line.

Examination should reveal the following:

1. Underdevelopment of the pedicles, which is often shown on oblique views also, or posterior displacement as revealed by George's line (a line drawn along the posterior bodies of the vertebrae) (Figs. 13.59 through 13.64).

2. Flattening of the lumbar lordosis on visual examination.

3. Spasm over the paravertebral musculature, which is very tender to touch, gluteus maximus spasm and tenderness, and an adductor that is spastic and tender to touch are possible.

Treatment should consist of the following:

1. Apply very gentle traction with the use of the Zenith-Cox table. As you may have noticed previously in handling this subluxation entity, thrusting into it can often be very painful to the patient. With the use of the Zenith-Cox table, very ex-

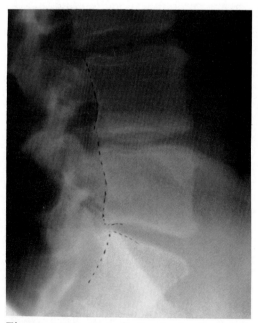

**Figure 13.60.** Retrolisthesis. L5 is posterior on the sacrum, as revealed by George's line.

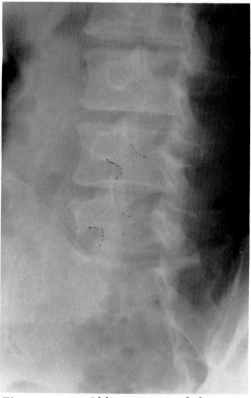

**Figure 13.61.** Oblique view of the same patient as in Figure 13.60. The pedicle of L5 seems less sagitally developed than that of L4 or L3.

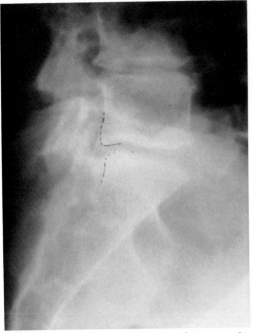

**Figure 13.62.** Retrolisthesis of L5 on the sacrum. There is loss of the L4-L5 and L5-S1 disc spaces.

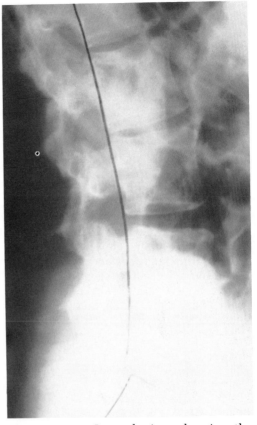

**Figure 13.64.** Lateral view showing the loss of lumbar lordosis commonly seen in retrolisthesis, in the same patient as in Figure 13.62.

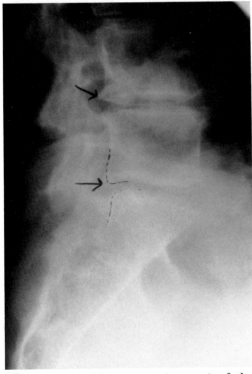

**Figure 13.63.** Note spurs (*arrows*) of the posterior body plates at L4 and L5.

cellent relief is afforded without the need for thrusting into the severe spasm accompanying this subluxation and possibly causing further damage.

2. Balance the muscles, as needed, according to the instructions given later in this chapter.

3. Apply deep Nimmo-type goading over the paravertebral levels in the lumbar area.

4. Apply acupressure over K1 and B54, as shown in the treatment of sciatica, which will afford rapid relief from pain.

## SACRUM INFERIORITY

Sacrum inferiority is usually found in patients with spasm of the piriformis muscle and with weakness of the opposite piriformis muscle.

Diagnosis of this entity can be determined from the following findings:

1. The innominates are fairly or completely level.

2. The sacrum is oblique in position between the innominates and is inferior on one side.

Treatment should consist of the following:

1. Treat the side of sacral base inferiority and lean for a spastic piriformis muscle (see section entitled "Piriformis Muscle"). External rotation of the thigh and foot on this side should be found.

2. Treat the side of sacral base superiority for a relatively weak piriformis muscle, as described later in this chapter.

3. Maintain a notch contact on the side of the inferiority of the sacrum in a cephalad direction for 30 seconds, during which time the patient is asked to slowly inhale and exhale. Then apply a thrust cephalad to the inferior sacrum. (See sketch below.)

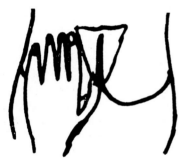

4. Check and treat for hamstring muscle spasm on the side of the inferiority. The lateral hamstring muscles are tested by forcing the flexed knee into extension in a medial direction; the medial hamstring muscles (semimembranosus and semitendinosus), by forcing the flexed knee into extension in a lateral direction.

Remember that the piriformis muscle often is pierced by the common peroneal branch of the sciatic nerve; therefore, spasm of the muscle can cause or aggravate sciatica.

## MUSCLE EVALUATION AND TREATMENT

It seems reasonable to trace the development of disc weakness and protrusion to early muscle weakness or spasm causing altered motoricity of the low back. In treatment of a disc protrusion, we must first concern ourselves with the extreme pain of the patient due to the nerve root compression. This necessitates the use of the Cox technic for reduction. Following reduction, we retrace the etiology by evaluating the muscles for weakness or spasticity and correct the muscles in order to establish a stable low back and to avoid future disc problems.

### GENERAL MUSCULAR CONDITION

Following reduction of the protruded nuclear material via Cox technic, we proceed with the evaluation of the musculature. The patient is asked to stand with his feet 4 inches apart. As we examine the patient, we look for the following:

1. Height of the iliae. Mark the high and low side. We are primarily interested in the side of pain.

2. Internal or external rotation of the foot or feet.

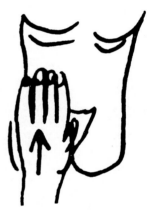

3. Relative internal or external flare rotation of the iliae.

4. Height of occiput. Mark the high side.

5. Anteroposterior lumbar curvature for lordotic decrease or increase.

6. Lean of the lumbar spine laterally.

We, of course, admit that congenital anomalies of the low back precipitate instability and lead to altered motoricity. We assert, however, that muscle balancing can afford the stability needed to render these anomalies asymptomatic.

Next the patient is asked to walk across the room. We look for internal or external rotation of the feet.

Then we study the individual muscles

and groups of muscles, such as the adductor, piriformis, gluteal, psoas, multifidus, and rotatores, quadriceps, and abdominal muscles.

## ADDUCTOR MUSCLES

### Gracilis Muscle

The gracilis or "tie-down" muscle of the pelvis permits anterior and posterior rotation of the ileum. Its origin is in the pubic bone near the symphysis pubis (Fig. 13.65). Its insertion is in the medial tibia below the condyle. Its nerve supply is the L3 and L4 nerve roots.

Functional alterations result in extreme tenderness and weakness of muscles in patients with sciatica. Ilium rotation often accompanies sciatica, and weakness of the gracilis allows the pelvis to rotate posteriorly.

Treatment of gracilis weakness consists of 10 to 20 seconds of deep goading at its origin and insertion.

According to Goodheart (1), the gracilis and sartorius muscles are indicators of the condition of the adrenal gland. In all cases of repeated posterior ilium subluxations, consider adrenal depletion from stress as the etiology. The use of the neurolymphatic reflexes or adrenal protomorphogen is helpful in the treatment of this condition.

Remember these factors about the gracilis muscle:

1. Weakness of the gracilis muscle results in a posterior ilium.

2. Adrenal insufficiency causes weakness of the gracilis and sartorius muscles. Stress, therefore, is involved.

3. The inguinal ligament is sore over its lower half in cases of sciatica and posterior ilium.

Test for gracilis weakness by pressing downward and outward on the patient's leg at the ankle while stabilizing the thigh as shown in Figure 13.66.

### Adductor Group Including Longus, Brevis, and Magnus Muscles

We have found that the adductor group is the specific key treatment area in patients with sciatic neuralgia caused by disc protrusion. Treatment of these muscles allows relief of pain much as acupressure provides control of pain. Therefore, the adductor group is the most important and the first muscle group we treat in controlling sciatica in patients with a disc lesion.

Its origin is in the pubis, ischium, and ramus (Fig. 13.67). Its insertion is in the medial femur in the linea aspera and femoral condyle. Its nerve supply is the 3rd and 4th lumbar nerve roots and a branch of the *sciatic* nerve. (*This is my idea of the reflex pattern allowing the relief of sciatica.*)

I have never treated a patient with sciatica caused by disc protrusion without finding some degree of adductor soreness. I test for this in the following way:

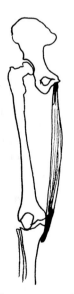

**Figure 13.65.** Illustration of gracilis muscle.

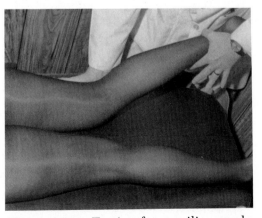

**Figure 13.66.** Testing for gracilis muscle strength.

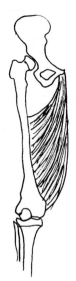

**Figure 13.67.** Illustration of the origin and the insertion of the adductor muscle group.

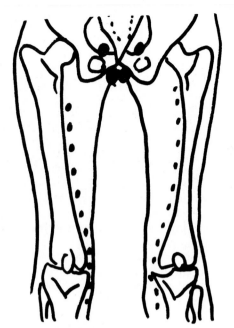

**Figure 13.68.** Illustration of origin and insertion points of the adductor muscles, which are used for goading.

1. Palpation of the muscle will reveal adductor soreness.

2. Weakness can be evaluated by having the patient lie supine, holding the legs tightly together. The patient is asked to keep his legs together while I grasp both legs just below the knee and try to force one leg apart (the other leg is being stabilized with my other hand). Due to pain, often the test cannot be performed in any other patient position.

Treatment of the adductor group consists of firm rotatory pressure being applied at its insertion along the medial femur for 20 to 30 seconds (Fig. 13.68). This pressure may bruise someone with capillary fragility, but this is of no significance. Constant pressure with the index area of the hand is applied to the pubic and ischial origins for 15 to 20 seconds while pressure over the inguinal ligament is maintained.

## GLUTEAL MUSCLES

The gluteus maximus arises from the ilium behind the ilial gluteal line, the posteroinferior sacrum, and the sacrotuberous ligament to insert into the iliotibial band. It acts to extend and laterally rotate the thigh.

The gluteus medius arises from the il-ium crest area to insert into the greater trochanter. It acts as an internal rotator and abductor of the thigh.

The gluteus minimus arises from the outer ilium and sciatic notch to insert into the greater trochanter. It acts as a medial rotator and abductor of the thigh (Figs. 13.69, 13.70, and 13.71).

Gluteus maximus spasm causes the il-ium to externally rotate and posteriorly deviate (posterior ilium). Gluteus maximus spasm causes the foot to rotate outward.

Sixty percent of patients with a L5-S1 disc lesion have weakness and visible atrophy of the gluteus maximus muscle on the side of these lesions; this is called the gluteal skyline sign (2).

Gluteus medius and minimus weakness allows external rotation of the leg and foot as well as elevation of the ilium. Spasm of the gluteus medius and minimus causes internal rotation of the feet. *Therefore, external rotation of the leg and foot represents gluteus maximus spasm and/or gluteus medius and minimus weakness.*

*Elevation of the ilium represents weakness of the gluteus medius and minimus muscles, as is seen in posterior ilium.*

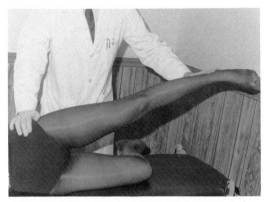

**Figure 13.69.** Testing for weakness of the gluteus medius muscle. Push the thigh forward and down.

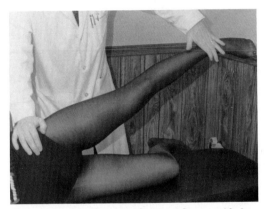

**Figure 13.70.** Testing for weakness of the gluteus minimus muscle. Push the thigh backward and down.

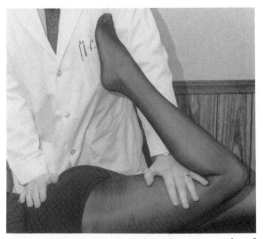

**Figure 13.71.** Testing for the strength of the gluteus maximus muscle.

Treatment for gluteus maximus spasm and/or gluteus medius and minimus weakness consists of the following:

1. Apply deep pressure into the belly of the gluteus maximus muscle for relaxation.
2. Goad the origins and insertions of the gluteus minimus and medius muscles.
3. Check for weak abdominalis muscles as shown in Figure 13.72. These muscles are antagonists to the gluteals. Treat by pressure to the origin and insertions.
4. Goodheart (1) neurolymphatic reflexes can be used in strengthening these muscles.

A typical anterior ilium pattern may be seen with gluteus maximus weakness and/or medius and minimus spasm.

Treatment consists of the following:

1. Goad the origin and insertion of the gluteus maximus muscles.
2. Apply pressure to the belly of the medius and minimus muscles.

The anterior and posterior ilium patterns may be seen with sciatic conditions. These two specific entities have been dis-

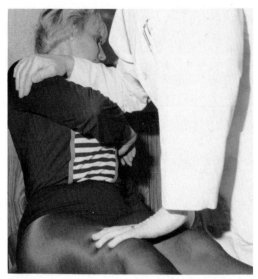

**Figure 13.72.** Testing for abdominal muscle strength. The patient sits upright to 70° and rotates at the waist while pressure is applied on the chest to push the patient supine. Stabilize the patient at the thighs so that the patient's legs don't raise from the table.

cussed in detail previously. They are treated after the disc protrusion has been reduced.

## PIRIFORMIS MUSCLE

This flat muscle originates at the front of the sacrum, inserting into the greater trochanter and acting as an external rotator of the thigh. It is intimate with the gluteus medius at its anatomical insertion.

Testing of the piriformis muscle is accomplished by grasping the patient's leg and ankle a shown in Figure 13.73, with the thigh externally rotated. Medial ankle pressure is applied laterally while the thigh is stabilized.

Weakness of the piriformis muscle results in internal rotation of the thigh and foot and a "knock knee" appearance. Strengthening of this muscle is usually accomplished by applying pressure on its insertion at the greater trochanter.

Spasm of the piriformis muscle externally rotates the thigh and foot and is relieved by pressure in the belly of the muscle from outside or by pressure applied from inside by rectal entrance.

The piriformis muscle is capable of sacral motion independent of the innominate by causing the sacrum to be inferior and posterior on the side of spasticity and relatively anterior and superior on the weak side.

### Occiput Height

We wish to stress that weakness of the posterior and anterior cervical spine muscles occurs with low back and pelvic weakness. A high occiput can occur on the side of gluteus medius and minimus muscle weakness and/or piriformis muscle weakness.

The cervical muscles should be balanced and any weakness in the low back should be strengthened.

## PSOAS MUSCLE

In acute sciatica, treatment of the psoas muscle is not helpful in controlling pain (Fig. 13.74). Later, after the pain has lessened, it can be treated for weakness by firm pressure at its insertion at the lesser trochanter and for spasm by lateral side-bending and flexion on the Zenith-Cox table. Goodheart (1) reflexes are utilized in the treatment of any kidney pathology.

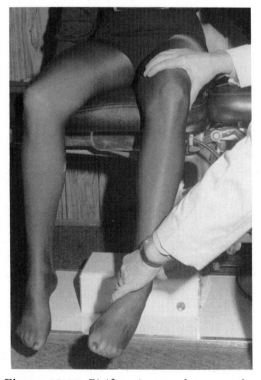

**Figure 13.73.** Piriformis muscle strength test.

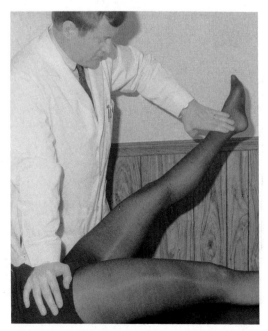

**Figure 13.74.** Psoas muscle strength test.

## QUADRICEPS MUSCLES

Treatment of the quadriceps muscles is not important in cases of acute disc lesions. Treatment of these muscles is important, however, in cases of anterior and posterior innominate lesions.

In cases of anterior ilium lesions, the quadriceps are spastic; in cases of posterior ilium lesions, they are weak.

Testing for weakness of the quadriceps muscles is accomplished as shown in Figure 13.75. Press down on the ankle while stabilizing the thigh.

Treatment of the quadriceps muscles is accomplished as follows: If there is spasm, pressure is applied into the belly of the rectus femoris and vastus lateralis, medialis, and intermedius muscles. If there is weakness, goading of the origin and insertions is done. Remember: it is weakness of the vastus group that leads to cartilage problems of the knee joint.

## HAMSTRING MUSCLES

The hamstring muscles are important in cases of disc lesion, as weakness of the hamstring muscles occurs along with the gluteus maximus and calf muscles with S1 dermatome involvement.

Testing for hamstring muscle weakness is accomplished as shown in Figure 13.76. The medial hamstrings (semitendinosus and semimembranosus) are tested by having the patient resist a force applied laterally on the ankle. The lateral hamstring (biceps femoris) is tested by having the patient resist a force applied medially on the leg.

Treatment of the hamstrings is accomplished as follows: If there is spasm, pressure is applied into the belly of the muscles for 20 seconds. If there is weakness, goading of the origins and insertions is done for 15 seconds.

## MULTIFIDUS AND ROTATORES MUSCLES

Multifidus muscles are important in extension and rotation of the vertebral column. Their origin is in the mammillary processes in the lumbar region. Their insertion is in the spinous processes of one, two, three, or four vertebrae above.

Rotatores muscles are important in rotation of the vertebral column. Their origin is in the transverse process. Their

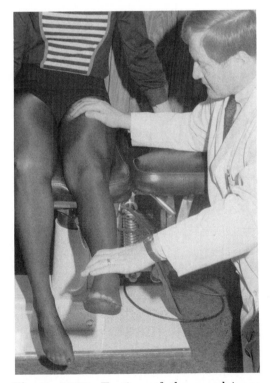

**Figure 13.75.** Testing of the quadriceps muscles. Press down on the leg at the ankle while stabilizing the thigh. (The quadriceps muscles may also be tested by flexing the knee and having the patient attempt extension of the knee joint.)

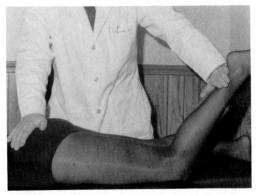

**Figure 13.76.** Testing of the hamstring muscle group. Have the patient forcefully resist extension of the knee joint as a force is applied on the leg at the ankle. Also ask the patient to attempt flexion of the knee joint while forced resistance is placed on the leg at the ankle.

insertion is in the lamina of the vertebra above.

Treatment of the multifidus and rotatores muscles is accomplished with deep Nimmo-type goading or application of pulsating sinusoidal current which brings about relaxation of these deep spinal muscles.

*In all cases of sciatica, these muscles are checked and treated accordingly. Specific conditions of the low back may be found in conjunction with sciatica, and each will* *necessitate correction following reduction of the disc protrusion by the Cox technic in order to insure stability of the low back in the future and to prevent a recurrence.*

## References

1. Goodheart G: *Applied Kinesiology (The Neurolymphatic Reflex and Its Relationship to Muscle Balancing)*, ed 3. Private publication, 1970, pp 15–18, 36, 37, and 45.
2. Katznelson A, Nerubay J, Lev-el A: The gluteal skyline sign. *Spine* 7(1):74, 1982.

*Genius may be described as the spirit of discovery — It is the eye of the intellect, and the wing of thought — It is always in advance of its time — The pioneer for the generation it precedes.*

*—Simms*

# Nutrition of the Intervertebral Disc

Direct vascular contacts, vascular buds, exist between the marrow spaces of the vertebral body and the hyaline cartilage of the end plates of the vertebra and are important for the nutrition of the disc (1). Until a person reaches the early 20s, the intervertebral disc receives nutrients via the epiphyseal end plates. Following their closure, however, a thinning of the hyaline cartilage between the nucleus and the vertebral body and an ingrowth of granulation tissue, which becomes important in the nutrition of the disc, occur. There is a diffusion of solutes both from the cancellous bone of the vertebral body into the nucleus through the end plate as well as from the anterior and posterior annulus fibrosus. Oxygen and glucose enter primarily through the former route, whereas the sulfate radical enters primarily through the anterior and posterior annulus fibrosus.

According to Naylor et al. (2), studies of the components of the disc by use of chemical analysis, x-ray crystallography, and electron microscopy have shown that in disc degeneration a fall in the total sulfate (both chondroitin sulfate and keratin sulfate) occurs with age. Happey, Wiseman, and Naylor (2a) have shown that there is a gradual diminution of the sulfate content of the disc with aging and degeneration and that the prolapsed nucleus pulposus usually contains values of sulfate less than half those of the normal disc. Keep in mind that the posterior annular fibers have the poorest nutrition, although they are subjected to the greatest strain by a bulging turgor-filled nucleus pulposus.

Robles (3), in an extensive study of the nutrition of the disc, used electron microscopy and atomic spectrometry to measure the mineral salts and water content of the annulus fibrosus and nucleus pulposus. He found that the disc, which is deprived of vessels, receives nutrients by the diffusion of plasma filtrates from the surrounding structures. The intervertebral disc is supplied by the vertebral epiphysis until a person reaches the age of approximately 25. After fusion of the epiphysis, the vessels join those of the vertebral bodies. Certain vascular loops reach the cartilaginous structures of the vertebral plates and that area above where the disc tissue is formed. It has been suggested that by the process of diffusion, these loops form nutrient channels from the cancellous bone of the vertebral body into the adjacent disc.

The nucleus pulposus demonstrates a hydrophilia which is an osmotic force that brings about a diffusion of fluid from the vertebral body into the nucleus. The nucleus pulposus demonstrates twice the hydrophilic capacity of the remaining disc. Nutrient channels are formed from the vertebral bone into the disc, and a high rate of mineral salt flow is noted within these channels.

It has been demonstrated by the use of atomic spectrometry that there are five mineral constituents, namely potassium, calcium, magnesium, iron, and sodium, that flow into the disc. Only one of these elements, sodium, is found in increased concentration within the nucleus.

It is interesting how Robles determined the flow of nutrients from the vertebral body into the disc. He injected dye into the nucleus and observed it to flow through the nutrient channels.

Urban et al. (4) found diffusion to be the main mechanism of transport of small solutes into the intervertebral disc. About 40% of the end-plate area was found to be permeable to small solutes in experiments on dogs. The amount of solute entering via the end plate was shown to be less for negatively charged solutes, such as the sulfate ion, than for the neutral solutes, such as glucose, because of charge exclusion in the region of the nucleus.

This route of nutrition is important, as many authors believe that there is a correlation between the impermeability of the central region of the end plate and disc degeneration. The only solute whose metabolism has been studied at all is the sulfate ion. In the dog it has been shown that there is a turnover of sulfate in the nucleus pulposus in about 500 days. Consequently, Nachemson (1) believes ruptured discs take a long time, if ever, to heal.

The in vivo procedure used to study sulfate metabolism was performed on dogs. They were anesthetized and given injections of radioactive sulfate tracers. Blood samples were collected at regular intervals until the dogs were killed at regular intervals of 1 hour to 6 hours after the initial injection. The spines were dissected as quickly as possible, usually within 5 to 10 minutes after death, and plunged into liquid nitrogen. Liquid nitrogen was poured onto the discs to stop diffusion from occurring during the measuring and cutting operations that followed. Urban et al. (4) reports that the cell density in the peripheral regions of the annulus and near the end plate is about 3 to 4 times higher than that in the rest of the disc. From the values determined in their study, it appears that the cells in the periphery of the disc are taking up sulfate and, hence, producing proteoglycan less actively than those in the center of the disc. The cells in the surface layers of the articular cartilage likewise are less active in producing proteoglycans than are those in the deeper zones.

We can see that there is a loss of sulfate from discs as they undergo degenerative change. It has been postulated that nutritional deficiencies could lead to disc degeneration. If the end plate were blocked, there could be a buildup of waste products or a nutritional deficiency that could predispose the disc to degenerative change (5). Consequently, we use Discat,[1] which incorporates manganese sulfate along with five other trace minerals, in the treatment of low back pain. No studies have been done on the benefits of such treatment, however, although nutritional prevention of low back pain via such nutrients should be considered and may provide another avenue of treatment for low back pain.

According to Nachemson (as reported in Ref. 6), exercise improves the delivery of nutrients to the spinal discs, perhaps delaying the deterioration that eventually afflicts all backs.

## References

1. Nachemson A: The lumbar spine, an orthopaedic challenge. Spine 1(1):59–69, 1976.
2. Naylor A, Happey F, Turner RL, Shentall RD, West DC, Richardson C: Enzymic and immunological activity in the intervertebral disc. Orthop Clin North Am 6:1, 1975.
2a. Happey F, Wiseman A, Naylor A: Biochemical aspects of intervertebral discs in aging and disease. In Jayson M (ed): Lumbar Spine and Back Pain. New York, Grune & Stratton, 1976, p 318.
3. Robles J: Study of disc nutrition. Rev Chir Orthop 60:5, 1974.
4. Urban JPG, Holm S, Maraudas A: Diffusion of small solutes into the intervertebral disc: an in vivo study. Biorheology 15:203–223, 1978.
5. Ogota D, Whiteside L: Nutritional pathways of the intervertebral disc. Spine 6(3):211–215, 1981.
6. Brody JE: The origins of backache: studies begin to explain the crippling pain of millions. NY Times January 12, 1982.

---

[1] A tablet of Discat contains 150 mg manganese sulfate, 150 mg calcium, 50 mg potassium, 75 mg magnesium, 4 mg iron, 10 mg zinc, and 50 mg perna canaliculus.

*Your Practice Is a Way of Life. It Makes Your Life Worthy and Beautiful. No Stream Can Rise Higher than Its Source and You Can Give No Better to Your Practice than You Are. Always Make Yourself the Quality You Would Have for Your Practice. Your Practice Is a Mirror Image of Yourself.*

*—James M. Cox, D.C.*

CHAPTER 15

# Statistical Data on the Diagnosis, Treatment, and Response of 576 Consecutive Low Back and Sciatic Patients to Chiropractic Manipulation[1]

JAMES M. COX, D.C., D.A.C.B.R.
SCOTT SHREINER, PH.D.[2]

## ABSTRACT

A chiropractic multicenter observational pilot study to compile statistics on the examination procedures, diagnosis, types of treatments rendered, results of treatment, number of days of care, and number of treatments required to arrive at a 50% and a maximum clinical improvement was carried out on 576 patients with low back and/or leg pain. The purpose of the study was to determine the congenital and developmental changes in patients with low back and/or leg pain, the combinations of such anomalies, the accuracy of orthodox diagnostic tests in assessing low back pain, the ergonomic factors affecting onset and, ultimately, the specific difficulty factors encountered in treating the various conditions seen in the average chiropractor's office. For all conditions treated, the average number of days to attain maximum improvement was 43 and the average number of visits was 19. It was concluded that this study provided useful data for assessment of routine chiropractic office-based diagnosis and treatment of related conditions. Further controlled studies, however, are necessary for validation of specific parameters.[1]

Chiropractic manipulation is primarily carried out in a clinical or private office setting devoid of institutionalization. This can have both positive and negative results. The positive results are that it does

---

[1] Reproduced with permission from J. M. Cox and S. Shreiner: "Chiropractic Manipulation in Low Back Pain and Sciatica: Statistical Data on the Diagnosis, Treatment and Response of 576 Consecutive Cases." *Journal of Manipulative and Physiological Therapeutics* 7(1):1–11, 1984.

Twenty-three chiropractic physicians contributed to this study: John Muilenberg, Mĩchael Rodriquez, R. Frank Stevens, D. T. Watkinson, Joseph Curcio, Tuck Kantor, David Belknap, Douglas W. Brown, Harold B. Allen, Joseph Katter, Paul Markey, Allen Parry, Jeffrey Brower, Kirk Steketee, Charles Neualt, Douglas Forsstrom, James M. Cox, Larry Widmer, Kathleen Fromelt, Dan Komesch, Richard Lauber, Gary Errigo, and Michael Howard.

This project is funded through a research grant from the Foundation for Chiropractic Education and Research to the International Academy on Chiropractic Low Back Pain Study.

Submit reprint requests for the report *Chiropractic Results of 576 Low Back Cases* to: James M. Cox, D.C., Low Back Pain Clinic, 3125 Hobson Road, Fort Wayne, Indiana 46805.

[2] Assistant Director of Computing and Data Processing and Sociologist, Indiana University-Purdue University at Fort Wayne, Fort Wayne Indiana.

minimize cost factors to patients, since hospital care is not utilized. Furthermore, it demands that the chiropractic physician in private practice develop his clinical diagnostic skills to as high a degree as possible so as to arrive at the most accurate clinical diagnosis without the use of invasive procedures such as are used in hospital settings. The negative result is that it restricts chiropractic treatment to patients who are ambulatory, thus capable of coming to the office for care. This certainly limits the type of patient seen in chiropractic care, all but eliminating those patients who must be institutionalized because of severe low back and/or sciatic pain.

Interest in the nonsurgical care of low back and leg pain has become prominent in the world today, primarily because learned surgeons, realizing that the success of surgery is directly related to the selection of the patient, believe that the best of conservative care should be attempted before resorting to surgery. Some even go so far as to state that 2 to 3 months of conservative care should be given before surgery is utilized.

Accurate assessment of the various conditions of low back pain being treated by the chiropractor and of the effects of this treatment are best accomplished by review of data from the private practices of chiropractors. Therefore, the International Academy on Chiropractic Low Back Pain Study, Inc., a nonprofit research institution, sought and found 22 doctors of chiropractic throughout the United States and 1 in Canada who were willing to utilize and fill out the prescribed examination form shown in Table 15.1 on 20 consecutive low back and/or sciatic patients seen in their offices. The findings from these examination forms were collected by the principle investigator of this study, J. M. C., and placed on a computer at Indiana University-Purdue University in Fort Wayne, Indiana for collection and study. The consultant for this project is Scott Schreiner, Ph.D., Sociologist and Assistant Director of Computing and Data Processing at this University.

Chiropractic colleges teach strong curriculum in the congenital abnormalities of the low back. Correct assessment of the

role of these anomalies in low back pain is going on today. This chapter focuses, therefore, on the incidence of such anomalies, the combination of these anomalies, and ultimately their response to chiropractic manipulative therapy.

The insurance industry and the chiropractic profession have long discussed the length of time and number of visits needed to produce satisfactory clinical results in patients with low back pain. This chapter, therefore, also focuses on two important questions that have arisen from these discussions: What are the specific diagnoses in patients seeking chiropractic care, and for each condition treated, what is the average visitation frequency and days of care required to arrive at 50% versus maximum chiropractic relief? These findings are given for each type of anomaly of the lumbar spine.

This paper should have relevance to the chiropractic profession and third party payors. We believe that it is the most comprehensive collection of data from clinical chiropractic practice that has been done today. Furthermore, it is hoped that this will be a basis for future collection of such data; the International Academy on Chiropractic Low Back Pain Study plan to pursue this to an even greater extent in the future.

## MATERIALS AND METHODS

Table 15.1 is the 293 variable questionnaire used by each participating doctor to record the results of the examination and treatment of 20 or more consecutive patients with low back pain who were treated at the doctor's office. Each patient filled out an Informed Consent Form after the project had been completely explained to them.

This fixed choice form provides for easy coding of these data which are then analyzed using the Statistical Package for the Social Sciences (SPSS).

Some points concerning this examination form need clarification. The statistics and findings that can be derived from these 293 variables are numerous. For that reason, some questions that you may consider important and that this study could answer may not be covered in this

**Table 15.1.**
**Low Back Examination Form for Clinical Evaluation and Statistical Research of Low Back and Disc Disorders**

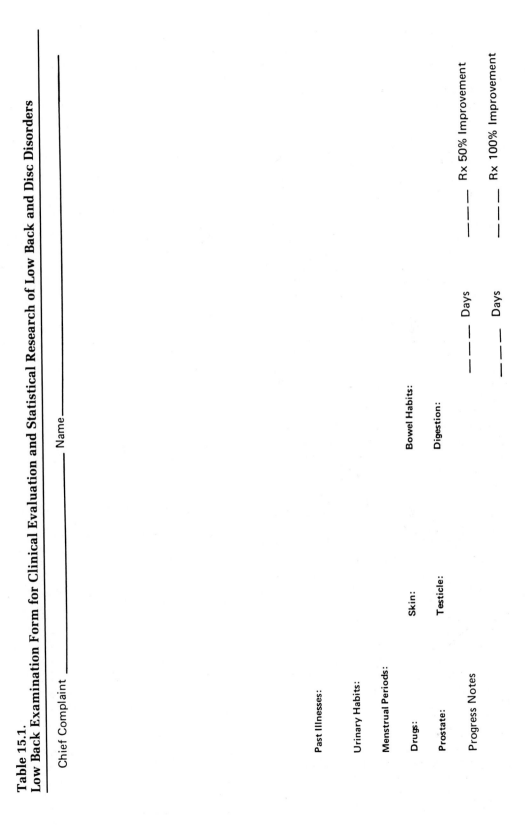

Chief Complaint _____ Name _____

Past Illnesses:

Urinary Habits:

Menstrual Periods:

Drugs:                          Skin:                          Bowel Habits:

Prostate:                       Testicle:                       Digestion:

Progress Notes

— — — Days        — — — Rx 50% Improvement

— — — Days        — — — Rx 100% Improvement

## Table 15.1—Continued

| BASIC PATIENT INFORMATION |
| --- |

NOTE: Be sure to right justify your numbers.

I.D. No. _ _ _ _ _ NAME _ _ _ _ _ _ _ _ _ _ _ _ _ CASNUM _ _ _ _

DOCNAM _ _ _ _ _ DATEXM _ _ / _ _ / _ _ OCCUPATION _ _ _ _ _ _ _ _
                         mo. da. yr.

| REFER BY _ | RACE _ | SEX _ AGE _ _ | MARSTA _ | HT _ IN _ | BODY TYPE _ |
| --- | --- | --- | --- | --- | --- |
| 1=M.D. | 1=Caucasian | 1=Male | 1=Single | WT _ _ _ lbs. | 1=Ectomorph |
| 2=D.C. | 2=Negro | 2=Fe Not Preg. | 2=Married | | 2=Mesomorph |
| 3=D.O. | 3=Japanese | 3=Fe 1st Tri | 3=Divorced | | 3=Endomorph |
| 4=Self | 4=Chinese | 4=Fe 2nd Tri | 4=Widowed | | 4=D/K |
| 5=Family | 5=Indian | 5=Fe 3rd Tri | | | |
| 6=Another Pt. | | Fe w/ _ births | | | |
| 7=Other | | | | | |

| HABITS |
| --- |

| SMOKER _ | STRESS _ | EXRTYPE _ _ |
| --- | --- | --- |
| 1=No | 1=No Stress | 1=None |
| 2=<1pk/day | to 9=Maximum | 2=Jog/Run |
| 3=1-2pks/day | | 3=Bowling |
| 4=2-3pks/day | | 4=Golf |
| 5=>3 pks/day | | 5=Racquetball |
| 6=D/K | | 6=Tennis |
| | | 7=Situps |
| | | 8=Swimming |
| | | 9=Walking |
| | | 10=Dancing |
| | | 99=Other |

| EXRPRD _ | EXFREQ _ | EXPOIN _ | WATLIF _ | FREQLF 30 lb. _ |
| --- | --- | --- | --- | --- |
| 1=None | 1=None | 1=None | 1=<10 lbs. | 1=1/hr |
| 2=<10 min. | 2=Daily | Heart and Breathing | 2=11-30 lbs. | 2=1/day |
| 3=11-30 min | 3=2-3 times week | 2=Slight ↑ | 3=31-50 lbs. | 3=1/wk |
| 4=31-60 min | 4=2-3 times month | 3=Mod. ↑ | 4=51-100 lbs. | 4=1/mo |
| 5=1-2 hrs. | 5=2-3 times year | 4=Great ↑ | 5=>100 lbs. | 5=1/yr |
| 6=>2 hrs. | | | | |

TIMSIT/day _ _ hrs.    TIMSTA/day _ _ hrs.

**Table 15.1—Continued**

## COMPLAINTS AND HISTORY

### COMPLA __ __ , __ __ , __ __ , __ __

order of descending importance

| | |
|---|---|
| 01=low back pain | 11=bloating |
| 02=leg pain | 12=headache |
| 03=constipation | 13=flatulence |
| 04=urinary difficulties | 14=incontinence-urinary |
| 05=testicular pain | 15=incontinence-bowel |
| 06=impotence | 16=eneuresis |
| 07=menstrual problems | 17=urethral stricture |
| 08=diarrhea | 18=nephritis |
| 09=groin pain | 19=cystitis |
| 10=abdominal pain | 20=prostatitis |

| |
|---|
| 21=prostatic hypertrophy |
| 22=neck pain |
| 23=thoracic pain |
| 24=thoracolumbar pain |
| 25=upper extremity pain |
| 26=foot pain |
| 27=tailbone pain |
| 28=coital pain |
| 29=other |

### CANSUR __ __
### PRESUR __ __ , __ __
### (NON-Ca) __ __ , __ __

**DIGESTIVE**
01=Esophagus
02=Stomach
03=Duodenum
04=Sm. Bowel
05=Colon
06=Rectum
07=Appendix
08=Pancreas

**CARDIOVASCULAR**
09=Heart
10=Great Vessels
11=Upper Ext. Vasc.
12=Lower Ext. Vasc.
13=Spleen
14=Lymphatics
15=Tonsils
16=Adenoids
17=Lymphatics (other)

**REPRODUCTIVE**
18=Uterus
19=Ovary
20=Ovarian Duct
21=Tubal Ligation
22=Vas Deferens
23=Testicle
24=Prostate
25=Genitalia

**ENDROCRINE**
26=Thyroid
27=Parathyroid
28=Pituitary
29=Adrenal
30=Thymus

**RESPIRATORY**
31=Lung Parenchyma
32=Trachea
33=Bronchi
34=Sinus
35=Kidneys
36=Ureter
37=U. Bladder
38=Urethra

**EXCRETORY**
39=Skin
40=Mucosa
41=Glands (sweat, sebaceous)
42=Mammary Glands

**URINARY**
35=Kidneys
36=Ureter
37=U. Bladder
38=Urethra

**SKELETAL**
47=Upper Extremity
48=Lower Extremity
49=Spine
50=None
51=Hernia

**NERVOUS**
43=Brain
44=Spinal Cord
45=Periph. N.S.-Upper
46=Periph. N'S.-Lower

52=Gall Bladder
53=Oral
54=Hemorrhoids
55=Adhesions

### PDXCON __ __ , __ __ , __ __

| | |
|---|---|
| 01=Abd. Aneurysm | 26=Muscular Dystrophy |
| 02=Appendicitis | 27=Nephritis |
| 03=Arthritis-Degen. | 28=Ovarian Ds. |
| 04=Arthritis-Infectious | 29=Polio |
| 05=Arthritis-Rheumatoid | 30=Prostatic Hypertrophy |
| 06=Celiac Ds. | 31=Prostatitis |
| 07=Colon-Spastic | 32=Ptosed Urinary Bladder |
| 08=Colon-Irritable | 33=Renul Calculi |
| 09=Colon-Crohn's Ds. | 34=Salpingitis |
| 10=Cystitis | 35=S.T.D.(Sex transmitted Ds.) |
| 11=Diabetes | 36=Scoliosis |
| 12=Diverticulosis | 37=Short leg |
| 13=Dysmenorrhea | 38=Ulcers |
| 14=Endometriosis | 39=Urethritis |
| 15=Fistula-Rectovag. | 40=Ureteral Stricture |
| 16=Fistula Urethrovag. | 41=Uterine Prolapse |
| 17=Gallstones | 42=Uterine Tumor |
| 18=Hemorrhoids | 43=Other (see history) |
| 19=Hypertension-Essent. | 44=Hiatal Hernia |
| 20=Hypertension-Malig. | 45=None |
| 21=Irreg. Menses | 46=Shingles |
| 22=Malignancy | 47=Gout |
| 23=Malposition Uterus | |
| 24=Miscarriage | |
| 25=Multiple Sclerosis | |

**Table 15.1—Continued**

## PAIN INFORMATION

**DATSYM**
/ mo. / da. / yr.
99=D/K

**PANRAT __**
1 minimal
to
9 maximal

**TIMCOM**
____ DAYS
9999=D/K

**PAN FRE __**
1=Constant
2=Intermittent

**PANTYP __**
1=Sharp
2=Dull Ache
3=Throbbing
4=Traction
5=Other
6=D/K 7=Burning

**PANONS ___**
1=Insidious
2=Acute/Traumatic
8=N/A
9=D/K

**INJACT __**
1=Straight Bending w/o lifting
2=Straight Bending w/lifting
3=Rotation, Bending w/lifting
4=Rotation Bending w/o lifting
5=Fall
6=Accident
7=No Activity Known

**SPORIN __ __**
01=Bowling
02=Golf
03=Tennis
04=Swimming
05=Weight Lift
06=Racquetball
07=Basketball
08=Football
09=Baseball
10=Dancing
11=Soccer
12=Rowing
13=Wrestling
14=Run/Jog
15=Other
99=No Sport Involved

**PREVBP __**
1=Immediate injury
2=Hours before injury
3=Days before injury
4=Weeks before injury
5=Months before injury
6=Years before injury
7=None
9=D/K

**WERINJ __**
1=At Work
2=At Home
3=In Motor Vehicle
4=Recreation Area
5=In Store, Restaurant
6=Another Household
8=Other
9=D/K

**PANLIF __**
1= <10 lbs.
2=11-30 lbs.
3=31-50 lbs.
4=51-80 lbs.
5=81-100 lbs.
6=101-200 lbs.
7=>200 lbs.
8=Not involved w/lifting
9=D/K

**NITPAN __**
1=NO
2=Yes
3=D/K

**PANSUC __**
1=No
2=Yes

**PN PREG __**
1=Not Pregnant, N/A
2=Yes 1st Trimester
3=Yes 2nd Trimester
4=Yes 3rd Trimester
5=Puerperium

**DERMAT __**
1=S1 Dermatome
2=L5 Dermatome
3=L4 Dermatome
4=L3 Dermatome
5=L5,S1 Dermatome
6=L4,L5 Dermatome
7=None
8=D/K
9=N/A

**PANLOC __**
1=Rt. Leg
2=Lf. Leg
3=Both Legs
4=Alternating Legs
5=Low Back
6=LB., Rt. Lg.
7=LB., Lf. Lg.
8=LB., Both Legs
9=D/K

**PANLEG __**
1=Before back pain
2=Simultaneous w/LBP
3=After LBP
4=None Present
5=D/K
6=No LBP, only Leg.

**PANEXT ___**
1=Buttock 2=Thigh
3=Knee 4=Calf
5=Ankle 6=Foot
7=Toes 8=Not present
9=D/K

**ABNSKN __ __**
1=Numbness
2=Hypoesthesia
3=Formication
4=Tingling
5=Hyperesthesia
6=Burning
7=Foot Falls Asleep
8=None Present
9=D/K

**Table 15.1—Continued**

**SENSTM ___**
1=Simultaneously
2=1 week
3=1-2 wk.
4=2-4 wk.
5=4-8 wk.
6=3-6 mos.
7=6-12 mos.
8=Not Present
9=D/K

**PANWAL ___**
1=No
2=L.Leg
3=Rt Leg
4=Both Legs
5=D/K
6=Low Back

**PANAGG ___,___,___**
1=Coughing
2=Sneezing
3=Straining at stool
4=Bending, Lifting
5=Sitting
6=None of above
7=Laying
8=Standing
9=D/K

**POSTEX ___,___**
1=Sitting
2=Standing
3=Recumbent
4=Kneeling
5=Hyperxtens
6=D/K
7=Flexion
8=Twisting
9=None

**POSREM ___,___**
1=Sitting
2=Standing
3=Recumbent
4=D/K
5=None

## MEDICAL HISTORY

**MYELOG ___**
1=Yes-Positive
2=Yes-Negative
3=No
4=Inconclusive
5=D/K

**POMYSM ___**
1=Headache
2=Arachnoiditis
3=Nausea
4=L.B.P.
5=L.P.
6=None
9=Myelog. not performed

**POMYTI ___**
1=No Symptoms
2=$<$1 wk.
3=1-2 wks.
4=2-4 wks.
5=1-3 mos.
6=3-6 mos.
7=6-12 mos.
8=$>$1 year
9=Myelo. not performed

**ODDPRO ___**
1=Epidural Venography
2=Discography
3=1 and 2
4=Electromyography
5=Gas Myelography
6=CAT Scan
7=None performed
9=D/K

**NMBKSU ___** SAMSUL ___
1=Yes
2=No
3=D/K
4=None of above
5=No Surgery

**TMBKSU ___,___,___**
888=D/K
999=No Surgery

Record Answer in months.

**BAKSUR ___**
1=Laminectomy
2=Fusion
3=Microsurgery
4=Screw Fixation
5=Harrington Rod
6=Other
7=D/K
8=No Surgery

**SHTRBS ___**
$<$1 year
1=Worsening
2=No Change
3=25% improved
4=50% improved
5=75% improved
6=100% improved
7=D/K
9=No Surgery

**LGTRBS ___**
$>$1 year
1=Worsening
2=No Change
3=25% improved
4=50% improved
5=75% improved
6=100% improved
7=D/K
9=No Surgery

**TREMOS ___,___**
1=Manipulation
2=Epidural injection
3=Chemonucleolysis
4=Closed Reduction
5=Rhizolysis
6=P.T.
7=Meridian Therapy
8=None
9=Other

**PREVPT ___**
1=Hot and Cold
2=High Volt Gal.
3=Low Volt Gal.
4=Ultrasound
5=Intermittent Traction
6=Massage
7=Trigger Point
8=Brace
9=None

**PREVTR ___**
1=M.D.
2=D.C.
3=D.O.
4=M.D. and D.C.
5=M.D., D.C., D.O.
6=None
7=D/K

**OTHERP ___**
1=LBP School
2=TNS
3=Counselling
4=Biofeedback
5=None
6=D/K
7=1 and 2
8=1,2 and 3
9=1,2,3, and 4

**RELTHE ___**
Change from therapies'
1=Worse
2=No Change
3=25% improvement
4=50% improvement
5=75% improvement
6=100% improvement
7=No Therapies given
9=D/K

**MEDICA ___**
1=Anti-inflammatory
2=Pain Relievers
3=Muscle Relaxers
4=Minor Tranquilizers
5=B-12
6=None Taken
8=Other
9=D/K

**RELMED ___**
1=Worse
2=No Change
3=25% improved
4=50% improved
5=75% improved
6=100% improved
7=D/K
9=None taken

**Table 15.1—*Continued***

## FAMILY HISTORY OF BACK PROBLEMS

| PREVCH __ | HARMYU __ | FAMSCI __ | FAMLBP __ | FAMSUR __ |
|---|---|---|---|---|
| 01=SOT | 1=Yes | 01=NONE | 01=NONE | 01=NONE |
| 02=Gonstead | 2=No | 02=Father | 02=Father | 02=Father |
| 03=Diversified | 3=D/K | 03=Mother | 03=Mother | 03=Mother |
| 04=Logan Basic | 4=N/A | 04=Brother | 04=Brother | 04=Brother |
| 05=Activator | | 05=Sister | 05=Sister | 05=Sister |
| 06=Cox | | 06=Father, Mother | 06=Father, Mother | 06=Father, Mother |
| 07=Pettibone | | 07=Father, Brother | 07=Father, Brother | 07=Father, Brother |
| 08=Meric | | 08=Father, Sister | 08=Father, Sister | 08=Father, Sister |
| 09=Ward | | 09=Mother, Brother | 09=Mother, Brother | 09=Mother, Brother |
| 10=Side posture | | 10=Mother, Sister | 10=Mother, Sister | 10=Mother, Sister |
| 11=Best | | 11=Brother, Sister | 11=Brother, Sister | 11=Brother, Sister |
| 12=Barge | | 12=2 or more brothers | 12=2 or more brothers | 12=2 or more brothers |
| 13=AK | | 13=2 or more sisters | 13=2 or more sisters | 13=2 or more sisters |
| 14=Masters | | 14=2 or more brothers or sisters | 14=2 or more brothers or sisters | 14=2 or more brothers or sisters |
| 15=Thompson | | 15=D/K | 15=D/K | 15=D/K |
| 16=Reinert | | | | |
| 17=Nimmo | | | | |
| 18=None | | | | |
| 19=Other | | | | |
| 99=D/K | | | | |

## PHYSICAL EXAMINATION

| BLDPRS __ __ / __ __ __ | HRTRAT __ __ __ /min. | HRTRHY __ | HRTSON __ | LUNGEX __ | ABDOEX __ | PHYSCO __ |
|---|---|---|---|---|---|---|
| | | 1=Normal | 1=Absent | 1=Normal | 1=Normal | 1=Poor |
| | | 2=Abnormal | 2=Present | 2=Abnormal | 2=Abnormal | 2=Average |
| | | | | | | 3=Good |
| | | | | | | 4=Excellent |

## Table 15.1—*Continued*

### Examination - Sitting

**MINORS**
1=Positive
2=Negative
3=D/K
4=N/A

**BECTRW**
1=L.B.P.
2=Rt. L.P.
3=1,2
4=Lf. L.P.
5=1,4
6=NEG.
7=Both Legs
8=D/K
9=N/A

**VALSAL**
1=L.B.P.
2=Rt. L.P.
3=1,2
4=Lf. L.P.
5=1,4
6=NEG
7=Both Legs
8=D/K
9=N/A

**VAL BEC**
1=L.B.P.
2=Rt. L.P.
3=1,2
4=Lf. L.P.
5=1,4
6=NEG
7=Both Legs
8=D/K
9=N/A

**PPUPLL**
1=L1-L2
2=L2-L3
3=L3-L4
4=L4-L5
5=L5-S1
6=S1-S2
7=None
8=D/K
9=N/A

**PERCUS**
1=L1
2=L2
3=L3
4=L4
5=L5
6=S1
7=D/K
8=N/A
9=Negative

**KEMPS**
1=Rt. Pos.
2=Lf. Pos.
3=Both Pos.
4=Neg.
5=D/K

**FOTSYM**
1=Low Arch
2=High Arch
3=Bunions
4=Hammer Toe
5=Neuroma
6=Morton's Syn.
7=Plantar Wart
8=None
9=D/K

### Examination - Standing

**NERIBO**
1=Rt.
2=Lf.
3=Both
4=NEG
5=D/K
6=N/A

**LEWNST**
1=L.B.P.
2=SI
3=L.P.
4=Both 1,3
5=NEG
6=D/K
7=N/A

**GAIT**
1=Normal
2=Rt. Limp
3=Left Limp
4=Other
5=D/K
6=N/A

**SPTILT**
1=Rt.
2=Lf.
3=None
4=D/K
5=N/A

**LORDOS**
1=Normal
2=Loss
3=Increase
4=D/K
5=N/A

**PPUPLA**
1=L1-L2
2=L2-L3
3=L3-L4
4=L4-L5
5=L5-S1
6=S1-S2
7=None
8=D/K
9=N/A

### MOTION DEGREES

FLEXON ___ /90___
EXTNSN ___ /30___
RLATFX ___ /20___
LLATFX ___ /20___
RROTAT ___ /30___
LROTAT ___ /30___

PAIN  1=Yes  b=no

**TOWALK**
1=Rt. Weak
2=Lf. Weak
3=B Weak
4=Neg
5=D/K
6=N/A

**HEELWK**
1=Rt. Weak
2=Lf. Weak
3=Both Weak
4=Neg.
5=D/K
6=N/A

**HISHOL**
1=RT.
2=LF.
3=LEVEL
4=D/K

### Examination - Supine

**LINDRS**
1=LBP
2=Rt. L.P.
3=1,2
4=Lf. L.P.
5=1,4
6=Neg.
7=Both Legs
8=D/K
9=N/A

**HAMSTR**
1=Rt. $<60°$
2=Rt. $>60°$
3=Lf. $<60°$
4=Lf. $>60°$
5=Both $<60°$
6=Both $>60°$
7=Neg.
8=D/K

**ST.LEG**
STLGRR___° $60°$
STLGRL___° $60°$
00=Neg.
99=N/A

**BRAGRD**
1=Rt. Pos.
2=Lf. Pos.
3=Both
4=Neg.
5=D/K
6=N/A
7=Hamstring Tightness
8=Gastroc Tightness

**Location**
PSLGRR--
PSLGRL--
1=LBP
2=LP
3=Both
4=None

**WELEGR**
1=Pos.
2=Neg.
3=D/K
4=N/A

**MEDHPR**
1=L.B.P.
2=Rt. L.P.
3=1,2
4=Lf. L.P.
5=1,4
6=Neg.
7=D/K
8=N/A

**PATRIK**
1=Rt. pos.
2=Lf. pos.
3=Both pos.
4=Neg.
5=D/K
6=N/A

**GANSLN**
1=Rt. L.B.P.
2=Lf. L.B.P.
3=Rt. S.I.
4=Lf. S.I.
5=Rt. LBP, SI.
6=Lf. LBP, SI.
7=Neg.
8=D/K
9=N/A

**Table 15.1—Continued**

## Examination - Supine Cont.

| COXSIN | AMOSS | MUSCLE STR | LEG M.M. | MILGRM | REFLEXES | SENSORY |
|---|---|---|---|---|---|---|
| 1=Rt. Pos. | 1=Pos. | DORFLX ___ | RITTHI ___ mm. | 1=Rt. | RANKRF ___ | RHYPRS ___ |
| 2=Lf. Pos. | 2=Neg. | PLANFX ___ | LFTTHI ___ mm. | 2=Lf. | LANKRF ___ | LHYPRS ___ |
| 3=Neg. | 3=D/K | GRATOF ___ | RTCALF ___ mm. | 3=Both | RKNERF ___ | RHYPOS ___ |
| 4=D/K | 4=N/A | GRATOX ___ | LFCALF ___ mm. | 4=Neg. | LKNERF ___ | LHYPOS ___ |
| 5=N/A | | FOTEVR ___ | blank=No reply | 5=D/K | 1=↑↑ 2=↑↑↑ | 1=None 2=L4,L5 |
| | | 1=Both Normal | 777=D/K | 6=N/A | 3=↓dec 4=Absent | 3=L3 4=L4 |
| | | 2=Rt. Dim. Lf. Nor. | 888=N/A | | 5=D/K 6=N/A | 5=L5 6=S1 |
| | | 3=Lf. Dim. Rt. Nor. | 25.4mm/inch | | | 7=S2 8=L5S1 |
| | | 4=Both Weak | | | | 9=D/K |
| | | 5=D/K | | | | |
| | | 6=N/A | | | | |

## Examination-Prone

| CIRCULATION | MOSES | NACLAS | YEOMAN | ELYS | PRONLF |
|---|---|---|---|---|---|
| FEMART ___ | 1=Rt. Pos. | 1=Rt. Pos. | 1=Rt. Pos. | 1=Rt. Pos. | 1=Inc. LBP |
| POPART ___ | 2=Lf. Pos. | 2=Lf. Pos. | 2=Lf. Pos. | 2=Lf. Pos. | 2=Inc. LP |
| POTART ___ | 3=Both | 3=Both Pos. | 3=Both Pos. | 3=Both Pos. | 3=Dec. A.J. |
| DOPART ___ | 4=Neg | 4=Neg. | 4=Neg. | 4=Neg. | 4=Alter Derm. |
| 1=Both equal | 5=D/K | 5=D/K | 5=D/K | 5=D/K | 5=Dec. Flexion |
| 2=Rt. Dim. Lf. Normal | 6=N/A | 6=N/A | 6=N/A | 6=N/A | 6=No Change |
| 3=Lf. Dim. Rt. Normal | | | | | 7=D/K |
| 4=Both Dim. | | | | | 8=N/A |
| 5=D/K 6=N/A | | | | | |

## NON-ORGANIC PHYSICAL SIGNS

| PANPOF | SHTLEG | LIBMAN | TENSKN | MANKOF | BURN BC | FLIPTS | PLANFX | FLXHIP |
|---|---|---|---|---|---|---|---|---|
| 1=Rt. | 1=Lf. | 1=Lo Pain | 1=Specific | 1=Pos | 1=Pos | 1=Pos | 1=Pos | 1=Pos |
| 2=Lf. | 2=Rt. | 2=Hi Pain | 2=Non-Anatomic | 2=Neg | 2=Neg | 2=Neg | 2=Neg | 2=Neg |
| 3=Both | 3=Even | 3=D/K | 3=D/K | 3=D/K | 3=D/K | 3=D/K | 3=D/K | 3=D/K |
| 4=D/K | 4=D/K | 4=N/A | 4=N/A | 4=N/A | 4=N/A | 4=N/A | 4=N/A | 4=N/A |
| 5=N/A | Amt. Short ___ | | | | | | | |
| 6=NEG. | | | | | | | | |

**Table 15.1—*Continued***

## XRAY INTERPRETATION - SPINAL MECHANICS

**AXILOD_**
1=LBP
2=Neg
3=D/K
4=N/A

**ROTSOP _**
1=LBP
2=Neg
3=D/K
4=N/A

**SPTILT_**
SPITLR____
SPITLL____
SCOLIR____
SCOL1L____
1=L1 2=L2
3=L3 4=L4
5=L5 6=None
7=D/K 8=N/A
9=Yes

**SCOSEV_**
1=Mild $<10°$
2=Mod 10-30°
3=Severe $>40°$
4=D/K
5=N/A
6=None

**SACANG __°**

**LUMANG __°**

FACSYN
1=L4-L5
2=L5-S1
3=Not present
4=D/K
5=N/A

VNAKST
1=Stable
2=Unstable
3=N/A

**FACFAC_,_,_**
1=Coronal Facets L5,S1
2=Coronal Facets L4,L5
3=Sagittal Facets L5,S1
4=Sagittal Facets L4,L5
5=Tropism L5,S1
6=Tropism L4,L5
7=Disc Lesion Side of
   Oblique Facet
8=D/K
9=N/A

**LEGSHT _**
1=Rt. Short $<$5mm
2=Rt Short 5-10mm
3=Rt Short $>$10mm
4=Lf. Short $<$5mm
5=Lf. Short 5-10mm
6=Lf. Short $>$10mm
7=No Difference
8=D/K
9=N/A

**PATHOL_**
1=Osteoporosis
2=Fracture
3=Malignancy
4=Deg. Hip. Disease
5=A.S.
6=Benign Tumor
7=Infection
8=Other
9=N/A

## Congenital Anomaly

**SPIBIF_**
1=L1
2=L2
3=L3
4=L4
5=L5
6=S1
7=S2
8=D/K
9=None

**SPONLY _,_**
1=L1
2=L2
3=L3
4=L4
5=L5
6=S1
7=None
8=D/K
9=N/A

**SPONLI _,_,_ %**
Level
1=L1
2=L2
3=L3
4=L4
5=L5
6=D/K
7=N/A
8=None

**SACTRV _**
1=Rt. True
2=Rt. False
3=Lf. True
4=Lf. False
5=Bilat. True
6=Bilat. False
7=D/K 8=N/A
9=Not present

**LUMTRV_**
1=Rt. True
2=Rt. False
3=Lf. True
4=Lf. False
5=Bilat. True
6=Bilat. False
7=D/K 8=N/A
9=Not present

**SAGDSC _,_,_**

**SAGVBD _,_,_**
L2, L3, L4, L5

INCRST
1=L4 Body
2=L5 Body
3=D/K 4=N/A

L5TRAN
1=Less 2=Greater
3=Equal 4=D/K
5=N/A
rel to L3

## ACQUIRED ABNORMALITIES

**PSUDSP _,_**
1=D.S.A.
2=Trauma
3=Elongated Pars
4=L3
5=L4
6=L5
7=D/K
8=N/A
9=None

**SHMRLN_**
1=L1
2=L2
3=L3
4=L4
5=L5
6=2 or more levels
7=None
8=D/K
9=N/A

**NARDIS _,_,_**

**SPONDL _,_,_**

**ARTFAR _,_,_**

**ARTFAL_**
1=L1-L2 2=L2-L3
3=L3-L4 4=L4-L5
5=L5-S1 6=None or slight
7=D/K 8=N/A

**RETROL _**
1=L1
2=L2
3=L3
4=L4
5=L5
6=2 or more levels
7=None
8=D/K
9=N/A

**Table 15.1—*Continued***

## CORRELATIVE DIAGNOSIS OF LOW BACK PAIN

**D.D. Disc** ___,___
01= L5-S1, 02= L4-L5, 03= L3-L4, 04= L2-L3, 05= L1-L2, 06= L5-L6, 07= S1-S2, 08= Rt. Medial, 09= Rt. Lateral, 10= Rt. Subrhizal, 11= Lf. Medial, 12= Lf. Lateral, 13= Lf. Subrhizal, 14= D/K, 15= Not involved, 16= Uncertain

**SEC DIS** ___,___
**(if involved)**
01= L5-S1, 02= L4-L5, 03= L3-L4, 04= L2-L3, 05= L1-L2, 06= L5-L6, 07= S1-S2, 08= Rt. Medial, 09= Rt. Lateral, 10= Rt. Subrhizal, 11= Lf. Medial, 12= Lf. Lateral, 13= Lf. Subrhizal, 14= D/K, 15= Not involved, 16= Uncertain

| | | |
|---|---|---|
| **Diag L1** ___,___,___ | 01 Annular Tear (Cat. I) | 08 Lumbar Spine Stenosis (Cat. VIII) |
| **Diag L2** ___,___,___ | 02 Nuclear Bulge (Cat. II) | 09 Iatrogenic Back Pain (Cat. IX) |
| **Diag L3** ___,___,___ | 03 Nuclear Protrusion (Cat. III) | 10 Functional Low Back Pain (Cat. X) |
| **Diag L4** ___,___,___ | 04 Nuclear Prolapse (Cat. IV) | 11 Lumbar Spine Sprain and Strain (Cat. XI) |
| **Diag L5** ___,___,___ | 05 Discogenic Spondyloarthrosis (Cat. V) | 12 Subluxation (Cat. XII) |
| **Diag L6** ___,___,___ | 06 Facet Syndrome (Cat. VI) | 13 Tropism (Cat. XIII) |
| **Diag S1** ___,___,___ | 07 Spondylolisthesis (Cat. VII) | 14 Transitional Segment (Cat. XIV) |
| | | 15 Other Pathologies (Cat. XV) |

**SILESN** ___
Was a sacroiliac lesion present when the disc was reduced or with L.B.P. only? If so, was it - 1-Rt. Ant. ilium, 2-Rt. Post. ilium, 3-Lf. Ant. ilium, 4-Lf. Post. ilium, 5-Not found, 6-D/K, 7-N/A?

**CORSLG** ___
Was a short leg over 6 mm. corrected after relief of symptoms? 1 = Yes, Rt. 2 = Yes, Lf., 3 = No, 4 = D/K, 5 = N/A

**Table 15.1—*Continued***

**CHIPRO** | — |

PRESENT CHIROPRACTIC PROCEDURE

01=Cox, 02=SOT, 03=Gonstead, 04=Logan, 05=Meric, 06=Activator, 07=Diversified, 08=Ward, 09=Pettibone, 10=Side Posture, 11=Thompson, 12=Barge, 13=Best, 14=Masters, 15=Reinert, 16=AK, 17=Nimmo, 18=Other

**PHYSTH** | —,— |
| —,— |
| —,— |

01=Hot, 02=Cold, 03=Hot and Cold, 04=High Volt Gal., 05=Low Volt Gal., 06=Ultrasound, 07=Intermittent Traction 08=Massage, 09=Trigger Points, 10=Acupuncture, 11=Accupressure, 12=None, 13=Bracing, 14=Sinusoidal current, 15=Arch Supports

**PTRESP** | — |

1=Excellent - 90% subjective relief, returned to regular job w/o need of further care.

2=Very good - 75% subjective relief, returned to regular job avoiding pain producing movements, with occasional discomfort not requiring regular treatment.

3=Good - 75% subjective relief, returned to regular job, but requires regular treatment by manipulation or mild analgesics.

4=Fair - 50% subjective relief, must change work duties so as to avoid aggravation of condition. Has pain requiring occasional care.

5=Poor - 50% or less relief of pain. Must avoid physical work and has pain on any lifting, bending, sitting, twisting.

6=Surgery - referred for

7=D/K

8=Patient stopped care or did not begin our treatment regime.

9=Examined but not treated.

**TIMR50** | —— |

Days to reach 50% improvement

**RXAR50** | —— |

Number of treatments to achieve 50% improvement

**TIMRMI** | —— |

Days to reach maximum improvement.

**RXARMI** | —— |

Number of treatments to achieve maximum improvement.

**FOLLUP** | — |

2-5 yr. follow-up. Same response as PTRESP.

chapter. It is hoped that future papers on specific questions will be forthcoming.

From this examination form we will be able to determine what exercise program a patient does or does not follow in the production of (and the relief from) low back pain. The amount of time that one sits per day can be determined. Previously diagnosed conditions that might indicate previous involvement with low back pain are determined on the first visit so that in the future, relief following manipulative care might be determined. The significance of body type in the etiology of low back pain can also be determined. The influence of such things as age, sex, marital status, and race on the production of low back pain can also be determined. Whether or not a person has had previous back pain and its correlation with the severity of the present symptoms can be determined. Pain aggravation by walking, Déjérine's triad, and positions that exacerbate or cause a remission of back pain are determined. If a person has had a myelogram, what postmyelographic symptoms, if any, has he experienced? If he has had back surgery, what type of surgery was performed and what were the short- and long-term results prior to seeking manipulative care? What types of physical therapy and what types of medications were administered, and what were the effects of these? Is there a familial incidence of back pain? If previous chiropractic treatment had been administered, what type of treatment was it and did it cause any harm?

The examination procedures called for on this form are designed to cover the basic pathologies of the low back. These procedures include the neurological signs of the deep reflexes and sensory change. Atrophy and muscle strength determinations are made. The Straight leg raise, Lindner's sign, Patrick's sign, and range of motion are determined. Antalgic posture, pain on palpation, and evidence of an increase in intradiscal pressure are determined.

The x-ray examination delineates the congenital anomalies, such as tropism, stenosis, short leg, spinal tilt, scoliosis, spondylolisthesis, spondylolysis, and transitional vertebrae, and the acquired abnormalities, such as discogenic spondyloarthrosis and subluxation pattern.

Ultimately, the diagnosis may be determined from these data. The diagnosis specifically determines whether the disc lesion is an annular tear, a nuclear bulge, a nuclear protrusion, a nuclear prolapse, or a condition such as discogenic spondyloarthrosis, facet syndrome, spondylolisthesis, lumbar spine stenosis, iatrogenic surgical or chiropractic-induced back pain, functional low back pain, sprain and strain, subluxation, tropism, transitional segment, or some other pathology. It may well be that the final diagnosis could be a combination of two or more of these diagnoses.

Categories I through IV are diagnoses based on the classification system of White and Panjabi (1) which was an update of Charnley's (2) hypothesis of 25 years ago. Charnley's work is a classical theoretical presentation on the mechanism, diagnosis, and treatment of various combinations of back pain and sciatica. From his work as the basis, I have divided disc involvement into the following four categories, fully aware of the often uncertain and overlapping conditions causing low back pain.

## Category I—Annulus Fibrosus Injury

This patient presents with the typical low back pain syndrome; i.e., he presents usually early in life complaining of low back pain following some flexion, twisting, or combined movement. No leg pain is usually present, and relief is obtained usually within a few days. This type of pain may be recurring with progressive worsening of symptoms.

Clinically, there are muscle spasm and a loss of lordosis; there are no abnormal findings seen on straight leg raising, Kemp's sign is positive, and there are no altered motor or sensory changes of the lower extremities. Any leg pain is transient and not subjectively severe.

X-rays will probably reveal no change of discal space or signs of discogenic spondylosis.

This patient responds well to distraction manipulation and is usually quite happy with the clinical results.

In Category I, the patient has undergone tearing, cracking, or severe sprain of the annular fibers, causing irritation of the sinuvertebral nerve and resultant back pain.

## Category II—Nuclear Bulge

Category II represents progression of Category I with the nucleus pulposus bulging into the tears and cracks of the annulus, causing further irritation of the sinuvertebral nerve and early and minimal irritation of the nerve roots exiting from the cauda within the vertebral canal.

The Category II patient presents with a worsening of low back pain and with minimal leg pain.

X-rays may show some early thinning of the disc space with some discogenic spondylotic change which may be minimal.

The patient may have paresthesias of the lower extremities but no frank altered deep reflexes.

At this stage, there is minimal irritation of the nerve root into the lower extremity. Examination reveals a more positive straight leg raise sign, Kemp's sign, and other orthopedic signs for early disc protrusion.

Clinically, this patient with prolonged exacerbation of low back pain and with leg symptomatology requires a longer treatment period than does the patient in Category I. At this stage, it is important that the patient wear a lumbosacral support in order to stabilize the low back for healing. Sitting must be strictly avoided in order to reduce the intradiscal pressure and allow the annulus to heal. At this stage, the use of exercises to open the dorsal intervertebral disc spaces are most helpful and nutrition with Discat should be incorporated into the overall treatment.

The articular facets have also become pain-producing entities because of the disruption of the articular cartilage and subluxation resulting from the loss of normal mobility of the motion segment. Thus, the backs of Category II patients contain two pain-producing entities, the annulus fibrosus and the articular facet.

## Category III—Nuclear Protrusion

Frank protrusion of nuclear material into the annulus is evident in the Category III patient. This patient can have severe antalgia, marked lower extremity pain, and altered deep motor and sensory abnormalities.

He may have difficulty in straightening from a flexed position and a marked loss of lumbar lordosis. He requires prolonged periods of time for treatment, and ambulation is limited because of pain on weight bearing.

His ranges of motion in the low back are markedly limited, and Kemp's sign is definitely positive, depending upon the medial or lateral relationship of the disc bulge to the nerve root.

X-rays show antalgia and possible discal change.

Category III is a progression of Category II. The patient must remain recumbent and wear a back support. At the outset of treatment the patient will need to make up to 2 to 3 visits/day for maximum relief from pain.

## Category IV—Nuclear Prolapse

The Category IV patient presents primarily with lower extremity pain and with minimal to absent low back pain. Nuclear material has completely torn through the annulus and lies within the canal as a free fragment irritating the nerve root and perhaps the cauda equina severely. Now the possibility of surgery becomes one of clinical differential diagnosis as to its necessity. If this patient does not show a 50% improvement within 3 weeks, the possibility of surgery is imminent. The patient may also experience constipation and incontinence.

Annular tear and bulge are theoretical diagnoses. According to Murphy (3), however, the sequence of events as involves production of pain in the lumbar region is as follows: There is an incomplete tear of the annulus, allowing nuclear protrusion, which stretches the annulus and posterior longitudinal ligament causing midline back pain. If the tear is lateral, the nuclear protrusion compresses the nerve root, resulting in buttock and leg pain. A patient with sudden cessation of low back pain and onset of leg pain has an extruded disc fragment and requires surgery. Today we would consider this patient to have a protruding disc, which would ultimately become a complete tear of the annulus, allowing prolapse of the nucleus.

For a patient to be considered to have nuclear protrusion or prolapse, three of the five following findings are necessary (4).

1. Leg pain rather than back pain is the dominant symptom. One leg only is affected and the pain follows a typical sciatic (or femoral) nerve distribution.

2. Paresthesiae are localized to a dermatomal distribution.

3. Straight leg raising is reduced by 50% of normal, and/or pain crosses over to the symptomatic leg when the unaffected leg is elevated, and/or pain radiates proximally or distally with digital pressure on the tibial nerve in the popliteal fossa.

4. Two of the four neurological signs are present, i.e., wasting, motor weakness, diminished sensory appreciation, and diminution of reflex activity.

5. A contrast study is positive; the visualized lesion corresponds to the clinical level.

The incidence of sacroiliac lesion or short leg following relief of sciatic pain is determined and recorded on the examination form.

The chiropractic procedure employed in the treatment of a particular patient's condition is recorded and any physical therapy is then administered and recorded.

Finally, the patient response to treatment (from excellent to need for surgery) is determined, and this gradation of response is recorded on the examination form.

Ultimately, the number of treatments and the days of treatment necessary to achieve 50% improvement and maximum improvement is determined for each of these conditions. This approach provides

both a subjective and an objective determination of the patient's response to treatment, based actually on the percentage of subjective relief felt by the patient and on the objective relief as evidenced primarily by four tests—straight leg raise, Kemp's, Déjérine's triad, and range of motion (5).

For each participating doctor, a code book which completely explained each question, the possible answers that the patient could make, and the method of reporting the answer on the examination form was made available and was used.

## RESULTS

The results that follow are based on the treatment of 576 patients by 23 different chiropractors in different geographic areas of the United States and Canada.

### Basic Patient Information

*Referrals.* Ten patients were referred to the chiropractor by a medical doctor; 50, by another chiropractor; 1, by an osteopath; 198, by the patients themselves; 74, by their families; 137, by other patients; and 66, by some other source. For 40 patients, the source of referral was unknown.

*Race.* Of these 576 patients, 550 were Caucasian, 17 were Negro, 1 was Japanese, 1 was Chinese, and 2 were American Indian. For 5, the race was unknown and/or unrecorded.

*Age.* The mean age for these patients was 43.4 years. The youngest was 13 and the oldest was 86 years of age.

*Sex.* Of these 576 patients, 331 were male and 233 were females; 2 of the females were in the first trimester of pregnancy and 1 was pregnant but the trimester was unrecorded.

*Marital Status.* There were 109 single patients, 386 married patients, 37 divorced patients, and 23 widowed patients.

*Height.* The average patient height for 370 known cases was 67 inches, with a minimum height of 33 inches and a maximum height of 83 inches recorded.

*Weight.* The average weight for 366 known cases was 165.8 lbs., with a minimum weight of 94 lbs. and a maximum weight of 295 lb recorded.

*Body Type.* Of these 576 patients, 90

were ectomorphs, 320 were mesomorphs, and 108 were endomorphs; information on 58 was missing.

## Habits

*Smoker.* Fifty-eight percent did not smoke, 14% smoked less than 1 pack/day, 12% smoked 1 to 2 packs/day, 2% smoked 2 to 3 packs/day, and 0.2% smoked 3 packs/day or more. Data on the other 13.4% were unknown and/or missing.

*Stress.* Each patient was asked to evaluate the stress in his life on a scale of 1 to 9, with 1 being no stress and 9 being maximum tolerable stress. Their answers were then recorded: 5% rated it at 1, 5% at 2, 12% at 3, 15% at 4, 24% at 5, 12% at 6, 10% at 7, 10% at 8, and 7% at 9. Data were missing on 144 patients.

*Period of Time in Exercise.* Of these 576 patients, 207 did no exercise, 32 exercised less than 10 minutes, 96 exercised from 11 to 30 minutes, 71 exercised from 31 to 60 minutes, 36 exercised from 1 to 2 hours, and 11 exercised more than 2 hours per workout. Data were missing on 122 patients.

*Frequency of Exercise Workout.* There were 207 who did no exercise, 105 who exercised daily, 115 who exercised 2 to 3 times weekly, and 3 who exercised 2 to 3 times a month. Data were missing on 118 patients.

*Heaviest Weight Normally Lifted During the Day.* Forty-five percent of patients lifted less than 10 lb/day, 29% lifted 11 to 30 lb/day, 12% lifted 31 to 50 lb/day, 8% lifted 51 to 100 lb/day, and 4% lifted more than 100 lb/day; data were missing on 25%.

*Frequency of Lifting Approximately 30 lb.* Twenty-seven percent of patients lifted 30 lb once an hour, 25% lifted it once a day, 18% lifted it once a week, 15% lift it once a month, and 13% lift it once a year; and data were missing on 159.

## Chief Complaint

The most common chief complaint was low back pain in 464 patients, and the second chief complaint was leg pain in 78 patients. The second most common chief complaint was low back pain in 65 and leg pain in 258.

## Pain Information

*Description of Pain.* Of those patients who reported having pain, 302 stated that the pain was constant and 216 stated that it was intermittent. On a scale of 1 to 9, with 1 being the least intense and 9 being the most intense pain, the average pain intensity recorded was as 6. The pain was reported as being insidious by 246 patients and as being acute and traumatic by 283. There were 47 who did not describe the pain in these terms.

*Activity Causing Injury.* Of 544 patients, 210 did not know of any activity causing their injury, 45 reported bending without lifting as the cause, 58 reported bending while lifting as the cause, 97 reported rotating at the waist while bending and lifting as the cause, 47 reported rotating and bending while not lifting as the cause, and 46 reported that the pain started after a fall, and 41 reported that the injury was due to an accident. We further correlated each low back diagnosis with the activity reported to have caused the injury. Interestingly, patients with discogenic spondyloarthrosis generally did not know what activity caused their injury, while patients with disc lesions could distinctly link the pain to a specific bending, lifting, and/or rotation injury.

*Sport Involved.* Sixty-three patients stated that they were participating in a sport when the onset of pain occurred, with running and jogging being the most commonly listed sports associated with low back pain or leg pain.

*Prior Back Pain.* There were 244 patients who stated that they had had previous incidences of back pain for years prior to their present complaint, 147 who stated that they had had no previous back pain, and 52 who stated that they had had weeks or months of prior pain. The home was the most common location where the injury occurred, followed by the work place. Although 269 patients stated that lifting was not involved with their injury, among those who stated that lifting was involved at the onset of injury, 83 lifted less than 10 lb, 82 lifted 11 to 30 lb, 28 lifted 31 to 50 lb, 15 lifted 51 to 80 lb, 15 lifted 81 to 100 lb, 16 lifted 101 to 200 lb, and 7 lifted over 200 lb. Two hundred fifty-five patients stated that they had no night pain along with the back pain, whereas 250 stated that they had had night pain. Eighteen of 576 patients had considered suicide due to the low back pain.

*Location of Pain and Dermatome Affected.* Of the patients having dermatome pain, 112 had pain involving the S1 dermatome, 65 had pain involving the L5 dermatome, 23 had pain involving the L4 dermatome, 15 had pain involving the L3 dermatome, 73 had pain involving the L5 and S1 dermatomes, and 12 had pain involving the L4 and L5 dermatomes. Fifty-two patients had pain in the right leg; 40, pain in the left leg; 25, pain in both legs; 1, alternating leg pain; 211, low back pain only; 80, low back and right leg pain; 114, low back and left leg pain; and 48, both low back and bilateral leg pain. Leg pain preceded back pain in 20 patients, back and leg pain occurred simultaneously in 94 patients, and leg pain occurred after low back pain in 222 patients. The leg pain was described as sharp by 224, as dull by 167, as throbbing by 32, and as a traction or burning by 12. The leg pain was described as extending to the buttock by 276, to the thigh by 208, to the knee by 185, to the calf by 134, to the ankle by 90, to the foot by 62, and into the toes by 35 patients. The most common skin sensation was numbness, followed by tingling, burning, and the feeling of being asleep.

Walking aggravated the low back pain in 138 patients, the left leg pain in 66, the right leg pain in 53, and pain in both legs in 24, whereas it did not aggravate low back or leg pain in 233 patients. Déjérine's triad was positive and aggravated the back and leg pain in 51% of the patients and was negative in 49%. Sitting exacerbated the symptoms in 347 patients, flexion at the waist, in 163; standing, in 149; hyperextension at the waist, in 84; and recumbency, in 22. Recumbency caused a remission of the symptoms in 390 patients; standing, in 58; and sitting, in 51.

## Medical History

*Previous Diagnostic and Treatment Results.* Of 576 patients, 56 had a myelogram performed previously, with 32 of the myelograms being positive, 21 negative, and 3 inconclusive. Eleven patients had CAT scans, 13 had electromyography, 3 had discography, and 1 had an epidural venogram.

Prior treatment had been rendered by a medical doctor in 168 patients, a doctor of chiropractic in 90 patients, a doctor of osteopathy in 13 patients, by both a medical doctor and a doctor of chiropractic in 69 patients, and by a medical doctor, a doctor of osteopathy, and a doctor of chiropractic in 8 patients; 205 reported having had no previous treatment.

Of those taking medication, 121 reported no change, 33 reported a 25% improvement, 31 reported a 50% improvement, 7 reported a 75% improvement, and 13 reported a 100% improvement; 8 believed that they were worse after taking the medication than before.

Twenty-seven patients had had low back surgery, with 21 having had a laminectomy; 4, a fusion; 1, microsurgery; and 1, an undefined procedure. At 1-year follow-up, 6 patients felt worse, 4 felt no change, 3 felt a 25% improvement, 3 felt a 50% improvement, 3 felt a 75% improvement, and 3 felt a 100% improvement; on 5, there was no report.

Of those patients receiving prior nonsurgical treatment, 153 had had manipulation; 10, epidural injections; 2, chemonucleolysis; 5, closed reduction; 87, physical therapy; and 8, acupuncture. Previous therapy had consisted of applications of heat and cold in 83 patients, of high-voltage galvanic current in 17, of low-voltage galvanic current in 13, of ultrasound in 60, of traction in 32, of massage in 21, of trigger point goading in 10, and of bracing in 31. Five patients had been to Low Back Pain School, 8 had worn transcutaneous electrical nerve stimulator (TENS) units, 4 had had psychological counseling, 5 had had biofeedback therapy, and 2 had had a combination of these treatments. Of those reporting the results of these therapies, 21 stated they were worse, 125 reported no change, 25 reported a 25% improvement, 20 reported a 50% improvement, and 25 reported a 75% to 100% improvement. Of the patients who had taken medication for their low back pain, 44 had taken anti-inflammatory drugs; 99, pain relievers; 55, muscle relaxants; 4, tranquilizers, 2, vitamin $B_{12}$; and 16, some other type of medication. Of those who had taken medication, 8 felt that they were worse after being medicated, 121 reported no change, 33 reported a 25% improvement, 31 reported a 50% improvement, 7 reported a 75% improvement, 13 reported a 100% improvement; on 29, there was no report. Of 194 patients who stated that a specific chiropractic technic had been applied prior to seeing the doctors involved in this project, 38 felt that they had been in someway harmed through chiropractic manipulation.

## Physical Examination

Following a general physical examination, 59 of the 576 patients were listed in poor physical condition; 145, in average condition; 204, in good condition; and 92, in excellent condition; the physical condition of 76 was not reported.

Specific tests were then performed. The following are the percentage of positive findings to each of these tests: Minor's sign, 40% Bechterew's sign, 55%; Valsalva maneuver, 45%; Valsalva maneuver with Bechterew's sign, 55%; Néri's sign, 15%; Lewin's sign, 20%; limp, 25%; spinal tilt, 49%; loss of lumbar lordosis, 40%; percussion, 36%; Kemp's sign, 73%; toe walk, 6%; heel walk, 8%; Lindner's sign, 33%; hamstring tightness, 50%; straight leg raise reduced to an average of 57°, 44%; well leg raise sign, 16%; Gaenslen's sign, 14%; Patrick's sign, 17%; Cox's sign, 17%; Amoss' sign, 33%; Milgram's sign, 32%; diminished right ankle jerk, 15%; diminished left ankle jerk, 16%; hyperesthesia, 15%; hypoesthesia, 26%; diminished circulation, 10%; Moses' sign, 8%; Nachlas' sign, 8%; Yeoman's sign, 28%; Ely's sign, 24%; prone lumbar flexion increasing low back pain, 55%; leg pain, 10%; decreased ankle jerk, 4%; altered dermatome pain, 5%; decreased flexion, 1%; pain in the popliteal fossa, 28%; short leg, 26%; medial hip rotation, 21%; limitation of range of motion to an average of 58° on flexion, 20° on extension, 17° on right and left lateral flexion, and 26° on rotation; the muscle strength changes such as weakness on dorsiflexion of the foot, 9%; plantar flexion of the foot, 4%; great toe flexion, 8%; great toe extension, 12%; and foot eversion, 5%. Déjérine's triad was positive in 51% of patients and negative in 49%.

Based upon the above statistics, the tests utilized most often to measure a patient's response to chiropractic manipulation were the straight leg raise, Kemp's sign, range of motion, and Déjérine's triad. Other tests found positive were added, of course, to these four in each individual case.

## X-ray Interpretation and Spinal Mechanics

***Findings on X-ray Examination.*** X-rays revealed the following: 33% of the patients had right spinal lean, and 35%, a left spinal lean. Sixty-seven patients had a right scoliosis, and 66, a left scoliosis, with 70% of these curves being under 10°, 28% being from 10° to 30°, and 2% being more than 40° as determined by Cobb's angle. The average sacral angle was 36° with a minimum of 4° and a maximum of 67°. The average lumbar lordosis angle was 38°, with a low of 2° and a high of 78°.

***Planes of Articulation.*** At L5-S1, 61% of the facets were bilaterally coronal, 10% were bilaterally sagittal, and 24% revealed tropism; there were no records on the missing 5%. At the L4-L5 level, 48% of the facets were coronal, 15% were sagittal, and 16% revealed tropism.

***Short Leg.*** On the initial examinations, 7% of patients in antalgic lean had a right short leg of less than 5 mm, 6% had a right short leg of 5 to 10 mm, and 5% had a right short leg of more than 10 mm. Eight percent of patients had a left short leg of less than 5 mm, 7% had a left short leg of 5 to 10 mm, and 4% had a left short leg of more than 10 mm, and 38% showed no difference in leg length; leg length was not recorded in 25%.

***Facet Syndrome.*** Of 212 patients, x-ray revealed facet syndrome in 62 (29%) at L4-L5 and in 150 (71%) at L5-S1. Of these 212 patients, 149 were listed as stable and 60 were listed as unstable by Van Akkerveeken measurement; the condition was not reported in 3.

Thirty-nine patients were found to have spina bifida, 16 patients had spondylolysis at L4, and 25 had spondylolysis at L5.

## Congenital Anomaly

*Spondylolisthesis.* There were 5.9% of patients who had spondylolisthesis; 2 patients had spondylolisthesis at the L3 level; 11, at the L4 level; and 19, at the L5 level. The maximum slippage was 45%. These were cases of true spondylolisthesis with pars interarticularis separation. There were also 14 patients who had pseudospondylolisthesis; 8 had it at the L4 level; 3, at the L5 level; and 3, at the L3 level.

*Transitional Segment.* Seven percent of the patients had sacralization, and 6% had lumbarization at the transitional L5-S1 zone.

*Pathologies.* Eight percent of patients were reported to have osteoporosis; 1% each were reported to have fracture, degenerative hip disease, ankylosing spondylosis, tumor, and infection. Forty-eight patients had Schmorl's nodes in the lumbar spine at one or more levels. Two hundred eighty-two patients had narrowing of the L5 disc; 107, of the L4 disc; 53, of the L3 disc; 34, of the L2 disc; and 35, of the L1 disc. Spondylosis was found at L5 in 120 patients, at L4 in 96 patients, at L3 in 71 patients, at L2 in 47 patients, and at L1 in 31 patients. Facet arthrosis was documented in 144 patients at L5, in 89 at L4, in 61 at L3, in 36 at L2, and in 25 at L1. Retrolisthesis subluxation of L5 was found in 10% of patients and of L4 was found in 7%.

## Correlative Diagnosis of Low Back Pain Patients

Tables 15.2 and 15.3 reveal the breakdown of conditions occurring at the L4 and the L5 level, respectively, by diagnosis as determined in these 576 cases. (The total responses may exceed 576 because one patient may have had more than one condition.) Of 126 L5 nuclear protrusions or prolapses, 61 occurred on the right side and 65 occurred on the left side. Of those that occurred on the right, 28 involved the medial discs and 33 involved the lateral discs; of those that occurred on the left, 35 involved the medial discs and 30 involved the lateral discs. Of 75 instances of nuclear protrusion or prolapse occurring at L4, 37 occurred on the right side and 38 occurred on the left side. Of those occurring on the right side, 14 involved the medial discs and 23 involved the lateral discs; of those occurring on the left side, 21 involved the medial discs and 17 involved the lateral discs.

Table 15.4 reveals the incidence of a disc lesion and an accompanying anomaly in 237 cases.

Table 15.5 shows the incidence of an L4 disc lesion and discogenic spondyloarthrosis at the L5 level. It also shows the incidence of Bertolotti's syndrome (an L5 transitional segment and L4 disc protrusion.) The respective percentages are also revealed. In 46% of the cases of L4 disc lesion, there was degeneration at the L5 disc.

Table 15.6 reveals the incidence of an L5 disc lesion and a combination of anomalies in 237 cases.

Tables 15.7 and 15.8 reveal the presence of Déjérine's triad in cases of L4 and L5 disc lesions, respectively. Please note that Déjérine's triad occurs in fewer cases of nuclear bulge or protrusion at L5 than it occurs in cases of nuclear prolapse at L5. Déjérine's triad occurs in more cases of nuclear bulge or protrusion at L4, however, than it occurs in cases of nuclear prolapse at L4.

Tables 15.9 and 15.10 reveal the locations of pain in cases of L4 and L5 spondylolisthesis, respectively.

*Stenosis.* Table 15.11 reveals the presence or absence of intermittent claudication symptoms in patients with stenosis. Fourteen percent of patients with stenosis had retrolisthesis subluxation of L5 when the stenosis occurred at that level, and another 12% had retrolisthesis at 2 or more levels when stenosis was present at these levels.

*Dermatome and Disc Correlation.* Table 15.12 reveals the dermatome involved in 126 correlatively diagnosed cases of L5 disc lesions.

*Leg Pain Related to Back Pain.* Table 15.13 shows the correlation of the onset

**Table 15.2.**
**Breakdown of Conditions Occurring at L4, by Diagnosis**

| Dichotomy Label | Name | No. of Responses[a] | % of Responses | % of Cases |
|---|---|---|---|---|
| Annular tear | X1 | 11 | 2.8 | 4.1 |
| Nuclear bulge | X2 | 31 | 7.9 | 11.5 |
| Nuclear protrusion | X3 | 79 | 20.3 | 29.3 |
| Nuclear prolapse | X4 | 9 | 2.3 | 3.3 |
| Discogenic spondyloar-throsis | X5 | 72 | 18.5 | 26.7 |
| Facet syndrome | X6 | 59 | 15.1 | 21.9 |
| Spondylolisthesis | X7 | 15 | 3.8 | 5.6 |
| Stenosis | X8 | 22 | 5.6 | 8.1 |
| Iatrogenic | X9 | 2 | 0.5 | 0.7 |
| Sprain and strain | X11 | 32 | 8.2 | 11.9 |
| Tropism | X13 | 33 | 8.5 | 12.2 |
| Transitional segment | X14 | 25 | 6.4 | 9.3 |
| Total | | 390 | 100.0 | 144.4 |

[a] Value tabulated equals 1.

**Table 15.3.**
**Breakdown of Conditions Occurring at L5, by Diagnosis**

| Dichotomy Label | Name | No. of Responses[a] | % of Responses | % of Cases |
|---|---|---|---|---|
| Annular tear | Y1 | 50 | 6.3 | 10.9 |
| Nuclear bulge | Y2 | 61 | 7.6 | 13.3 |
| Nuclear protrusion | Y3 | 107 | 13.4 | 23.4 |
| Nuclear prolapse | Y4 | 19 | 2.4 | 4.1 |
| Discogenic spondyloar-throsis | Y5 | 122 | 15.3 | 26.6 |
| Facet syndrome | Y6 | 204 | 25.5 | 44.5 |
| Spondylolisthesis | Y7 | 20 | 2.5 | 4.4 |
| Stenosis | Y8 | 73 | 9.1 | 15.9 |
| Iatrogenic | Y9 | 3 | 0.4 | 0.7 |
| Sprain and strain | Y11 | 79 | 9.9 | 17.2 |
| Tropism | Y13 | 42 | 5.3 | 9.2 |
| Transitional segment | Y14 | 19 | 2.4 | 4.1 |
| Total | | 799 | 100.0 | 174.5 |

[a] Value tabulated equals 1.

**Table 15.4.**
**Incidence of a Disc Lesion and an Accompanying Anomaly in 237 Cases**

| Level of Lesion | Anomaly | No. | % |
|---|---|---|---|
| L5 | Discogenic spondyloarthrosis | 19 | 13 |
| L5 | Facet syndrome | 39 | 5 |
| L5 | Spondylolisthesis | 5 | 3 |
| L5 | Stenosis | 25 | 17 |
| L5 | Tropism | 19 | 13 |
| L5 | Transitional segment | 3 | 2 |

**Table 15.5.**
**Incidence of a Disc Lesion and One Anomaly in 237 Cases**

| Level of Lesion | Anomaly | | No. | % |
|---|---|---|---|---|
| | Level | Type | | |
| L4 | L5 | Discogenic spondyloarthrosis | 25 | 46 |
| L4 | L5 | Transitional segment | 4 | 7.3 |

**Table 15.6.**
**Incidence of a Disc Lesion and a**
**Combination of Anomalies in 237 Cases**

| Level of Lesion | Anomalies | No. |
|---|---|---|
| L5 | Tropism Stenosis | 2 |
| L5 | Tropism Facet syndrome | 6 |
| L5 | Stenosis Facet syndrome | 13 |
| L5 | Tropism Facet syndrome Stenosis | 2 |

**Table 15.7.**
**Presence of Déjérine's Triad in Cases of**
**L4 Disc Lesion**

| Type of Lesion | % |
|---|---|
| Nuclear tear | 46 |
| Nuclear bulge | 65 |
| Nuclear protrusion | 62 |
| Nuclear prolapse | 89 |

**Table 15.8.**
**Presence of Déjérine's Triad in Cases of**
**L5 Disc Lesion**

| Type of Lesion | % |
|---|---|
| Nuclear tear | 48 |
| Nuclear bulge | 64 |
| Nuclear protrusion | 66 |
| Nuclear prolapse | 37 |

**Table 15.9.**
**Location of Pain in 15 Cases of L4**
**Spondylolisthesis**

| Location | No. |
|---|---|
| Right leg | 1 |
| Left leg | 1 |
| Both legs | 1 |
| Low back | 5 |
| Low back and right leg | 1 |
| Low back and left leg | 3 |
| Low back and both legs | 3 |

**Table 15.10.**
**Location of Pain in 20 Cases of L5**
**Spondylolisthesis**

| Location | No. |
|---|---|
| Right leg | 4 |
| Left leg | 1 |
| Low back | 7 |
| Low back and right leg | 5 |
| Low back and left leg | 1 |
| Low back and both legs | 2 |

**Table 15.11.**
**Presence or Absence of Intermittent**
**Claudication in 73 Patients with**
**Stenosis**

| Location of Pain (if any) | No. |
|---|---|
| None | 30 |
| Left leg | 11 |
| Right leg | 7 |
| Both legs | 2 |
| Don't know | 11 |
| Low back | 12 |

**Table 15.12.**
**Dermatome Involved in 126 Cases of L5**
**Disc Lesions**

| Level of Lesion | No. |
|---|---|
| S1 | 64 |
| L5 | 7 |
| L5-S1 | 23 |
| L4 | 2 |
| L4-L5 | 4 |
| L3 | 3 |
| Don't know | 23 |

and leg pain is found more often in cases of disc protrusion.

*Sacroiliac Lesions.* In 11% of patients who had low back pain without leg pain, a sacroiliac subluxation was found following relief of the disc lesion.

*Short Leg.* In 11% of patients, following maximum relief of their mechanical low back problems, a 6-mm or more short leg that required correction was found.

## Treatment and Response

Table 15.14 reveals the responses of the 576 patients to chiropractic manipulation.

of leg pain with the onset of back pain in cases of disc protrusion and prolapse. It has been written that leg pain is found more often in cases of disc prolapse, whereas the combination of both back

**Table 15.13.**
**Onset of Leg Pain in Relation to Back Pain in Cases of Disc Protrusion and Prolapse**

| | % of Cases at L4 Level | | % of Cases at L5 Level | |
|---|---|---|---|---|
| | Before Back Pain | After Back Pain | Before Back Pain | After Back Pain |
| Protrusion | 26 | 51 | 22 | 65 |
| Prolapse | 34 | 55 | 33 | 56 |

**Table 15.14.**
**Response to Chiropractic Manipulation in 576 Patients**

| Response | No. | % |
|---|---|---|
| Excellent | 275 | 50 |
| Very good | 74 | 14 |
| Good | 60 | 11 |
| Fair | 36 | 6 |
| Poor | 22 | 4 |
| Surgery | 17 | 3 |
| Stopped, not started[a] | 57 | 10 |
| Examined but not treated | 7 | 1 |

[a] Treatment was stopped or was never started.

Table 15.15 reveals the chiropractic procedures utilized in the treatment of these patients.

The definition of response is given in Table 15.1 under "Basic Patient Information."

Tables 15.16 through 15.19 provide a breakdown of patient responses to specific conditions at the L4-L5 and L5-S1 levels, respectively (Tables 15.16 and 15.17, for responses of patients with L4-L5 lesions; and Tables 15.18 and 19, for responses of patients with L5-S1 lesions).

Table 15.20 reveals the response of patients with various anomalies and a disc lesion at L5 to chiropractic treatment.

## Length of and Need for Treatment

Patient response to treatment was measured both subjectively and objectively. Subjectively, the patient was asked to note when he felt a 50% improvement from his pain or when he returned to normal, i.e., obtained maximum relief from pain. Objectively, Kemp's sign, range of motion, Déjérine's triad, and straight leg raise, along with other pertinent positive findings in each case, were used to measure the objective relief from

**Table 15.15.**
**Chiropractic Procedures Used in the Treatment of 576 Patients**

| Procedure | No. | % |
|---|---|---|
| Cox | 529 | 94 |
| Gonstead | 3 | 0.5 |
| Meric | 6 | 1.1 |
| Side posture | 10 | 1.8 |
| Diversified | 13 | 2.3 |
| Thompson | 1 | 0.2 |

pain. In either case, the number of visits, days, and treatments needed to obtain relief were recorded.

Tables 15.21 and 15.22 show the number of treatments and days of treatment necessary to obtain 50% or maximum improvement, respectively, in 576 patients regardless of diagnosis. Maximum improvement is defined as the return of the patient to his pre-pain state or that point at which treatment no longer renders relief from pain for the patient. Usually, the maximum amount of time that any of these patients are treated is 3 months, as it is believed that maximum relief from pain is attained by this time.

Tables 15.23 and 15.24 provide breakdowns of the data from these 576 cases by the number of treatments (Table 15.23) and the number of days of treatment (Table 15.24) needed to obtain 50% and maximum relief from pain.

Table 15.25 shows the response of patients who had had back surgery to chiropractic treatment for recurring back pain.

Tables 15.26 through 15.33 provide a breakdown of the cases by the type of lesion and the number of treatments and the days of treatment necessary to achieve improvement.

**Table 15.16.**
**Response of Patients with Conditions at L4-L5 to Chiropractic Treatment, by Number and Percent of Specific Lesion**

| | Annular Tear | | Nuclear Bulge | | Nuclear Protrusion | | Nuclear Prolapse | | Discogenic Spondyloarthrosis | | Facet Syndrome | | Spondylolisthesis | | Stenosis | | Tropism | |
|---|---|---|---|---|---|---|---|---|---|---|---|---|---|---|---|---|---|---|
| | No. | % | No. | % | No. | % | No. | % | No. | % | No. | % | No. | % | No. | % | No. | % |
| Excellent | 6 | 67 | 21 | 67 | 23 | 32 | 4 | 44 | 29 | 41 | 28 | 52 | 5 | 39 | 8 | 40 | 14 | 45 |
| Very good | 2 | 22 | 3 | 10 | 12 | 16 | 1 | 11 | 14 | 20 | 6 | 11 | 2 | 15 | 4 | 20 | 4 | 13 |
| Good | 1 | 11 | 1 | 3 | 9 | 12 | 2 | 22 | 5 | 7 | 3 | 6 | 1 | 8 | 1 | 5 | 2 | 7 |
| Fair | | | 1 | 3 | 8 | 11 | 1 | 11 | 9 | 13 | 8 | 15 | 2 | 15 | 2 | 10 | 3 | 10 |
| Poor | | | 1 | 3 | 5 | 7 | | | 2 | 3 | 2 | 4 | | | 1 | 5 | 2 | 7 |
| Surgery | | | | | 4 | 6 | | | | | 1 | 2 | | | | | 1 | 3 |
| Don't know | | | | | | | | | | | | | | | | | | |
| Stopped, not started[a] | | | 4 | 13 | 10 | 14 | 1 | 11 | 10 | 14 | 5 | 9 | 3 | 23 | 4 | 20 | 4 | 13 |
| Examined but not treated | | | | | 2 | 3 | | | 1 | 1 | 1 | 2 | | | | | 1 | 3 |
| Total | 9 | | 31 | | 73 | | 9 | | 70 | | 54 | | 13 | | 20 | | 31 | |

[a] Treatment was stopped or was never started.

**Table 15.17.**
**Response of Patients with Disc Lesions at L4-L5**

| Response | No. | % |
|---|---|---|
| Excellent | 52 | 43 |
| Very good | 16 | 13 |
| Good | 14 | 12 |
| Fair | 10 | 8 |
| Poor | 6 | 5 |
| Surgery | 4 | 3 |
| Stopped, not started[a] | 16 | 13 |
| Examined but not treated | 2 | 2 |
| Total | 120 | |

[a] Treatment was stopped or was never started.

**Table 15.18.**
**Response of Patients with Conditions at L5-S1 to Chiropractic Treatment**

| | Annular Tear | | Nuclear Bulge | | Nuclear Protrusion | | Nuclear Prolapse | | Discogenic Spondyloarthrosis | | Facet Syndrome | | Spondylolisthesis | | Stenosis | | Tropism | | Transitional Segment | |
|---|---|---|---|---|---|---|---|---|---|---|---|---|---|---|---|---|---|---|---|---|---|
| | No. | % | No. | % | No. | % | No. | % | No. | % | No. | % | No. | % | No. | % | No. | % | No. | % |
| Excellent | 36 | 77 | 30 | 52 | 46 | 45 | 3 | 16 | 51 | 45 | 107 | 55 | 6 | 32 | 35 | 53 | 17 | 44 | 11 | 61 |
| Very good | 2 | 4 | 9 | 16 | 15 | 15 | 6 | 32 | 17 | 15 | 24 | 12 | 4 | 21 | 9 | 14 | 7 | 18 | 3 | 17 |
| Good | 3 | 6 | 11 | 19 | 9 | 9 | 1 | 5 | 10 | 9 | 25 | 13 | 5 | 26 | 8 | 12 | 2 | 5 | 1 | 6 |
| Fair | 1 | 2 | 4 | 7 | 6 | 6 | 1 | 5 | 18 | 16 | 13 | 7 | 3 | 16 | 5 | 8 | 6 | 15 | 2 | 11 |
| Poor | 2 | 4 | | | 1 | 1 | 3 | 16 | 4 | 4 | 6 | 3 | | | 1 | 2 | 1 | 3 | | |
| Surgery | | | | | | | 2 | 11 | | | 1 | 0.5 | | | 2 | 3 | 1 | 3 | | |
| Don't know | | | | | 11 | 11 | | | | | | | | | | | | | | |
| Stopped, not started[a] | 3 | 6 | 4 | 7 | 13 | 13 | 3 | 16 | 12 | 11 | 15 | 8 | 1 | 5 | 6 | 9 | 5 | 13 | 1 | 6 |
| Examined but not treated | | | | | 1 | 1 | | | 1 | 1 | 4 | 2 | | | | | | | | |
| Total | 47 | | 58 | | 102 | | 19 | | 113 | | 195 | | 19 | | 66 | | 39 | | 18 | |

[a] Treatment was stopped or was never started.

**Table 15.19.**
**Response of Patient with Disc Lesions at L5-S1 to Chiropractic Treatment**

| Response | No. | % |
|---|---|---|
| Excellent | 110 | 50 |
| Very good | 32 | 15 |
| Good | 23 | 11 |
| Fair | 12 | 6 |
| Poor | 6 | 3 |
| Surgery | 13 | 6 |
| Stopped, not started[a] | 22 | 10 |
| Examined but not treated | 1 | 0.5 |
| Total | 219 | |

[a] Treatment was stopped or was never started.

**Table 15.20.**
**Response of 288 Patients with Various Anomalies and a Disc Lesion at L5 to**
**Chiropractic Treatment**

| Response | Count | No. of Patients with the Following Anomalies and Lesions | | | | |
|---|---|---|---|---|---|---|
| | | Disc Lesion, Tropism, Stenosis | Disc Lesion, Tropism, Facet Syndrome | Disc Lesion, Stenosis, Facet Syndrome | Disc Lesion, Tropism, Facet Syndrome, Stenosis | Total No. |
| Excellent | 1. | 1 | 3 | 5 | 1 | 10 |
| | | 10.0[a] | 30.0 | 50.0 | 10.0 | 47.6[d] |
| | | 50.0[b] | 50.0 | 41.7 | 100.0 | |
| | | 4.8[c] | 14.3 | 23.8 | 4.8 | |
| Very good | 2. | 1 | 1 | 2 | 0 | 4 |
| | | 25.0[a] | 25.0 | 50.0 | 0.0 | 19.0[d] |
| | | 50.0[b] | 16.7 | 16.7 | 0.0 | |
| | | 4.8[c] | 4.8 | 9.5 | 0.0 | |
| Good | 3. | 0 | 0 | 2 | 0 | 2 |
| | | 0.0[a] | 0.0 | 100.0 | 0.0 | 9.5[d] |
| | | 0.0[b] | 0.0 | 16.7 | 0.0 | |
| | | 0.0[c] | 0.0 | 9.5 | 0.0 | |
| Fair | 4. | 0 | 1 | 0 | 0 | 1 |
| | | 0.0[a] | 100.0 | 0.0 | 0.0 | 4.8[d] |
| | | 0.0[b] | 16.7 | 0.0 | 0.0 | |
| | | 0.0 | 4.8 | 0.0 | 0.0 | |
| Poor | 5. | 0 | 0 | 1 | 0 | 1 |
| | | 0.0[a] | 0.0 | 100.0 | 0.0 | 4.8[d] |
| | | 0.0[b] | 0.0 | 8.3 | 0.0 | |
| | | 0.0[c] | 0.0 | 4.8 | 0.0 | |
| Stopped, not started[e] | 8. | 0 | 1 | 2 | 0 | 3 |
| | | 0.0[a] | 33.3 | 66.7 | 0.0 | 14.3[d] |
| | | 0.0[b] | 16.7 | 16.7 | 0.0 | |
| | | 0.0[c] | 4.8 | 9.5 | 0.0 | |
| Column | | 2 | 6 | 12 | 1 | 21 |
| Total | | 9.5 | 28.6 | 57.1 | 4.8 | 100.0 |

[a] Percent of each problem to specific response (read across row).
[b] Percent of each column problem to specific response (read down column).
[c] Percent of total row percent, i.e., percent of each problem to specific response.
[d] Percent of total column, i.e., percent of response row to total responses.
[e] Treatment was stopped or was never started.

**Table 15.21.**
**Number of Treatments and Days of Treatment Necessary to Achieve a 50% Improvement in 576 Patients Regardless of Diagnosis**

|         | Days | Treatments |
|---------|------|------------|
| Mean    | 14.4 | 9.5        |
| Median  | 10.1 | 6.5        |
| Minimum | 1    | 1          |
| Maximum | 140  | 120        |

**Table 15.22.**
**Number of Treatments and Days of Treatment Necessary to Achieve Maximum Improvement in 576 Patients Regardless of Diagnosis**

|         | Days | Treatments |
|---------|------|------------|
| Mean    | 42.8 | 18.6       |
| Median  | 30.1 | 13.7       |
| Minimum | 1    | 1          |
| Maximum | 420  | 201        |

**Table 15.23.**
**Number of Treatments Necessary to Achieve 50% Improvement and Maximum Improvement in 576 Patients**

| No. of Treatments | 50% Improvement | | Maximum Improvement | |
|-------------------|-----------------|---|---------------------|---|
|                   | No. of Patients | % | No. of Patients | % |
| Less than 10      | 452 | 79  | 294 | 51  |
| 10–20             | 94  | 16  | 146 | 25  |
| 20–30             | 15  | 3   | 73  | 13  |
| 30–40             | 6   | 1   | 28  | 5   |
| 40–50             |     | 0   | 16  | 3   |
| 50–60             | 4   | 1   | 6   | 1   |
| 60–80             | 3   | 0.5 | 5   | 1   |
| 80–100            |     | 0   | 2   | 0.3 |
| More than 100     | 2   | 0.3 | 6   | 1   |

**Table 15.24.**
**Number of Days of Treatment Necessary to Achieve 50% Improvement and Maximum Improvement in 576 Patients**

| No. of Days | 50% Improvement | | Maximum Improvement | |
|-------------|-----------------|---|---------------------|---|
|             | No. of Patients | % | No. of Patients | % |
| Less than 10 | 356 | 62  | 194 | 34 |
| 10–20        | 130 | 23  | 83  | 14 |
| 20–30        | 56  | 10  | 85  | 15 |
| 30–45        | 17  | 3   | 61  | 11 |
| 45–60        | 9   | 2   | 45  | 8  |
| 60–90        | 7   | 1   | 72  | 13 |
| More than 90 | 1   | 0.2 | 36  | 6  |

**Table 15.25.**
**Response of 34 Patients Who Had Had Back Surgery to Chiropractic Treatment for Recurring Back Pain**

|                  | No. of Patients | |
|------------------|-----------|------------|
|                  | 1 Surgery | 2 Surgeries |
| Excellent        | 4         | 6          |
| Very good        | 4         | 3          |
| Good             | 1         | 4          |
| Fair             | 2         | 1          |
| Poor             | 4         | 0          |
| Surgery          | 2         | 0          |
| Stopped treatment | 3        | 0          |
|                  | 20        | 14         |

**Table 15.26.**
**Cases of Discogenic Spondyloarthrosis in Relation to the Number of Treatments and the Days of Treatment Necessary to Achieve Improvement**

| Level of Lesion | Total No. of Cases | No. of Cases Requiring the Following No. of Days to 50% Improvement | | | | | | |
|---|---|---|---|---|---|---|---|---|
| | | Less than 10 | 10–20 | 20–30 | 30–45 | 45–60 | 60–90 | More than 90 |
| L4 | 72 | 43 (60%) | 15 | 10 | 1 | 3 | 0 | 0 |
| L5 | 122 | 71 (58%) | 27 | 18 (15%) | 1 | 3 | 2 | 0 |

| Level of Lesion | Total No. of Cases | No. of Cases Requiring the Following No. of Days to Maximum Improvement | | | | | | |
|---|---|---|---|---|---|---|---|---|
| | | Less than 10 | 10–20 | 20–30 | 30–45 | 45–60 | 60–90 | More than 90 |
| L4 | 72 | 20 (28%) | 12 | 11 | 6 | 7 | 12 (17%) | 4 |
| L5 | 122 | 39 (32%) | 16 | 22 (18%) | 13 | 11 | 15 (12%) | 6 (5%) |

| Level of Lesion | Total No. of Cases | No. of Cases Requiring the Following No. of Treatments to 50% Improvement | | | | | | | | |
|---|---|---|---|---|---|---|---|---|---|---|
| | | Less than 10 | 10–20 | 20–30 | 30–40 | 40–50 | 50–60 | 60–80 | 80–100 | More than 100 |
| L4 | 72 | 56 (78%) | 12 | 1 | 1 | 0 | 2 | 0 | 0 | 0 |
| L5 | 122 | 96 (79%) | 17 | 3 (3%) | 1 | 0 | 1 | 1 | 0 | 1 |

| Level of Lesion | Total No. of Cases | No. of Cases Requiring the Following No. of Treatments to Maximum Improvement | | | | | | | | |
|---|---|---|---|---|---|---|---|---|---|---|
| | | Less than 10 | 10–20 | 20–30 | 30–40 | 40–50 | 50–60 | 60–80 | 80–100 | More than 100 |
| L4 | 72 | 32 (44%) | 21 | 10 | 4 | 4 (6%) | 1 | 0 | 0 | 0 |
| L5 | 122 | 59 (48%) | 35 | 15 (12%) | 6 | 4 | 1 | 1 | 0 | 1 |

**Table 15.27.**
**Cases of Spondylolisthesis in Relation to the Number of Treatments and the Days of Treatment Necessary to Achieve Improvement**

| Level of Lesion | Total No. of Cases | No. of Cases Requiring the Following No. of Days to 50% Improvement | | | | | | |
|---|---|---|---|---|---|---|---|---|
| | | Less than 10 | 10–20 | 20–30 | 30–45 | 45–60 | 60–90 | More than 90 |
| L4 | 15 | 8 (53%) | 3 | 2 | 2 | 0 | 0 | 0 |
| L5 | 20 | 10 (50%) | 7 | 2 | 1 | 0 | 0 | 0 |

| Level of Lesion | Total No. of Cases | No. of Cases Requiring the Following No. of Days to Maximum Improvement | | | | | | |
|---|---|---|---|---|---|---|---|---|
| | | Less than 10 | 10–20 | 20–30 | 30–45 | 45–60 | 60–90 | More than 90 |
| L4 | 15 | 5 (33%) | 1 | 2 | 0 | 2 | 5 (33%) | 0 |
| L5 | 20 | 6 (30%) | 3 | 5 (25%) | 1 | 1 | 3 (15%) | 1 |

| Level of Lesion | Total No. of Cases | No. of Cases Requiring the Following No. of Treatments to 50% Improvement | | | | | | | | |
|---|---|---|---|---|---|---|---|---|---|---|
| | | Less than 10 | 10–20 | 20–30 | 30–40 | 40–50 | 50–60 | 60–80 | 80–100 | More than 100 |
| L4 | 15 | 12 (80%) | 3 | 0 | 0 | 0 | 0 | 0 | 0 | 0 |
| L5 | 20 | 17 (85%) | 2 | 0 | 1 | 0 | 1 | 0 | 0 | 0 |

| Level of Lesion | Total No. of Cases | No. of Cases Requiring the Following No. of Treatments to Maximum Improvement | | | | | | | | |
|---|---|---|---|---|---|---|---|---|---|---|
| | | Less than 10 | 10–20 | 20–30 | 30–40 | 40–50 | 50–60 | 60–80 | 80–100 | More than 100 |
| L4 | 15 | 7 (47%) | 2 | 4 | 2 | 0 | 0 | 0 | 0 | 0 |
| L5 | 20 | 9 (45%) | 6 (30%) | 3 | 1 | 0 | 0 | 0 | 0 | 1 |

**Table 15.28.**

**Cases of Facet Syndrome in Relation to the Number of Treatments and the Days of Treatment Necessary to Achieve Improvement**

| Level of Lesion | Total No. of Cases | No. of Case Requiring the Following No. of Days to 50% Improvement | | | | | | |
|---|---|---|---|---|---|---|---|---|
| | | Less than 10 | 10–20 | 20–30 | 30–45 | 45–60 | 60–90 | More than 90 |
| L4 | 59 | 32 (54%) | 18 | 8 | 1 | 0 | 0 | 0 |
| L5 | 204 | 128 (63%) | 46 | 19 (9%) | 4 | 3 | 3 | 1 |

| Level of Lesion | Total No. of Cases | No. of Cases Requiring the Following No. of Days to Maximum Improvement | | | | | | |
|---|---|---|---|---|---|---|---|---|
| | | Less than 10 | 10–20 | 20–30 | 30–45 | 45–60 | 60–90 | More than 90 |
| L4 | 59 | 19 (32%) | 6 | 5 | 9 (15%) | 5 | 11 (19%) | 4 |
| L5 | 204 | 64 (31%) | 33 | 27 | 21 | 18 | 27 (13%) | 14 |

| Level of Lesion | Total No. of Cases | No. of Cases Requiring the Following No. of Treatments to 50% Improvement | | | | | | | | |
|---|---|---|---|---|---|---|---|---|---|---|
| | | Less than 10 | 10–20 | 20–30 | 30–40 | 40–50 | 50–60 | 60–80 | 80–100 | More than 100 |
| L4 | 59 | 47 (80%) | 9 | 2 | 1 | 0 | 0 | 0 | 0 | 0 |
| L5 | 204 | 161 (79%) | 31 | 6 | 2 | 0 | 2 | 2 | 0 | 0 |

| Level of Lesion | Total No. of Cases | No. of Cases Requiring the Following No. of Treatments to Maximum Improvement | | | | | | | | |
|---|---|---|---|---|---|---|---|---|---|---|
| | | Less than 10 | 10–20 | 20–30 | 30–40 | 40–50 | 50–60 | 60–80 | 80–100 | More than 100 |
| L4 | 59 | 30 (51%) | 9 | 12 (20%) | 4 | 1 | 0 | 1 | 1 | 1 |
| L5 | 204 | 102 (50%) | 46 | 27 (13%) | 13 | 5 | 4 | 2 | 2 | 3 |

**Table 15.29.**

**Cases of Sprain and Strain in Relation to the Number of Treatments and the Days of Treatment Necessary to Achieve Maximum Improvement**

| Level of Lesion | Total No. of Cases | No. of Cases Requiring the Following No. of Days to Maximum Improvement | | | | | | |
|---|---|---|---|---|---|---|---|---|
| | | Less than 10 | 10–20 | 20–30 | 30–45 | 45–60 | 60–90 | More than 90 |
| L4 | 32 | 13 (41%) | 7 | 2 | 3 | 4 (13%) | 3 | 0 |
| L5 | 79 | 26 (33%) | 15 | 12 | 11 | 6 | 7 (9%) | 2 |

| Level of Lesion | Total No. of Cases | No. of Cases Requiring the Following No. of Treatments to Maximum Improvement | | | |
|---|---|---|---|---|---|
| | | Less than 10 | 10–20 | 20–30 | 60–80 |
| L4 | 32 | 19 (59%) | 11 | 2 | 0 |
| L5 | 79 | 47 (60%) | 26 (33%) | 4 | 2 |

**Table 15.30.**

**Cases of Tropism in Relation to the Number of Treatments and the Days of Treatment Necessary to Achieve Maximum Improvement**

| Level of Lesion | Total No. of Cases | No. of Cases Requiring the Following No. of Days to Maximum Improvement | | | | | | |
|---|---|---|---|---|---|---|---|---|
| | | Less than 10 | 10–20 | 20–30 | 30–45 | 45–60 | 60–90 | More than 90 |
| L4 | 33 | 15 (46%) | 3 | 5 | 1 | 1 | 7 (21%) | 1 |
| L5 | 42 | 20 (48%) | 9 | 5 | 2 | 1 | 4 (10%) | 1 |

| Level of Lesion | Total No. of Cases | No. of Cases Requiring the Following No. of Treatments to Maximum Improved | | | | |
|---|---|---|---|---|---|---|
| | | Less than 10 | 10–20 | 20–30 | 30–40 | 40–50 |
| L4 | 33 | 21 (64%) | 5 | 4 | 3 | 0 |
| L5 | 42 | 30 (71%) | 5 | 3 | 3 | 1 |

**Table 15.31.**

**Cases of Transitional Segment in Relation to the Number of Treatments and the Days of Treatment Necessary to Achieve Maximum Improvement**

| | No. of Cases Requiring the Following No. of Days to Maximum Improvement | | | | | | |
|---|---|---|---|---|---|---|---|
| Less than 10 | 10–20 | 20–30 | 30–45 | 45–60 | 60–90 | More than 90 |
| 4 (21%) | 1 | 3 | 4 | 1 | 4 (21%) | 2 |

| | No. of Cases Requiring the Following No. of Treatments to Maximum Improvement | | |
|---|---|---|---|
| Less than 10 | 10–20 | 20–30 | 50–60 |
| 8 (42%) | 4 | 6 (32%) | 1 |

**Table 15.32.**

**Cases of Stenosis in Relation to the Number of Treatments and the Days of Treatment Necessary to Achieve Maximum Improvement**

| Level of Lesion | Total No. of Cases | No. of Cases Requiring the Following No. of Days to Maximum Improvement | | | | | | |
|---|---|---|---|---|---|---|---|---|
| | | Less than 10 | 10–20 | 20–30 | 30–45 | 45–60 | 60–90 | More than 90 |
| L4 | 22 | 8 (36%) | 0 | 3 | 3 | 0 | 5 (23%) | 3 (14%) |
| L5 | 73 | 21 (29%) | 6 | 10 | 13 | 7 | 11 (15%) | 5 |

| Level of Lesion | Total No. of Cases | No. of Cases Requiring the Following No. of Treatments to Maximum Improvement | | | | | | |
|---|---|---|---|---|---|---|---|---|
| | | Less than 10 | 10–20 | 20–30 | 30–40 | 40–50 | 50–60 | 60–80 |
| L4 | 22 | 10 (46%) | 4 | 4 | 1 | 1 | 1 | 1 |
| L5 | 73 | 35 (48%) | 20 | 8 | 6 (8%) | 2 | 1 | 1 |

**Table 15.33.**

**Cases of Nuclear Protrusion in Relation to the Number of Treatments and the Days of Treatment Necessary to Achieve Improvement**

| Level of Lesion | Total No. of Cases | No. of Cases Requiring the Following No. of Days to 50% Improvement | | | | | | |
|---|---|---|---|---|---|---|---|---|
| | | Less than 10 | 10–20 | 20–30 | 30–45 | 45–60 | 60–90 | More than 90 |
| L4 | 79 | 40 (51%) | 24 | 11 (14%) | 2 | 2 | 0 | 0 |
| L5 | 107 | 72 (67%) | 21 | 8 | 3 | 2 | 1 | 0 |

| Level of Lesion | Total No. of Cases | No. of Cases Requiring the Following No. of Days to Maximum Improvement | | | | | | |
|---|---|---|---|---|---|---|---|---|
| | | Less than 10 | 10–20 | 20–30 | 30–45 | 45–60 | 60–90 | More than 90 |
| L4 | 79 | 27 (34%) | 8 | 6 | 13 | 7 | 9 (11%) | 9 |
| L5 | 107 | 36 (34%) | 11 | 18 | 10 | 8 | 15 (14%) | 9 |

| Level of Lesion | Total No. of Cases | No. of Cases Requiring the Following No. of Treatments to 50% Improvement | | | | | | | | |
|---|---|---|---|---|---|---|---|---|---|---|
| | | Less than 10 | 10–20 | 20–30 | 30–40 | 40–50 | 50–60 | 60–80 | 80–100 | More than 100 |
| L4 | 79 | 49 (62%) | 19 | 4 | 3 | 0 | 2 | 1 | 0 | 1 |
| L5 | 107 | 86 (80%) | 13 | 5 | 1 | 0 | 1 | 1 | 0 | 0 |

| Level of Lesion | Total No. of Cases | No. of Cases Requiring the Following No. of Treatments to Maximum Improvement | | | | | | | | |
|---|---|---|---|---|---|---|---|---|---|---|
| | | Less than 10 | 10–20 | 20–30 | 30–40 | 40–50 | 50–60 | 60–80 | 80–100 | More than 100 |
| L4 | 79 | 34 (43%) | 13 | 20 (25%) | 3 | 3 | 4 (5%) | 0 | 0 | 2 |
| L5 | 107 | 54 (51%) | 28 (26%) | 4 | 6 | 7 (7%) | 2 | 4 | 1 | 1 |

## SUMMARY

The incidence of congenital anomalies does not appear to be any higher in those patients complaining of low back discomfort than in the normal population. The presence of such anomalies does not seem to produce less favorable treatment results. In the treatment of anomalies of the low back, fewer treatments were needed over longer periods of time, whereas in the treatment of the acute disc protrusions, more treatments were needed for relatively shorter periods of time. This is probably due to the more acute and severe pain associated with disc lesions than the pain associated with anomalies. Stenosis is an example of an anomaly requiring more days for healing than are required by other anomalies (Table 15.32). The quickest responding condition with the fewest number of treatments and days of treatment required was discogenic spondyloarthrosis with no sciatica (Table 15.26).

Note that there were fewer cases of nuclear protrusion and spondylolisthesis at L4 than there were at L5. Cases of disc protrusion and spondylolisthesis at L5 re-

sponded quicker to treatment (10 to 20 treatments) than did cases of disc protrusion and spondylolisthesis at L4, and cases of spondylolisthesis at L5 showed faster improvement (within 30 days) than did cases of spondylolisthesis at L4 (Table 15.27). Thus, L4 spondylolisthesis responded much slower and required more treatments than did L5 spondylolisthesis.

Figures 15.1 to 15.18 are cumulation percent curves of patient response to treatment of diagnosed conditions at the L4 and L5 levels, by days or number of treatments to maximum improvement. In general, if after a number of responses have been plotted the curve becomes increasingly exponential, treatment could be considered to be cumulative in effect; i.e., after a certain number of treatments, dramatic improvement could be expected. If the curve becomes linear or resembles a straight line, treatment could be considered to provide a steady but gradual improvement. Finally, in cases of decaying exponential curves, treatment could be considered to provide a rapid response for the majority of patients. Furthermore, these plots may be read so as to indicate the proportion of patients who

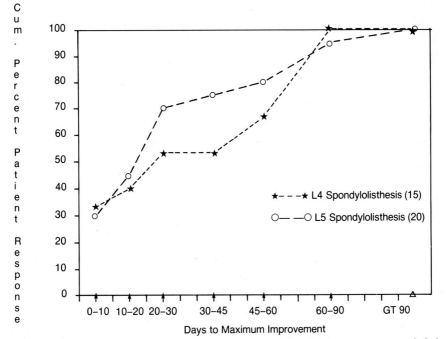

**Figure 15.1.** Days to maximum improvement curves by diagnosis: L4 spondylolisthesis and L5 spondylolisthesis.

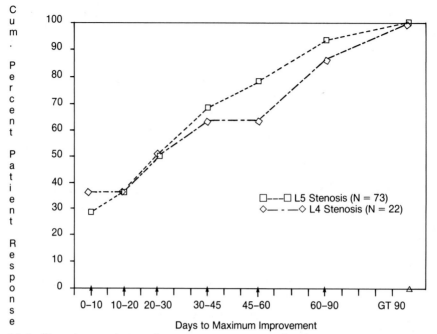

**Figure 15.2.** Days to maximum improvement curves by diagnosis: L4 stenosis and L5 stenosis.

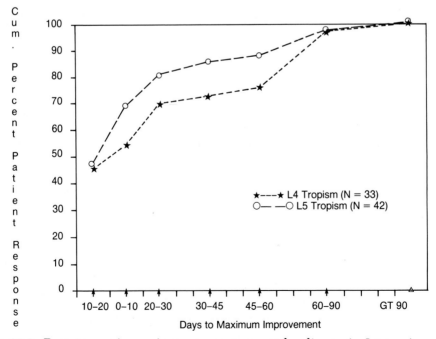

**Figure 15.3.** Days to maximum improvement curves by diagnosis: L4 tropism and L5 tropism.

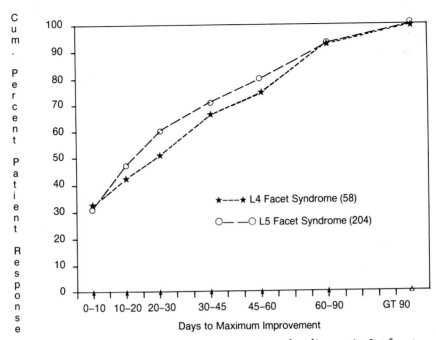

**Figure 15.4.** Days to maximum improvement curves by diagnosis: L4 facet syndrome and L5 facet syndrome.

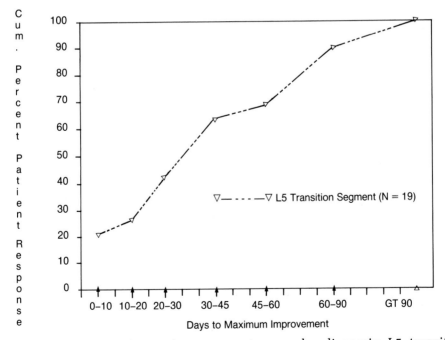

**Figure 15.5.** Days to maximum improvement curve by diagnosis: L5 transitional segment.

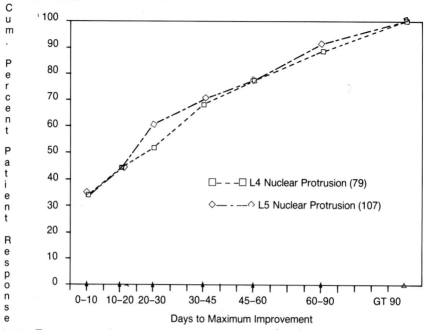

**Figure 15.6.** Days to maximum improvement curves by diagnosis: L4 nuclear protrusion and L5 nuclear protrusion.

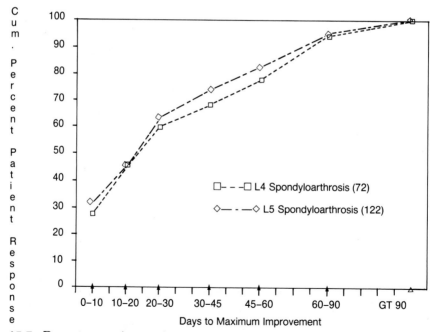

**Figure 15.7.** Days to maximum improvement curves by diagnosis: L4 spondyloarthrosis and L5 spondyloarthrosis.

achieved maximum improvement after a number of days or treatments. For example, in cases of nuclear protrusion a practitioner may reasonably expect 35% of his patients to show maximum improvement in 10 days or less. Finally, another important feature to be noted in these plots is the starting point of the curves which indicates the proportion of patients responding to initial treatment. For exam-

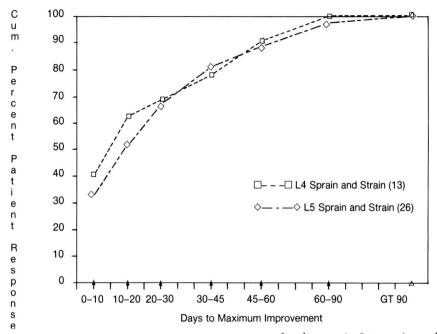

**Figure 15.8.** Days to maximum improvement curves by diagnosis: L4 sprain and strain and L5 sprain and strain.

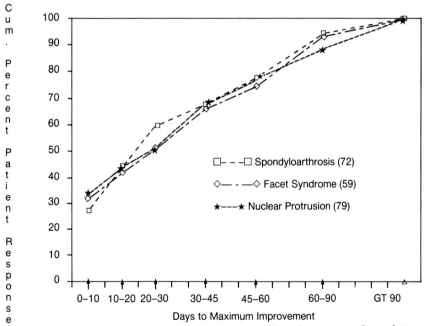

**Figure 15.9.** Days to maximum improvement curves by diagnosis of conditions at L4: spondyloarthrosis, facet syndrome, and nuclear protrusion.

ple, response to treatment for transitional segment is lowest at 21% in 10 days, whereas response to treatment for tropism is highest at 45% in 10 days. A final word

of caution should be mentioned here. When these curves represent a very small sample (less than 30), they may not represent adequately the response of patients

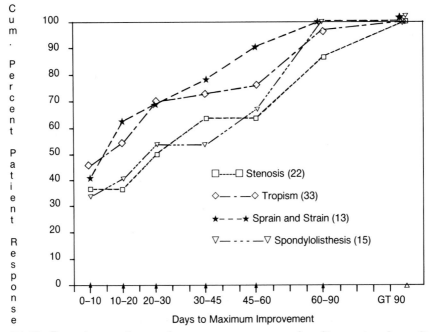

**Figure 15.10.** Days to maximum improvement curves by diagnosis of conditions at L4: stenosis, tropism, sprain and strain, and spondylolisthesis.

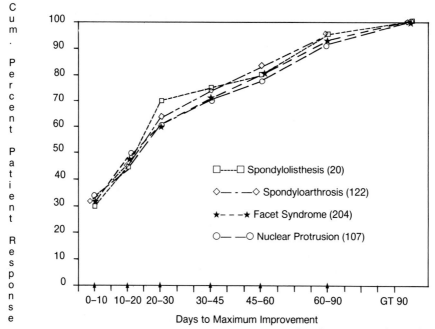

**Figure 15.11.** Days to maximum improvement curves by diagnosis of conditions at L5: spondylolisthesis, spondyloarthrosis, facet syndrome, and nuclear protrusion.

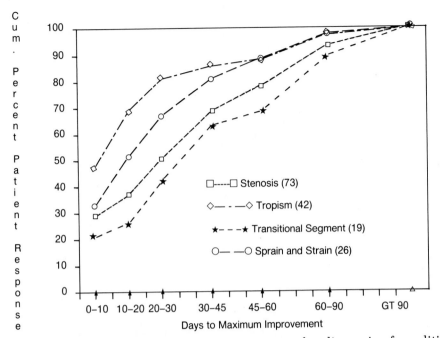

**Figure 15.12.** Days to maximum improvement curves by diagnosis of conditions at L5: stenosis, tropism, transitional segment, and sprain and strain.

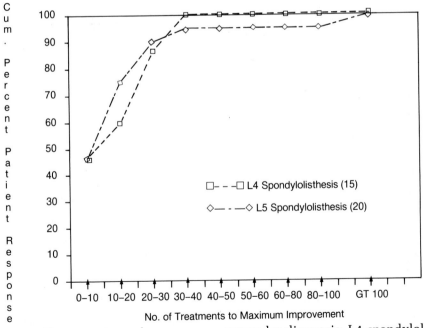

**Figure 15.13.** Treatment number response curves by diagnosis: L4 spondylolisthesis and L5 spondylolisthesis.

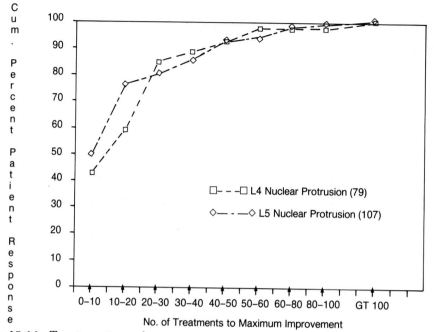

**Figure 15.14.** Treatment number response curves by diagnosis: L4 nuclear protrusion and L5 nuclear protrusion.

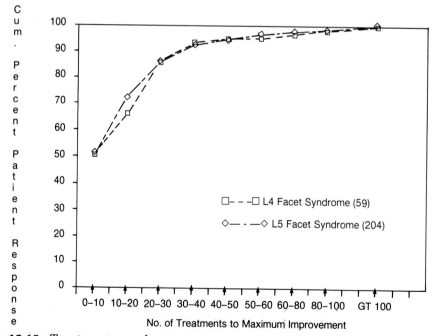

**Figure 15.15.** Treatment number response curves by diagnosis: L4 facet syndrome and L5 facet syndrome.

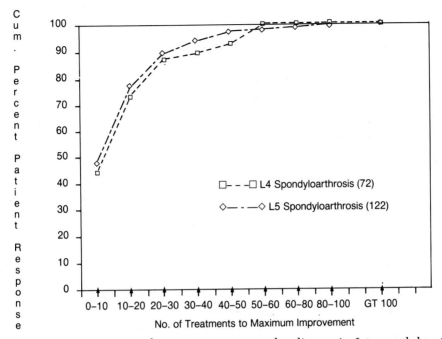

**Figure 15.16.** Treatment number response curves by diagnosis: L4 spondyloarthrosis and L5 spondyloarthrosis.

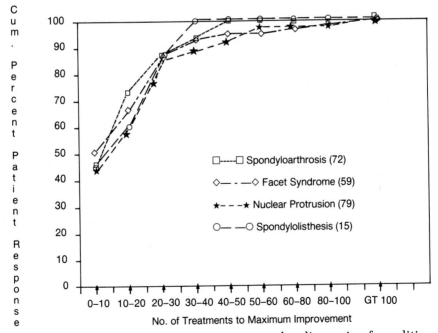

**Figure 15.17.** Treatment number response curves by diagnosis of conditions at L4: spondyloarthrosis, facet syndrome, nuclear protrusion, and spondylolisthesis.

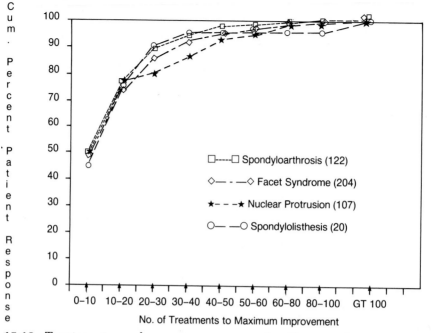

**Figure 15.18.** Treatment number response curves by diagnosis by conditions at L5: spondyloarthrosis, facet syndrome, nuclear protrusion, and spondylolisthesis.

in the general population seeking chiropractic treatment for back pain.

### Days to Maximum Response

In the first series of graphs, days to maximum improvement was plotted for nuclear protrusion, transitional segment, tropism, stenosis, sprain and strain, spondylolisthesis, and spondyloarthrosis. Linear response patterns are indicated for facet syndrome (L4 and L5), nuclear protrusion (L4 and L5), and transitional segment (L5 only). In these cases, the rates of response to treatment at both L4 and L5 levels closely parallel each other.

In cases of sprain and strain, spondyloarthrosis and, most clearly, tropism, response patterns illustrate decaying exponential curves that indicate a more rapid rate to maximum improvement. Patients treated for tropism, sprain and strain, and spondyloarthrosis show rapid improvement, with the majority (60% or more) achieving maximum improvement in 20 to 30 days.

These curves also indicate that there is little difference in cumulative patient responses to treatment for sprain and strain, spondyloarthrosis, nuclear protrusion, and facet syndrome between L4 and L5 levels. The response rate is better for the treatment of tropism at L5 than for the treatment of tropism at L4, and the response pattern for treatment of stenosis, which is 30 to 45 days, closely parallels the response pattern for the treatment of tropism, whereas the response pattern for treatment of stenosis at L5 is better, since it shows more rapid improvements in these patients.

An example of an exponential increase in improvement is found in the response pattern for treatment of L4 spondylolisthesis, in which improvement rates rapidly increase after 45 days. On the other hand, the response pattern for treatment of L4 spondylolisthesis shows a rapid initial improvement up to 30 days, at which point the curve flattens.

### Curves concerning the Number of Treatments to Maximum Improvement

Due to incompatible summary categories concerning the number of treatments, only patterns concerning the response to treatment for spondyloarthrosis, facet syndrome, nuclear protrusion, and spondylolisthesis were plotted. In all cases, these response curves clearly show the decaying exponential pattern, with maximum improvement clearly being present up to 30 treatments.

Response curves for treatment of L4 and L5 spondyloarthrosis show little difference, with about 90% of patients showing maximum improvement with 20 to 30 treatments. Response curves for treatment of L4 and L5 facet syndrome also show little difference, with 80% improvement achieved with 20 to 30 treatments and with a high of about 50% of the patients showing maximum improvement with 10 or fewer treatments. Response curves for treatment of L4 and L5 nuclear protrusion closely parallel each other after 20 to 30 treatments, but the response curve for treatment of L5 nuclear protrusion shows a more rapid improvement (more than 70%) at 10 to 20 treatments than does the response curve for treatment of L4 nuclear protrusion.

Response curves for treatment of spondylolisthesis at both L4 and L5 levels are similar, but the vast majority of patients achieve maximum improvement by 30 to 40 treatments. Patients with L5 spondylolisthesis also showed a faster response rate to treatment than did patients with L4-spondylolisthesis.

A comparison of the response curves for treatment of spondyloarthrosis, facet syndrome, nuclear protrusion, and spondylolisthesis at L4 shows that they are remarkably similar in the number of treatments; more than 80% of these patients showed maximum improvement with 20 to 30 treatments. Response curves for treatment of nuclear protrusion at both L4 and L5 show that patients with this diagnosis were the slowest to respond to treatment after 20 to 30 treatments.

## LOOKING AHEAD

Although this descriptive investigation into the response of patients to chiropractic treatment, by diagnosis and region, clearly illustrates what can be expected with the use of specific treatments, it just begins to scratch the surface of this research. Future research will involve exploring additional correlates of response to treatment. Such relevant factors as previous medical history and such demographic characteristics as age and sex are all hypothetical to treatment and improvement, but statistical investigation must wait until larger samples are gathered for each kind and level of lesion. At this time, correlation and regression analysis into these related factors may begin. Also at this time, the search for statistically significant differences in improvement rates can be explored.

## References

1. White AA, Panjabi MM: *Clinical Biomechanics of the Spine.* Philadelphia, JB Lippincott, 1978, pp 284–289.
2. Charnley J: Acute lumbago and sciatica. *Br Med J* 1:344, 1955.
3. Murphy F: Sources of pain in disc disease. *Clin Neurosurg* 15:343–351, 1968.
4. McCullough JA: Chemonucleolysis. *J. Bone Joint Surg* 59B:45–52, 1977.
5. Million WH, Haavik N, Baker KD, Jayson MV: Assessment of the progress of the back pain patient. *Spine* 7(3):204–212, 1982.

# Index